Drogenkonsum in Geschichte und Gesellschaft

Drug Use in History and Society

Herausgegeben von | Edited by

Prof. Dr. Heino Stöver

Dr. Ingo Ilja Michels

Band | Volume 8

Ulla Pape | Heino Stöver
Ingo Ilja Michels | Meryem Grabski [Eds.]

HIV and Hepatitis C in Central Asia and China

Understanding Vulnerabilities and Social Work Responses

Nomos

Gefördert vom DAAD aus Mitteln des Bundesministeriums für Wirtschaftliche Zusammenarbeit und Entwicklung (BMZ).

Funded by the DAAD with funds from the Federal Ministry for Economic Cooperation and Development (BMZ).

The Deutsche Nationalbibliothek lists this publication in the Deutsche Nationalbibliografie; detailed bibliographic data are available on the Internet at http://dnb.d-nb.de

ISBN 978-3-7560-1465-1 (Print)
978-3-7489-2002-1 (ePDF)

Onlineversion
Nomos eLibrary

1st Edition 2024

Table of contents

Additional Case Studies and Cross-Cutting Issues

Introduction

1. HIV and Hepatitis C in Central Asia and China: Understanding the Role of Social Work and NGOs in the Response to Infectious Diseases

Ulla Pape, Heino Stöver, Ingo Ilja Michels, Meryem Grabski

In 2015, the United Nations Member States adopted the Sustainable Development Goals (SDGs) for 2030. The SDGs are a global development framework consisting of seventeen interrelated goals, designed to serve as a 'shared blueprint for peace and prosperity for people and the planet, now and into the future' (United Nations n.d.). Good health and well-being are essential to sustainable development and are described in SDG 3. Within the framework of the SDGs, infectious diseases, including HIV/AIDS and hepatitis C, are an important target. SDG 3 specifies the target of 'ending the epidemics of AIDS, tuberculosis, malaria and neglected tropical diseases and combating hepatitis, waterborne and other communicable diseases' (United Nations n.d.).

In this book, we take a closer look at the development of the response to two major infectious diseases – HIV/AIDS and Hepatitis C – in Central Asia and China. In this introduction, we first provide an overview of the epidemiological trends and the responses in the countries of the region with a focus on China, Kazakhstan, Kyrgyzstan, and Uzbekistan. The country overview includes an analysis of the vulnerabilities that are associated with these diseases, especially among key populations. Secondly, we take a look at the development of HIV/AIDS and Hepatitis C prevention approaches among key populations, a field in which non-governmental organisations (NGOs) play a vital role. We analyse how social work services have developed, especially with regards to vulnerable populations, and to what extent social work actors and NGOs have been contributing to the response. Thirdly, we identify arenas for future action to improve services for key populations. The introduction concludes with a detailed overview of the chapters of this publication.

HIV/AIDS in Central Asia and China

Central Asia has long been a hotspot for high prevalence rates of HIV/AIDS, often associated with injecting drug use and incarceration (Bobrova et al. 2007; Thorne et al. 2010; LaMonaca et al. 2019; Deryabina et al. 2019; Golichenko 2020). In recent years, as a result of various factors, the HIV/AIDS epidemic in the countries of Central Asia has undergone significant changes, in particular with regards to HIV transmission and new infections in groups of different ages, genders, and social identities. The epidemiological situation in each Central Asian country remains complex and has its own specific characteristics.

A wide range of factors contribute to the region's HIV/AIDS epidemic, including poverty, unemployment, injecting drug use, sex work, labour migration, and a lack of public awareness about HIV transmission and prevention. The latest statistics show a decrease in injecting drug use and opioid use in all Central Asian countries. Recent developments suggest that unlike in the Russian Federation and Ukraine where 70% of HIV-registered infections are due to injecting drug use, in Central Asia, sexual transmission is now the leading cause of new infections (Zabransky et al. 2014; The Joint United Nations Programme on HIV/AIDS [UNAIDS] 2018; LaMonaca et al. 2019, InBeAIDS 2020). The SOLID project has developed a substantial body of research on HIV/AIDS and HCV in Central Asia and China. In the following section, we present the main epidemiological trends and responses in the individual countries.

Kazakhstan was the first country in Central Asia to record HIV infections. At the end of 1990, the Republican AIDS Center was established, followed by networks of regional centres across Kazakhstan (see Chapter 3, 'HIV/Aids and HCV in Kazakhstan' by Dinara Yessimova, Mariya Prilutskaya, Dalida Mukasheva, and Medet Kudabekov in this book). In 2017, it was estimated that 75% of people living with HIV in Kazakhstan were aware of their HIV status, of which only 59% were receiving antiretroviral treatment (ART). Over the past two decades, Kazakhstan has developed a concentrated HIV epidemic with a prevalence of 0.3% in the general population. In 2022, the absolute number of people living with HIV (PLWH) was between 35,000 and 38,000. HIV prevalence among key populations was significantly higher than in the general population: 7.6% among people who inject drugs (PWID), 1.3% among sex workers, 6.9% among men having sex with men (MSM), and 4.1% among people living in prisons. This represents a decrease in prevalence in all groups since 2019/2020. In

2019, HIV testing was conducted by 23 stationary laboratories distributed across all regions. There were no mobile laboratories in the Republic of Kazakhstan, but 23 mobile trust points that travel to the points with the highest concentration of key group representatives and conduct rapid testing.

In 2017, the Republican AIDS Center estimated that 11,207 PWID were living with HIV in Kazakhstan. Among them, 9,072 individuals (80.9%) were aware of their HIV-positive status. Nevertheless, only less than half of these individuals, namely 4,340 (38.7%) of them, were receiving ART. The estimated number of PWID is currently decreasing due to changing patterns of drug use in the country. Since the beginning of the epidemic, NGOs have been playing a key role in providing HIV/AIDS prevention and support to PLWH in Kazakhstan, which has been acknowledged by the international community. Kazakhstan's NGOs often collaborate with the Global Fund to access funding, technical expertise, and best practices. They actively engage with the Joint United Nations Programme on HIV/AIDS (UNAIDS) and other UN agencies to align their strategies with international standards and access data, research, and policy guidance.

In **Kyrgyzstan**, the character of the HIV/AIDS epidemic has changed as well (Pape 2019). For example, the numbers of sexual transmissions of HIV increased over the past decade from 787 cases in 2011 to 3,156 cases in 2018. New infections also occurred among women whose partners are injecting drug users (Deryabina et al. 2019) and women who engage in injecting drug use and sex work (Vélez-Grau et al. 2022). Similar statistics from Kazakhstan and Tajikistan show a steady decrease in the percentage of HIV transmissions that result from injecting drug use. The reasons for this stabilisation are not fully understood. It is unclear whether the decline in new HIV cases and the increase in heterosexual transmission rates are due to an underreporting of transmissions among PLWH and their partners (Deryabina et al. 2019).

The epidemiological situation in Kyrgyzstan regarding HIV and HCV infections presents a complex problem (see Chapter 4, 'HIV/Aids and HCV in Kyrgyzstan' by Jarkyn Shadymanova and Nurgul Musaeva in this book). Over the past decade, there has been an intensification of HIV and hepatitis C transmission not only among vulnerable groups with risky behaviours but also among the general population, leading to an increase in the number of people living with these infections. In Kyrgyzstan, the first case of HIV infection was recorded in 1987. In the following years, there was a continuous increase in the registration of new cases. According to WHO/

UNAIDS estimates, 12,231 people were living with HIV in Kyrgyzstan by the end of 2022. The number of women with HIV increased by 2.8% compared to the end of 2021. The percentage of people who inject drugs and live with HIV remained roughly the same, at 14.6% (compared to 14.3% in 2009). It is worth noting that the prevalence of viral hepatitis C was high among PLWH (50.4%).

In 2022, more than 36,000 representatives of vulnerable groups were provided with HIV testing, harm reduction services, care, and support programmes. HIV rapid testing is actively carried out in Kyrgyzstan among vulnerable groups (see Chapter 10, 'Analysis of Harm Reduction Programmes in HIV/AIDS Prevention in Kyrgyzstan: Experience, Problems, and Prospects' by Tynchtyk Estebes uulu in this book). These activities are developed with the support of the Global Fund, but also by the government of Kyrgyzstan. NGOs have played a significant role in Kyrgyzstan's response to the HIV epidemic. Often, they were the first to advocate for the need to implement prevention programmes, emphasising the importance of the epidemic at the political level. However, repressive drug control policies as well as careless attitudes and discrimination from medical workers push drug users, sex workers, and MSM away from support programmes. Discrimination particularly affects MSM, as homosexuality carries a particular stigma (Pape 2019). People who use drugs and live with HIV and/or HCV often face a double stigma that hinders them from accessing testing, treatment, and support.

According to the official data of the Ministry of Health, at the onset of 2023, a total of 52,420 people living with HIV were registered in **Uzbekistan**, the most populous country in Central Asia. Similar to other countries in the region, Uzbekistan's HIV epidemic has changed over the past two decades. At present, labour migrants are among the most affected population groups (see Chapter 9, 'Labour Migrants' by Azizbek Boltaev in this book). Since the first detection of HIV infection in Uzbekistan in 1987 until 1st January 2022, around 71,000 people living with HIV have been registered, of whom 23,000 have died due to AIDS. An analysis carried out in 2022 of HIV-infected individuals, segregated by gender, revealed that 55% of HIV cases pertain to males, while 45% pertain to females. Sexual transmission accounted for 79% of all registered cases of HIV, followed by parenteral (through injecting drug use) (12.7%) and mother-to-child (0.6%) transmission.

The HIV epidemic in Uzbekistan seems to being stabilising at approximately 3,000 new cases per year, but key populations, including MSM, people who inject drugs, and sex workers, remain at risk. These populations are at increased risk of HIV infection due to many factors, including stigma, discrimination, and lack of access to prevention and care services. In order to further enhance the role of NGOs as active participants and partners in the prevention of HIV infection (such as by providing syringes and needles to injection drug users), strengthen the protection of the rights and legitimate interests of people living with HIV, Uzbekistan needs to expand the scale of state support to NGOs.

At present, a small number of NGOs have been established in Uzbekistan to offer prevention services and social support for key populations (see Chapter 12, 'The role of public organizations and non-governmental organizations (NGOs) in addressing and supporting people with HIV' by Guzalkhon Zakhidova in this book). NGOs also make a significant contribution to the prevention of HIV infection. Communities living with and affected by HIV, including key populations, support programme development and implementation, the expansion of coverage, and improvements to the quality of health services.

Previous studies, such as the CADAP project (Central Asia Drug Action Programme [CADAP] 2020), have shown that the number of new HIV infections is increasing, especially in Kazakhstan, while at the same time the share of transmissions resulting from injecting drug use is decreasing. This trend can also be observed in other Central Asian countries, and it indicates that the epidemic has spread beyond key populations and is now affecting the general population (Pape 2019). Notably, the number of officially registered opioid users in Central Asia has been steadily declining over recent years. In 2013, 35,150 drug users (mostly opioid users) were registered in Kazakhstan, but in 2017 this number decreased to 23,020 (-35%).

In Kyrgyzstan the number of people who use drugs decreased from 9,024 in 2013 to 8,485 in 2017 (-6%), while in Tajikistan, the numbers changed only slightly, from 7,176 in 2013 to 6,947 (-3%) in 2017, nonetheless representing the regional trend (see also Azbel et al. 2017; Michels et al. 2017; Zabransky et al. 2014; Michels/Stöver 2022). Moreover, the number of opioid users treated in narcological clinics has been declining, while the number of patients in opioid substitution treatment (OST) has been slowly increasing, even though this increase is minimal, given the overall number of registered opioid users (Michels et al. 2020). Whether OST affects HIV prevalence rates is difficult to assess, but the overall range and the retention rates are either too low or too high to produce generalisable epidemiological effects.

A review of the available literature suggests that there is a visible gap in the information about the population living with HIV/AIDS, as well as treatment for this population group and injecting drug users in Central Asia. Still often referred to as transitional states, given the challenges in healthcare reforms that resulted from the collapse of the Soviet Union (Habibov 2016), the countries in Central Asia have developed in different ways, with vulnerable populations remaining the most disadvantaged (Scheil-Adlung/Kuhl 2011). This is especially the case in terms of public health concerns such as the HIV/AIDS epidemic, which remains concentrated in all Central Asian countries. This means that HIV has spread rapidly in one or more subpopulations but is not well established in the general population.

The data from national and international surveys suggest that poverty, unemployment, and an increase in the number of people who inject drugs and people engaged in sex work are the main contributing factors to the HIV/AIDS epidemic in Central Asia. The situation is exacerbated by the lack of public awareness about HIV transmission and prevention methods. The development of the epidemiological monitoring mainly undertaken by international prevention programmes reveals higher rates of HIV in Central Asia.

Data from national AIDS centres show that prevalence is high among so-called key populations, including PWID (29.8% in Kazakhstan and 23% in Kyrgyzstan). The HIV epidemic remains concentrated in all three countries, with HCV being most prevalent in Kyrgyzstan, where the numbers show an increase in 2017 compared to previous years (60.9%), and in Kazakhstan (68.7%). However, a recent increase in the mother-to-child transmission cases shows that the epidemic is spreading beyond the key population groups and into the general population.

In **China,** the HIV/AIDS epidemic has undergone various changes in terms of the routes of transmission over the past 40 years (Xu et al. 2021), even though the overall prevalence remains low. China has made remarkable achievements in HIV prevention and control. UNAIDS estimated that the number of HIV-infected individuals in China could reach 10 million by 2010 (Kaufmann/Jing 2002). However, China has been able to limit the epidemic to a prevalence of <0.1% as of the end of 2017 (NHC 2020; Liu et al. 2021). In 2018, according to the government, there were 1.25 million

PLWH in China, 69% of whom were aware of their HIV status and 83% of whom were accessing ART.

In the 1980s, the first HIV/AIDS outbreak occurred among PWID in the Dehong Prefecture, in the Yunnan Province, which is along the south-west border of the world's largest illicit drug production and distribution centre, the so-called 'Golden Triangle'. The HIV epidemic steadily spread from Yunnan to neighbouring provinces and then to nearly all of China's 31 provinces. In the early 1990s, the second HIV/AIDS outbreak occurred, alongside the emergence of illegal commercial blood collection stations in rural areas of central China. Successful efforts to curb injection drug use and illegal blood collection have led to the emergence of sexual transmission, both heterosexual and homosexual, as the major route for HIV infection in recent years (Xu et al. 2021).

According to official data, there are an estimated 2,561,000 injecting drug users in China, with an estimated HIV prevalence of 11.9% (304,000 people). Of these HIV-positive PWID, 59% had been tested for HIV antibodies in the previous twelve months. Furthermore, there is an HCV antibody prevalence among people who inject drugs of 49% and an HCV ribonucleic acid (RNA) prevalence of 35.8%, but no information regarding how many of the HCV-infected people received treatment (Hajarizadeh et al. 2023).

HIV and HCV epidemic patterns in China can be divided into two main categories. Initially, during the HIV epidemic in southern and south-western China, injecting drug use was the primary mode of transmission, accounting for the majority of infections between 1989 and 1995. However, this situation has since changed, with over 70% of newly reported HIV transmissions now resulting from heterosexual contact (see Chapter 2, 'HIV/Aids and HCV in China' by Hang Su, Yifan Xu, Huiting Lei, Shuxin Shao, and Jiang Du in this book).

China's response to HIV/AIDS has undergone significant transformations over the past 35 years. China has implemented a multitude of laws, policies, and guidelines to support the response to HIV/AIDS, demonstrating a strong commitment both politically and economically to dealing with HIV/AIDS. These achievements have led to a remarkable reduction in mortality from HIV/AIDS over the past two decades, and the number of patients on long-term sustained ART in China now exceeds 800,000. Nevertheless, challenges such as late diagnosis and linkage to care continue to be significant barriers, and the emergence of non-AIDS comorbidities represents a new area of concern in HIV care. The most significant challenge in eliminating HIV in China lies in identifying currently undiagnosed infections and ensuring that infected individuals are rapidly linked to treatment. Approximately 30% of HIV infections in China go undetected.

Since 2003, China has offered free HIV counselling and testing, along with free antiretroviral therapy. Multiple strategies can be employed to enhance HIV detection, such as implementing more intensive testing programmes that target high-risk groups. Consequently, the most plausible scenario is that by 2030, treatment coverage will have significantly increased, HIV transmission rates will have decreased, drug resistance will remain at low levels, and China will be on the verge of realising UNAIDS' second and third treatment targets. However, the foremost challenge will likely revolve around achieving UNAIDS' first treatment target by 2030.

Regarding the prevention and treatment of HIV/AIDS among injecting drug users, the Chinese Ministry of Public Security has cooperated with the Ministry of Health to gradually improve drug rehabilitation regulations over time. The regulations on HIV/AIDS prevention and treatment issued in 2006 and the Anti-Drug Law issued in 2008 allowed healthcare institutions to provide OST – in China, known as methadone maintenance treatment (MMT) – and clean needles to PWID for the purpose of reducing HIV transmission through needle-sharing behaviour. By June 2016, there were 33,486 participants in needle exchange programmes and 161,975 PWID receiving MMT. From 2006 to 2017, HIV incidence among MMT clients decreased from 0.95 per 100 person-years to 0.03 per 100 person-years. Moreover, results from a needle exchange programme showed that the proportion of needles being shared in the intervention group was lower than that in the control group (35.3% versus 62.3%). At the Guangdong site, the HIV incidence of the intervention group was significantly lower than that of their counterparts (12.9% versus 33.3%, $P < 0.011$) (Xu et al. 2021; Su 2022).

At present, the HIV/AIDS epidemic in China is concentrated among key populations, particularly among gay men and other MSM (UNAIDS 2021). Another study estimated that by October 2020, there were 1.045 million people actually reported living with HIV/AIDS across China (National Health Commission of China [NHC] 2020). The political commitment, social engagement, and international support that are jointly responsible for this remarkable achievement have rarely been evaluated or reviewed. UNAIDS provides country progress reports on the achievements of the UNAIDS strategy, more specifically on improvements that relate to achieving the UNAIDS '95-95-95' targets – namely, that 95% of all people living with HIV know their HIV status; 95% of all people with diagnosed HIV infection receive ART; and 95% of all people receiving ART achieve viral suppression (UNAIDS 2019).

In response to the first epidemic outbreak of HIV among injecting drug users and the second one through illegal commercial blood collection, China issued the Anti-Drug Law and launched the Blood Donation Act which almost ended the blood product-related infection. China has been providing free ART since 2003, which has covered more than 80% of the identified patients and achieved a viral suppression rate of 91% (UNAIDS 2019; Xu et al. 2021). To bend the curve of HIV/AIDS, China should consider constraining HIV spread through sexual transmission, narrowing the gaps in identifying HIV cases, and guaranteeing access to ART for all people in need.

Hepatitis C in Central Asia and China

With approximately 71 million people chronically infected worldwide, viral hepatitis is a global health concern (Botheju et al. 2019). Hepatitis C is a bloodborne virus that is transmitted through sharing needles, syringes, or other drug-injection equipment; from gestational parent to baby during pregnancy or at birth; or rarely through sexual contact (CDC n.d.). PWID are particularly vulnerable to HCV (Botheju et al. 2019). Transmission can occur through sharing needles, syringes, or preparation equipment or through blood contact (Center for Disease Control [CDC] n.d.).

Central Asia is one of the regions most affected by HCV infections, with Uzbekistan enduring one of the highest prevalence levels globally (Botheju et al. 2019). The spread of HCV in Central Asia is driven by injecting drug use and healthcare exposures (Botheju et al. 2019). In China, reported cases of HCV infections have been increasing since the beginning of the 21st century (Duan et al. 2014; Liu et al. 2021). Both in Central Asia and China, PWID are particularly affected by HCV. Overall, HCV infections, prevention, and treatment are not a focal point of social policy in Central Asia and China. Historically, viral hepatitis has been a serious public health problem in Central Asian countries, a situation that worsened after the end of the Soviet Union (Akmatov et al. 2023). Despite public health concerns, there is a lack of robust data on the epidemiology of viral hepatitis in both Central Asia and China (Liu et al. 2021; Akmatov et al. 2023).

For Kazakhstan, a recent meta study found that HCV prevalence ranged from 0.7% to 5.1% among the general population, with a median of 0.9%, and from 2.0% to 50.0% among populations at intermediate risk, with a median of 29.0% (Botheju et al. 2019). Among key populations, HCV prevalence is substantially higher: studies found an HCV prevalence of 40.3% in PLWH and 43.3%–90.2% among PWID, with a median of 60.3% (Botheju et al. 2019).

In Kyrgyzstan, the situation is similar to Kazakhstan. Among the general population, HCV prevalence ranged from 0.8% to 5.0%, with a median of 2.0%. Among PWID, HCV prevalence ranged from 17.0% to 60.4%, with a median of 46.4% (Botheju et al. 2019).

In Tajikistan, HCV prevalence ranged from 0.5% to 7.3% among the general population, with a median of 3.9%. Among PWID, HCV prevalence was between 24.9% and 67.1%, with a median of 32.6% (Botheju et al. 2019). Studies on Tajikistan have especially looked into risk factors for HCV transmission among PWID: daily injection, a history of incarceration, and living/working outside of Tajikistan in the past ten years were all associated with a higher risk of HCV infection (Botheju et al. 2019).

For Turkmenistan, no epidemiological studies on HCV are available (Botheju et al. 2019).

Uzbekistan has a particularly high prevalence of HCV. Among the general population, it was between 6.4% and 13.1%, with a median of 11.9%. Among PWID, HCV prevalence ranged between 20.9% and 63.8%, with a median of 51.7% (Botheju et al. 2019). There are an estimated 2.1 million people with a chronic HCV infection in Uzbekistan. This means that about 80% of people with a chronic HCV infection in Central Asia reside in Uzbekistan (Botheju et al. 2019). The high HCV prevalence in Uzbekistan is associated, among other things, with 'excessive practice of medical and non-medical invasive procedures, such as blood transfusion and bloodletting, in addition to poor infection control, inadequate blood screening, and use of unsafe medical injections' (Botheju et al. 2019).

This comparison of the countries of Central Asia shows a significant variation in HCV prevalence, with Uzbekistan being the most affected country in the region. The comparison of key populations shows that the prevalence of HCV is especially high among PWID, with 51.3% of the cohort being positive (Botheju et al. 2019). PWID are also vulnerable to HIV. From the high level of comorbidities, we can conclude that the two epidemics overlap. To make matters worse, there is hardly any treatment available for HCV patients, as treatment remains unaffordable (CADAP 2019).

In comparison to Central Asia, China is less affected by HCV. A 2016 study found that HCV prevalence was 1.3% among the general population (Petruzziello et al. 2016). The primary challenge in HCV management in China is a complex issue that involves identifying HCV-infected patients, ensuring their access to treatment options, and making treatment affordable. Furthermore, patient adherence and physician guidance could introduce additional variability in the eventual therapeutic outcomes. The absence of a comprehensive epidemiological monitoring system in China also presents additional hurdles in enhancing HCV management at a national level.

HIV and Hepatitis C Prevention and Care among Key Populations

HIV and HCV are described as dual epidemics that mainly affect key populations. The overlapping nature of the two epidemics stems from underlying behaviours and health disparities among disproportionately affected populations, primarily PWID (Moorman et al. 2023). The particular vulnerability of PWID is particularly evident in Central Asia and China, as tailored prevention programmes are not sufficiently available for PWID. International evidence shows that harm reduction services are key to prevent the transmission of HIV and HCV among PWID. Although the effectiveness of harm reduction has been proven in international research, the availability and coverage of harm reduction services in Central Asia and China is still low.

The reasons for the limited access to and low coverage of harm reduction programmes are of a political nature. There is a strong link between the lack of harm reduction services and conservative legislation that focuses on control and repression rather than on assistance and support for key populations. Key populations, and especially PWID, often face stigmatisation and discrimination in the healthcare system. They are also not seen as a priority by policymakers. Consequently, existing programmes are often limited to small-scale projects that are developed by local community organisations and financed by international donors. As a result, key populations often lack access to medical services, and HIV, tuberculosis (TB), and HCV coinfections are a widespread concern. According to a recent study, up to 50% of individuals, co-infected with HIV and multidrug-resistant TB

(MDR-TB) in Eastern Europe and Central Asia die within two years of treatment initiation (Kraef et al. 2022). Moreover, ART coverage for PLWH in the region is far below the UNAIDS 90% targets (Kraef et al. 2022). The overall policy approach has a negative effect on the situation of PWID and key populations in both Central Asia and China.

To improve the effectiveness of harm reduction efforts in Central Asia and China, the structural conditions must be changed. Local experts argue that there is a lack of prevention programmes for populations in Central Asia and China. For example, there is no outpatient counselling or support services for key populations. There is hardly any outreach work among PWID, except for a few programmes that are conducted by community organisations of former drug users. Secondly, social work is still in its infancy and is not equipped to work with people with drug use disorders. However, over the past decade, the involvement of international donors in the region's overall development has had a positive influence on the development of drug policies, treatment, and prevention of the spread of associated infectious diseases (Michels et al. 2017).

As a result of this international investment, modern and effective harm reduction approaches have been adapted by local NGOs and have generated social and professional initiatives aiming to engage the local governments to strive for more humane drug policies (Michels et al. 2017/2020). In its 'Bishkek Resolution', the CADAP project concluded that the 'consolidated work of non-commercial organizations, community-based organizations, governmental agencies, international organizations and donors' has made a significant impact on the development of social work with people who use drugs (CADAP 2018).

The same holds true for China. Although organised social work in China was established more than 30 years ago, the profession of social work did not play an explicit role in the grand scheme of 'socialist society' until the end of the 20th century (Xiong/Wang 2007; Dominelli 2020). This picture has changed significantly since then, as the country has begun to implement professional accreditation of social workers through training, social work degree programmes at universities, and professional assessment standards (Xiong/Wang 2007; Sherraden et al. 2020). With the expansion of social work schools, the China Association for Social Work Education (CASWE) has played a significant role in leading and promoting professional social work training and has had a profound influence both on formalising the curriculum and on improving the quality of social work teaching.

The lack of social support structures for key populations can be explained by the stigmatisation and marginalisation of these groups by both healthcare professionals and the general public. Existing laws, which oftentimes contradict each other in terms of implementation strategies, have also played a role in excluding key populations from service delivery. Moreover, NGOs are not involved in preparing applications for ART, which is often a strenuous process for patients. There are no job positions for social workers in inpatient facilities such as hospitals or AIDS centres in China. In addition, most NGO workers in the HIV/AIDS institutions have no social work education or training. Furthermore, if employed, social workers are paid low wages, making the profession unattractive for the majority of young graduates. For example, in AIDS centres and hospitals, the role of medical workers is more highly valued than that of social workers; equally, providing basic medical assistance is deemed more important than providing social assistance when it comes to 'social diseases' such as HIV/AIDS (see also Sultan/Mažeikienė 2019).

One important issue for improving access to services is dealing with stigma and discrimination. Anderson and Fenton (2022) argue that 'despite major advances, people with HIV still experience more multimorbidity and poorer health-related quality of life than people without HIV. They frequently face other intersecting forms of stigma, in relation to race, gender, sexual orientation, and migration status.' According to Anderson and Fenton (2022), service providers such as social workers and healthcare professionals are important for eliminating stigma so that healthcare becomes a safe environment for key populations. In Central Asia and China, several programmes have been initiated that address stigma and discrimination and thereby strive to improve access to services for key populations. In Kyrgyzstan, for example, special training courses have been developed that prepare social workers to provide services to PLWH.

The media plays a powerful role in shaping public perceptions of HIV/AIDS and HCV (see Chapter 11, 'Media Portrayal and Stigma' by Uladzimir Pikirenia in this book). However, media representations of HIV/AIDS are often inaccurate and stigmatising. These representations can have a negative impact on the lives of people living with HIV, making it more difficult for them to access the services they need and leading to social isolation and discrimination. Stigma has been driven by societal beliefs about the severity and contagiousness of HIV, perceptions that people who acquire HIV are blameworthy, and associations between HIV and behaviours that violate some individuals' behaviour variations, such as sex between men, having multiple partners, drug use, and sex work. These stereotypes can have a devastating impact on the lives of people living with HIV. They can lead to social isolation, discrimination, and even violence.

One of the most important areas in which the services of social workers are in demand is in the provision of psychosocial support for key populations. This entails open conversations, awareness raising, counselling, and facilitating access to social and medical institutions. NGOs can play a central role in the protection of rights and the provision of social support for PLWH. Worldwide, social workers fulfil a key role in providing services to key populations. However, the practice of involving social workers in prevention services for PWID is still new in Central Asia and China. The countries lack experience in developing social work services, despite the available evidence showing that injecting drug use, HIV, and HCV pose public health concerns.

Another indispensable basis for the development of prevention strategies is the availability of high-quality data. For Central Asia and China, however, there is not enough reliable data on the epidemiological development of HIV and HCV in key populations. It is therefore difficult to make a good assessment of vulnerability and to design well-coordinated prevention strategies. For example, a systematic *Lancet* review on the global, regional, and country-level coverage of testing and treatment for HIV and hepatitis C infection among PWID from November 2023 (Hajarizadeh et al. 2023) showed that data from recent HIV antibody testing were available for 67 countries and data on HCV antibody testing were available for 49 countries. Globally, an estimated 48.8% of PWID have been recently tested for HIV antibodies and 47.1% have at some point in time been tested for HCV antibodies. The authors concluded that HIV and HCV testing and treatment uptake among PWID was highly variable and suboptimal in most countries. Strategies to improve access to HIV and HCV testing and treatment for PWID and the availability of public health surveillance are urgently required.

Regarding Central Asia and China, hardly any data were included in this research; all that was available was estimations of the percentage of PWID who have ever been tested for HIV (11.5%) or HCV antibodies (10.7%) and data from only one of the five CA countries, but no data on the percentage of PWID with HIV or/and hepatitis C currently receiving HIV antiretroviral therapy or HCV treatment. Only Tajikistan was included in the study by Hajarizadeh et al. (2023), with an estimated 26,000 injecting drug users (mostly heroin users), of whom 61.3% had been tested for HCV antibodies and 46% had received treatment. This example shows that there is a need to improve the data situation regarding the overlapping HIV and HCV epidemics in Central Asia and China.

The Way Forward: How to Involve NGOs and Improve Services for Key Populations

The quality of life of people living with HIV or HCV is influenced by a number of factors, including general well-being, family status, emotional support, social contacts, environment, access to education, stigma, and discrimination, as well as the availability, accessibility, and affordability of both medical and social services (Jolley et al. 2012). In light of these factors, PLWH require comprehensive programmes that provide professional support by social workers and other social and medical service professionals. Given the fact that the role of social workers is mainly oriented at changing public opinion, building tolerance towards PLWH in society, and mobilising and activating affected people, outreach work and the use of peer-to-peer approaches have proven especially effective in the countries of Central Asia and China.

At present, social work is mostly carried out by outreach workers in places with key populations, such as prisons, street drug scenes, and other social spaces where marginalised people can be found. Both social work on the streets – with PWID and women involved in sex work – and mobile points (specially equipped vehicles for harm reduction services such as needle exchange programmes) can provide primary medical care, testing, and psychological and other preventive counselling. It is essential to develop partnerships between government agencies and NGOs, to provide financial support to NGO-led projects and to organise the financing of NGO-provided services through state contracts.

One of the aims of this book is to identify key factors emerging from close collaboration between local NGOs and project coordinators in each partnering country. We provide an overview of social work approaches in the region, including harm reduction, and drug treatment services. This includes an analysis of the situation of key populations, including people living in prison, MSM, transgender people, and sex workers. We also discuss medical services for HIV and HCV, HIV and TB comorbidity cases, the treatment and prevention of HIV, collaboration between public health authorities and social partners, implementation strategies of ART therapy,

HIV prevention in the penitentiary system, and finally the benefits of social work for people living with HIV/AIDS.

The findings suggest a need for further exploration of the interrelations between local and international NGOs, international donors, and governments. The provision of state-funded healthcare, harm reduction, and awareness-raising programmes depends on direct communication, the building of trust, and the role of effective and knowledgeable mediators. The following chapters show that the prevalence of HIV, HCV, and other infectious diseases associated with injecting drug use, sex work, and incarceration should be addressed at structural, social, and individual levels. These levels also enable the identification of the strategies necessary for working with key populations, based on indicators such as participation in the labour market, access to social protection, social and economic stratification, and individual biographies (Scheil-Adlung/Kuhl 2011). Our research findings suggest that social work with key populations requires well-organised management, a comprehensive approach to problem-solving strategies, systematic training of local social workers, increased engagement in the social support of vulnerable populations on a state level, and, as a result, the overall strengthening of interaction between all bodies responsible for HIV/AIDS and HCV prevention.

Overview of the Book

This publication presents information on the dual epidemics of HIV and HCV in Central Asia and China. Both epidemics disproportionally affect PWID who are affected by social marginalisation and discrimination. The aim of social work with this key population is to give clients access to medical and social services and to support and stabilise them so that they can make use of services. The development of social work with PWID is a complex process with many obstacles. The present publication shows the efforts that have been made to address the specific needs and vulnerabilities of PWID in Central Asia and China. The book is divided into two parts – country case studies and cross-cutting issues.

The first part of this publication includes five country studies that delve deeper into the development of HIV and HCV in the region of Central Asia and China. Each country case study comprises information about the epidemiological trends and the policy responses in the individual countries.

The first case study is Chapter 2, 'HIV and Hepatitis C in China' by Hang Su, Yifan Xu, and Jiang Du, which analyses the development of the HIV/AIDS and Hepatitis C epidemics and respective policy responses in China. The author argues that the country has made substantial progress in addressing the epidemics management, but there is still a significant journey ahead.

Chapter 3, 'HIV and Hepatitis C in Kazakhstan' by Dinara Yessimova, Mariya Prilutskaya, Dalida Mukasheva, Medet Kudabekov, and Sandugash Ismagulova provides a comprehensive account of the development of HIV/AIDS and HCV in Kazakhstan. The chapter studies the vulnerability in different population groups and gives a detailed account on the government response to the two overlapping epidemics. The argue that Kazakhstan needs multi-disciplinary teams, consisting of medical doctors and social workers, to effectively respond to HIV and HCV. The chapter concludes with an outlook on Kazakhstan's effort to reach the United Nations Sustainable Development Goals.

Chapter 4, 'HIV and Hepatitis C in Kyrgyzstan' by Jarkyn Shadymanova and Nurgul Musaeva shows that stigma and discrimination remains a main barrier in the response to the epidemics. The authors argue that addressing the complexities of HIV and HCV requires a comprehensive strategy encompassing medical, social, legal, and economic dimensions. According to Shadymanova and Musaeva, Kyrgyzstan has demonstrated a firm commitment to safeguarding its citizens' health by integrating HIV/AIDS and HCV initiatives into its long-term national development plan. Most importantly, Kyrgyzstan is committed to reach key populations, educate the public, and uphold partnerships with NGOs to sustain progress against HIV and HCV.

Chapter 5, 'HIV and Hepatitis C in Tajikistan' by Safarkhon Sattorov, Alijon Soliev, Umed Talbov, Sona Orbelyan, and Mykyta Trofymenko discusses the development of the two epidemics in Tajikistan. The authors argue that Tajikistan has made significant progress in its response to the HIV epidemic. The number of people covered by prevention, testing, and treatment services increased dramatically, which led to a decrease in the AIDS mortality rate. Tajikistan has also demonstrated its commitment to developing a system for responding to HCV by joining the Coalition for Global Hepatitis Elimination and requesting that the WHO conducts a hepatitis assessment in Tajikistan.

The last country case study is Chapter 6, 'HIV and Hepatitis C in Uzbekistan' by Uladzimir Pikirenia and Azizbek Boltaev, which examines the efforts to control HIV and HCV epidemics. The authors argue that the country faces significant challenges in the fight against HIV/AIDS and Hepatitis C. Stigma and discrimination continue to hinder access to and uptake of HIV testing and treatment services, particularly among key populations. In addition, the criminalization of behaviors associated with HIV transmission, such as drug use and sex work and MSM, exacerbates this issue, creating barriers to effective prevention and care.

The second part contains additional case studies and cross-cutting issues, such as stigma and discrimination that hamper the response to the HIV/AIDS and Hepatitis C epidemics in Central Asia and China. Other cross-cutting issues concern the role of NGOs in the response to HIV/AIDS and Hepatitis C, media reporting and the development of specific interventions such as harm reduction programmes.

Chapter 7, 'Stigma' by Hang Su, Yifan Xu, and Jiang Du, deals with HIV-related stigma in China. According to the authors, stigma significantly influences people's decisions and behaviours, diminishing their willingness to participate in HIV testing, treatment, and prevention efforts. The authors argue that efforts to reduce the burden of stigma should strategically target key risk factors associated with this issue. Specifically, interventions need to be tailored to populations experiencing heightened stigma, including urban residents and individuals with depression. Consequently, China needs to provide social support and education for the families of patients, thus strengthening connections with potential support networks. Furthermore, future strategies should focus on training health professionals and community leaders in empathy-building, stigma reduction, and discrimination elimination. This will contribute to creating a supportive clinical environment for individuals living with HIV and HCV in China.

Chapter 8, 'Opioid Antagonist Maintenance Treatment in Central Asia' by Uladzimir Pikirenia, Medet Kudabekov, Zhyldyz Bakirova, and Azizbek Boltaev, provides a comparative overview of the development of opioid antagonist maintenance treatment (OAMT) in Central Asia. The authors argue that OAMT is a key strategy in the response to HIV/AIDS and Hepatitis C among people who use drugs. Despite medical evidence, OAMT is not implemented in all countries of Central Asia. Only Kyrgyzstan and Tajikistan currently offer a full programme, whereas Kazakhstan has introduced a pilot programme. In contrast, OAMT is not available in Turkmenistan and Uzbekistan.

Chapter 9, 'Labor Migrants: Exploration of the New Driving Force of the HIV Epidemic in Uzbekistan' by Azizbek Boltaev turns to the vulnerable group of migrant workers in Uzbekistan. Nearly 5 million migrants from

Central Asia were living in the Russia by end of 2020, among which over 630,000 Uzbeks. Labour migrant regularly return to their home country. They are particularly vulnerable to HIV, as Russia has a much higher prevalence rate than the countries of Central Asia. Azizbek Boltaev shows that HIV prevalence among labour migrant is significantly higher than in the general population. It was 1.1% in 2021. There is a particularly high HIV prevalence among labour migrants from the cities Samarkand (4.8%), Nukus (1.7%), and Andijan (1.6%).

Chapter 10, 'Harm Reduction Programmes in HIV/AIDS Prevention in Kyrgyzstan: Experience, Problems, and Prospects' by Tynchtyk Estebes uulu discusses the development of harm reduction services in Kyrgyzstan. The author argues that harm reduction programmes provide information on safe drug use thereby contribute to reducing the spread of HIV among people who use drugs. By doing this, harm reduction programmes have a positive impact on public health and promote the social integration of people who use drugs. Furthermore, harm reduction helps to reduce stigma and discrimination. The chapter by Tynchtyk Estebes uulu also emphasizes the importance of a sociological approach in studying and improving the effectiveness of these programmes.

Chapter 11, 'Media Portrayal and Stigma: Analysing HIV/AIDS Coverage in Uzbekistan's Press' by Uladzimir Pikirenia presents another case study from Uzbekistan. The author analyses the way in which the HIV/AIDS epidemic is portrayed in Uzbek media. The chapter presents the findings of a study regarding the presentation of HIV/AIDS in the 14 most popular media outlets in Uzbekistan during November 2022 to October 2023. Many media articles make us of a stigmatizing language, particularly with regard to key population. A particularly troubling aspect of the media coverage is the emphasis on the criminal penalties faced by women under Article 113 of the Criminal Code, which penalises the transmission of HIV/AIDS. The author argues that journalists should be encouraged to follow guidelines for HIV reporting, ensuring that coverage is not only accurate but also respectful and free from stigmatising language.

Chapter 12, 'The Role of public organizations and non-governmental organizations in addressing and supporting people with HIV' by Guzalkhon Zakhidova, deals with the work of community-based organisations in supporting people living with HIV in Uzbekistan. The author paints a picture of the development of the most relevant civil society organisations in Uzbekistan that have developed services for key populations. The author argues that NGOs have become key actors in HIV prevention efforts and are playing a pivotal role in advocacy, programme development and support services.

Chapter 13, 'Innovative Approaches in Adolescent Sexual Education: Bridging the Gap between Awareness and Action in Uzbekistan' by Tatsiana Pikirenia, discusses the development of HIV prevention programmes among adolescents and schoolchildren. According to the author, it is essential to look at many problems through the eyes of teenagers and assess whether the surrounding infrastructure meets their needs and how programmes can be improved to prevent destructive forms of behaviour among young people. By targeting adolescents and schoolchildren with appropriate interventions, it's possible to significantly reduce their risk of HIV and STI transmission and support their overall health and well-being.

Chapter 14, 'Social and Psychological Assistance to Women Living with HIV in Kyrgyzstan' by Alla Bessonova, Asel Tentigenova, and Nurgul Musaeva, discusses the development of psychosocial support programmes for mothers with HIV in Kyrgyzstan who represent a particularly vulnerable group, especially those women who use or had been using drugs. The authors argue that it is necessary to strengthen support services in Kyrgyzstan, as mothers and children with HIV require special attention due to stigma and stereotyping.

Chapter 15, 'The Role of Social Work in the Prevention and Treatment of HIV/AIDS in Germany' by Larissa Steimle, Heino Stöver, Ingo Ilja Michels, and Daniel Deimel analyses the history of social work and HIV/AIDS in Germany. The authors show that social work plays a prominent role in supporting people affected by HIV/AIDS. To properly address the challenges posed by the epidemic social work in Germany are well advised to take an international perspective, by cooperating with and learning from different countries.

All in all, this book provides a comprehensive overview of the situation of HIV/AIDS and Hepatitis C in Central Asia and China, focusing on the specific vulnerabilities of people who inject drugs. The contributions show that the two overlapping epidemics present serious challenges for the region. Although important progress has been achieved, a lot of work still needs to be done in order to develop effective responses. The authors of this volume show approaches that can make a difference.

Bibliography

Akmatov, Manas K./Beisheeva, Nurgul J./Nurmatov, Asylbek Z./Gulsunai, Sattarova J./Saikal, Kylychbekova N./Derkenbaeva, Aisuluu A. et al. (2023): The Changing Epidemiology of Viral Hepatitis in a Post-Soviet Country – The Case of Kyrgyzstan. In: Pathogens 12, No. 8, p. 989.

Anderson, Jane/Fenton, Kevin (2022): HIV related stigma: a dangerous roadblock. In: BMJ 379, No. o2989. DOI: 10.1136/bmj.o2989.

Azbel, Lyuba/Rozanova, Julia/Michels, Ingo/Altice, Frederick L./Stöver, Heino (2017): A qualitative assessment of an abstinence-oriented therapeutic community for prisoners with substance use disorders in Kyrgyzstan. In: Harm Reduction Journal 14, No. 43, pp. 1–9.

Bobrova, Natalia/Sarang, Anya/Stuikyte, Raminta/Lezhentsev, Konstantin (2007): Obstacles in provision of anti-retroviral treatment to drug users in Central and Eastern Europe and Central Asia: A regional overview. In: International Journal of Drug Policy 18, No. 4, pp. 313–318.

Botheju, Welathanthrige S.P./Zghyer, Fawzi/Mahmud, Sarwat/Terlikbayeva, Assel/El-Bassel, Nabila/Abu-Raddad, Laith J. (2019): The epidemiology of hepatitis C virus in Central Asia: Systematic review, meta-analyses, and meta-regression analyses. In: Scientific Reports 9, No. 2090, pp. 1–15.

Center for Disease Control (CDC) (n.d.): Fact Sheet Hepatitis C and injecting drug use. www.cdc.gov/hepatitis/hcv/pdfs/factsheet-pwid.pdf, 12.02.2024.

Central Asia Drug Action Programme (CADAP) (2018): Resolution. International conference 'The role of community and social work in the sphere of drug use and prevention of infectious diseases', Bishkek, Kyrgyzstan, 24–25 January 2018.

Central Asia Drug Action Programme (CADAP) (2019): Regional Report on the Drug Situation in Central Asia. www.solid-exceed.org/resources/publication/regional-report-drug-situation-central-asia, 27.02.2024.

Central Asia Drug Action Programme (CADAP) (2020): Central Asia Drug Action Programme (CADAP) Phase 6. Final Report. March 2020. www.researchgate.net/publication/340453078_Central_Asia_Drug_Action_Programme_CADAP_Phase_6_Final_Report_A_European_Union_Assistance_Programme_for_Central_Asia, 27.02.2024.

Deryabina, Anna P./Patnaik, Padmaja/El-Sadr, Wafaa M. (2019): Underreported injection drug use and its potential contribution to reported increase in sexual transmission of HIV in Kazakhstan and Kyrgyzstan. In: Harm Reduction Journal 16, No. 1, pp. 2–7.

Dominelli, Lena (2020): Personal reflections on 30 years of social work development in China. In: China Journal of Social Work 13, No. 1, pp. 102–109.

Duan, Zhongping/Jia, Ji-Dong/Hou, Jinlin/Lou, Lillian/Tobias, Hillel/Xu, Xiao Yuan et al. (2014): Current Challenges and the Management of Chronic Hepatitis C in Mainland China. In: Journal of Clinical Gastroenterology 48, No. 8, pp. 679–686. DOI: 10.1097/MCG.0000000000000109.

Golichenko, Mikhail (2020): Documenting human rights violations is not enough to reform archaic drug policies in Eastern Europe and Central Asia. In: Bewley-Taylor, David R./Tinasti, Khalid (eds.): Research Handbook on International Drug Policy. Cheltenham: Edward Elgar Publishing, pp. 113–130.

Habibov, Nazim (2016): Effect of corruption on healthcare satisfaction in post-soviet nations: A cross-country instrumental variable analysis of twelve countries. In: Social Science and Medicine 152, pp. 119–124.

Hajarizadeh, Behzad/Kairouz, Abe/Ottaviano, Sophie/Ireland, Jeremy/Willing, Alex/Cunningham, Evan/Webb, Paige et al. (2023): Global, regional, and country-level coverage of testing and treatment for HIV and hepatitis C infection among people who inject drugs: a systematic review. In: The Lancet Global Health 11, No. 12, pp. e1885–e1898.

InBeAIDS (2020): Prevention of infectious diseases and treatment of HIV/AIDS and hepatitis among injecting drug users in Central Asia and the contribution of social work to the services for drug using people (InBeAIDS). Frankfurt am Main: Frankfurt University of Applied Sciences. DOI: 10.13140/RG.2.2.24808.62727.

Jolley, Emma/Rhodes, Tim/Platt, Lucy/Hope, Vivian/Latypov, Alisher/Donoghoe, Martin/Wilson, David (2012): HIV among people who inject drugs in Central and Eastern Europe and Central Asia: A systematic review with implications for policy. In: BMJ Open 2, No. 5, p. e001465.

Kaufman, Joan/Jing, Jun (2002): China and AIDS – the time to act is now. In: Science 296, No. 5577, pp. 2339–2340.

Kraef, Christian/Bentzon, Adrian/Skrahina, Alena/Mocroft, Amanda/Peters, Lars/Lundgren, Jens D./Chkhartishvili, Nikoloz et al. (2022): Improving healthcare for patients with HIV, tuberculosis and hepatitis C in eastern Europe: a review of current challenges and important next steps. In: HIV Medicine 23, No. 1, pp. 48–59.

LaMonaca, Katherine/Dumchev, Kostyantyn/Dvoriak, Sergii/Azbel, Lyuba/Morozova, Olga/Altice, Frederick L. (2019): HIV, Drug Injection, and Harm Reduction Trends in Eastern Europe and Central Asia: Implications for International and Domestic Policy. In: Current Psychiatry Reports 21, No. 7, p. 47.

Liu, Xue-Jiao/McGoogan, Jennifer M./Wu, Zun-You (2021): Human immunodeficiency virus/acquired immunodeficiency syndrome prevalence, incidence, and mortality in China, 1990 to 2017: a secondary analysis of the Global Burden of Disease Study 2017 data. In: Chinese Medical Journal 134, No. 10, pp. 1175–1180.

Michels, Ingo Ilja/Keizer, Bob/Trautmann, Franz/Stöver, Heino/Robelló, Ernest (2017): Improvement of Treatment of Drug use Disorders in Central Asia the contribution of the EU Central Asia Drug Action Programme (CADAP). In: Journal of Addiction Medicine and Therapy 5, No. 1, pp. 1–14.

Michels, Ingo Ilja/Stöver, Heino (2022): Drug Treatment, Culture and Social Policy in Central Asia and China. 3rd ed., Baden-Baden: Nomos.

Michels, Ingo Ilja/Stöver, Heino/Aizberg, Oleg/Boltaev, Azizbek (2020): Opioid Agonist Treatment for Opioid Use Disorder patients in Central Asia. In: Heroin Addiction and Related Clinical Problems 22, No. 1, pp. 33–46.

Moorman, Anne C./Bixler, Danae/Teshale, Eyasu H./Hofmeister, Megan/Roberts, Henry/Chapin-Bardales, Johanna/Gupta, Neil (2023): Hepatitis C Virus-HIV Coinfection in the United States Among People Who Inject Drugs: Data Needed for Ending Dual Epidemics. In: Public Health Reports. DOI: 10.1177/00333549231181348.

National Health Commission of China (NHC) (2020): Home page. www.nhc.gov.cn/jkj/new_index.shtml, 01.06.2021.

Pape, Ulla (2019): HIV/AIDS politics and policy in Eastern Europe and Central Asia. In: Oxford Research Encyclopaedia of Politics. DOI: 10.1093/acrefore/9780190228637.013.1314.

Petruzziello, Arnolfo/Marigliano, Samatha/Loquercio, Giovanna/Cozzolino, Anna/Cacciapuoti, Carmela (2016): Global epidemiology of hepatitis C virus infection: An up-date of the distribution and circulation of hepatitis C virus genotypes. In: World Journal of Gastroenterolgy 22, No. 34, pp. 7824–7840. DOI: 10.3748/wjg.v22.i34.7824.

Scheil-Adlung, Xenia/Kuhl, Catharina (2011): Social Security for All: Addressing inequities in access to health care for vulnerable groups in countries of Europe and Central Asia. Geneva: International Labour Office, Social Security Department.

Sherraden, Michael/Yuen-Tsang, Angelina W.K./Wang, Sibin/Khinduka, Shanti/Zou, Li/Deng, Suo/Gao, Jianguo et al. (2020): Re-emergence of social work in modern China: A perspective by Chinese and U.S. partners. In: China Journal of Social Work 13, No. 1, pp. 40–54. DOI: 10.1080/17525098.2020.1732534.

Su, Hang (2022): China: history of development of addiction treatment social work in China. In: Michels, Ingo Ilja/Stöver, Heino (eds.): Drug Treatment, Culture and Social Policy in Central Asia and China. 3rd ed., Baden-Baden: Nomos, pp. 53–72.

Sultan, Aysel/Mažeikienė, Natalija (2021): Living with HIV in post-Soviet states: Rejecting individual stigma through social activism. In: International Social Work 64, No. 3, pp. 386–398. DOI: 10.1177/0020872819858746.

The Joint United Nations Programme on HIV/AIDS (UNAIDS) (2018): Miles To Go. Closing Gaps Breaking Barriers Righting Injustices. www.unaids.org/sites/default/files/media_asset/miles-to-go_en.pdf, 12.02.2024.

The Joint United Nations Programme on HIV/AIDS (UNAIDS) (2019): Country progress report – China. Global AIDS Monitoring 2019. www.unaids.org/sites/default/files/country/documents/CHN_2019_countryreport.pdf, 26.02.2024.

The Joint United Nations Programme on HIV/AIDS (UNAIDS) (2021): China. Community-based organizations call for scaled up Internet-based HIV prevention services in China. 14th September 2021. www.unaids.org/en/keywords/china#:~:text=Community%2Dbased%20organizations%20call%20for,HIV%20prevention%20services%20in%20China&text=called%20for%20strengthen-,Networks%20of%20key%20populations%20and%20community%2Dbased%20organizations%20in%20China,Internet%2Dbased%20HIV%20prevention%20services, 26.02.2024.

Thorne, Claire/Ferencic, Nina/Malyuta, Ruslan/Mimica, Jadranka/Niemiec, Tomasz (2010): Central Asia: Hotspot in the worldwide HIV epidemic. In: The Lancet. Infectious diseases 10, No. 7, pp. 479–488. DOI: 10.1016/S1473-3099(10)70118-3.

United Nations (n.d.): The 17 Goals. www.sdgs.un.org/goals, 12.02.2024.

Vélez-Grau, Carolina/El-Bassel, Nabila/McCrimmon, Tara/Terlikbayeva, Assel/Primbetova, Sholpan/Mergenova, Gaukhar/Bussey, Erin et al. (2022): 'I never hoped for anything ... now I have other plans': The role of microfinance in HIV intervention for women who use drugs and engage in sex work in Kazakhstan. In: International Social Work 65, No. 4, pp. 663–677.

Xiong, Yuegen/Wang, Sibin (2007): Development of Social Work Education in China in the Context of New Policy Initiatives: Issues and Challenges. In: Social Work Education 26, No. 6, pp. 560–572.

Xu, Jun-Jie/Han, Meng-Jie/Jiang, Yong-Jun/Ding, Hai-Bo/Li, Xi/Han, Xiao-Xu/Lv, Fan et al. (2021): Prevention and control of HIV/AIDS in China: lessons from the past three decades. In: Chinese Medical Journal 134, No. 23, pp. 2799–2809.

Zabransky, Tomas/Mravcik, Viktor/Talu, Ave/Jasaitis, Ernestas (2014): Post-Soviet Central Asia: A summary of the drug situation. In: International Journal of Drug Policy 25, No. 6, pp. 1186–1194.

Country Case Studies

2. HIV and Hepatitis C in China

Hang Su, Yifan Xu, Jiang Du

1. Epidemiology of HIV in China

Development of the HIV Epidemic in China

In 1985, Peking Union Medical College Hospital in Beijing recorded the first instance of acquired immunodeficiency syndrome (AIDS) in China. Since then, the HIV/AIDS epidemic in China has escalated rapidly, particularly within the last decade. Over the past 35 years, the development of human immunodeficiency virus (HIV) infection in China has evolved significantly. Initially, HIV infections were concentrated among people who inject drugs (PWID). This was followed by outbreaks due to contaminated plasma collection in the mid-1990s, and today the virus is primarily spread through sexual contact. The annual count of newly diagnosed cases and HIV-related deaths has risen consistently since 2004, coinciding with a substantial expansion of both HIV testing and the introduction of antiretroviral therapy. The proportion of cases diagnosed at advanced disease stages has remained consistent throughout this period (Cao et al. 2020, p. 26).

The HIV/AIDS epidemic in China has unfolded in three distinct phases: 1) sporadic cases (1985–1988), involving 24 cases imported from overseas and four cases resulting from infected blood products; 2) endemic outbreaks (1989–1994), marked by incidents among injecting drug users (IDUs) in various border regions of Yunnan province; and 3) the expansion phase (1995 to the present day), characterised by increasing prevalence and broader geographical impact. Since the beginning of the third phase, the number of HIV/AIDS cases surged significantly. The annual number of newly reported cases in China soared from 2,705 in 2005 to 42,406 in 2019, a 15-fold increase. Meanwhile, HIV/AIDS-related deaths increased by only 25% from 40,711 in 2005 to 51,250 in 2019. Between January and October 2020, 112,000 individuals were diagnosed with HIV in China. By October 2020, the total reported cases of people living with HIV in China reached 1.045 million, representing a prevalence rate of less than 0.075% (Xu et al. 2021, p. 2800).

Epidemic patterns can be classified into two main categories. Initially, during the HIV/AIDS epidemic in southern and south-western China between 1989 and 1995, injecting drug use was the primary mode of transmission, accounting for the majority of infections. However, the situation has evolved, and currently, over 70% of newly reported HIV cases result from heterosexual contact. Male-male sexual contact has also emerged as a rising method of HIV transmission in present-day China, particularly in major urban centres like Beijing, Shanghai, Tianjin and other parts of Northern China (Wu et al. 2019, p. 463).

Vulnerable Groups

(1) People Who Inject Drugs (PWID)

Ruili County is a rural region in Yunnan province, which is in south-western China and is adjacent to Myanmar. In October 1989, in detoxification centres located in Ruili, Chinese scholars Ma and his team obtained blood samples from 175 individuals who were using drugs. Their objective was to screen for viral Hepatitis infections, which were spreading at that time due to the sharing of heroin injection equipment. Furthermore, they examined the residual specimens for HIV infections and detected 79 cases, resulting in an HIV prevalence rate of 45%. This study marked the initial confirmation of a significant HIV outbreak among PWID in China (Wu et al. 2019, p. 459).

Following the initial discovery of HIV cases among PWID in Ruili, Yunnan in 1989, the majority of early-phase HIV infections were concentrated within this specific region. Yunnan, located in southern China and positioned along a drug trafficking corridor known as the 'Golden Triangle', serves as a significant gateway for opiates and other illicit substances entering China from the China/Myanmar border. It's estimated that about one third of the drugs originating from this area were trafficked through China. Consequently, the increased availability of drugs in this region triggered a substantial surge in drug abuse. This, in turn, created an environment conducive to the spread of HIV infections, primarily through unsafe sexual practices and the sharing of injection equipment. During this period, the prevalence of HIV infection among PWID reached alarming levels, surpassing 80% in certain areas of Yunnan province (Wu et al. 2019, p. 461).

In 1995, new cases of HIV emerged within the community of PWID in Sichuan and Xinjiang provinces. Subsequently, the HIV/AIDS epidemic among PWID grew rapidly, particularly along the drug trafficking routes adjacent to the China/Myanmar border at first and later extending to the entire expanse of China. By 2002, every province in China had reported cases of HIV infection among PWID. It took less than 15 years for the virus to spread from Yunnan to all provinces in the nation, spreading from rural to urban areas and from border communities to central regions of the country (Wu et al. 2019, p. 461).

Between 2003 and 2005, there was a notable peak in both HIV prevalence and the number of newly diagnosed cases among PWID. However, since that period, HIV infections among PWID have consistently decreased across all provinces. Nationally, the prevalence of HIV infection among drug users fell from 7.5% in 2005 to 2% in 2018. The number of newly reported HIV cases among drug users also declined significantly, dropping from nearly 20,000 cases annually in 2005 to fewer than 4,000 cases per year by 2018. This sustained reduction in HIV infections among PWID can largely be attributed to the widespread implementation of harm reduction programmes on a national scale. These programmes include initiatives such as methadone maintenance treatment (MMT) and needle and syringe exchange programmes (NSP) (Wu et al. 2019, p. 461).

(2) Heterosexual Contact

In 2007, for the first time since the initial HIV outbreak among PWID in 1989, the number of newly diagnosed HIV infections resulting from heterosexual transmission exceeded the cases attributed to injection drug use. Since then, the proportion of HIV cases linked to heterosexual contact has continued to rise, reaching 50% in 2010, over 60% in 2011, and exceeding 70% in 2018.

Concurrently, the number of new infections among HIV-positive couples, where one partner is HIV-positive (people living with HIV, PLWH for short) and the other is not, also saw an increase. A study conducted among HIV-positive couples in Yunnan reported that the risk of HIV transmission was reduced by one third in uninfected partners of PLWH who were receiving antiretroviral therapy (ART), compared to those not receiving ART. Following the implementation of treatment as prevention among HIV-positive couples, the incidence of HIV transmission through marital sexual contact notably decreased, dropping from 2.6% in 2011 to 1.1% in 2018 (Wu et al. 2019, p. 462).

(3) Men Who Have Sex with Men (MSM)

Unlike many other countries where the HIV epidemic initially emerged within the men who have sex with men (MSM) community, China reported very few HIV cases among MSM until 2005. However, since then, the rate of HIV infections among this group has been significantly and continuously rising. In 2005, the reported prevalence was just 1.4%. Yet a national survey conducted in 61 cities across China from 2008 to 2009 revealed a national-level HIV prevalence of 5% among MSM. This prevalence continued to escalate to 8% in 2015, with some individual cities reporting even higher rates.

More recently, the estimated national HIV prevalence among MSM has reached 6.9%. The proportion of newly diagnosed cases among MSM also saw a drastic increase, rising from 0.3% in 2005 to 12% in 2010, reaching a peak of 28.2% in 2015, and then slightly declining to 23.3% in 2018. Since 2010, the prevalence of HIV among MSM has consistently been the highest infection rate among all key populations in China (Wu et al. 2019, p. 462).

(4) Female Sex Workers

Working at the National Center for AIDS/STD Control and Prevention (NCAIDS) in China, Cui and colleagues (2016, p. 1ff.) analysed sentinel surveillance data from 2010 to 2014 and discovered that the national HIV prevalence remained relatively stable during this period, fluctuating between 0.17% and 0.24%. Delving into the specifics, they surveyed all 499 surveillance sites catering to female sex workers (FSWs) in 2014. Their findings indicated that the prevalence at 473 of these sites remained below 1%, while 26 sites exhibited a higher prevalence, ranging from 1% to 5%.

In a separate study, Wang and associates (2014, p. 1ff.) conducted comprehensive nationwide cross-sectional surveys from 2008 to 2012, involving 827,079 FSWs. Their research revealed a national decline in HIV prevalence among FSWs, decreasing from 0.6% in 2008 to 0.3% in 2012. Notably, FSWs in lower-tier venues, characterised by fees less than 50 Chinese yuan (approximately 7–8 US dollars) per client and constituting 28.1% to 41.5% of all FSWs, demonstrated a higher HIV prevalence compared to their counterparts in higher-tier venues, such as karaoke bars, hotels, or nightclubs, where clients typically have a higher socioeconomic status (0.8% vs. 0.4% in 2008; 0.6% vs. 0.1% in 2012).

(5) Plasma Donors

Between late 1994 and early 1996, HIV outbreaks surfaced within impoverished rural communities across various provinces in central and eastern China, mainly among individuals who had previously donated plasma. The emergence of HIV infections among these former plasma donors (FPDs) in the mid-1990s caught the nation off guard. Initial epidemiological investigations suggested that this outbreak spanned the time period from late 1994 to early 1996 and had affected a considerable number of plasma donors and blood recipients. A 1996 survey conducted in a rural area in China revealed that the HIV prevalence among former commercial plasma donors stood at 12.5%. Regrettably, due to the sensitive nature of the issue, no comprehensive national surveys were undertaken during this period to assess the full extent of the HIV epidemic among commercial blood plasma donors in China. Occasional epidemiological studies with limited sample sizes indicated alarming rates of HIV infection among FPDs. For instance, out of 96 donors involved in underground plasma donation activities from 1998 to 1999, a staggering 74% tested positive for HIV infection.

The prevalence of HIV infection among FPDs, as revealed during the national HIV testing campaign, turned out to be significantly lower than anticipated. Just prior to the 2003 testing campaign, a scientific epidemiological study conducted in Shanxi yielded similar results. The study encompassed a substantial sample size, providing a reliable estimate of HIV prevalence. Among the 3,062 villagers who participated, 29.5% reported a history of selling whole blood or plasma. The overall HIV prevalence was estimated at 1.3%, with a slightly higher rate of 4.1% observed among plasma donors. Once again, these figures were much lower than previously assumed. The full scope of the HIV outbreak among former commercial blood plasma donors only became evident during the national HIV testing campaign conducted in 2004 and 2005. Approximately 69,000 HIV infections were linked to contamination during blood plasma collection or the transfusion of tainted blood products in China during the mid-1990s.

Following the HIV testing campaign, there was an expectation that most individuals infected through blood or plasma contamination had been identified and diagnosed, and that the remaining number of infected donors would be limited. However, the number of newly diagnosed HIV-positive individuals attributing their infection to blood or plasma contamination remained alarmingly high in the subsequent years, with over 7,000 new cases reported in 2006, 2007, and 2008, separately. After that, however, newly diagnosed HIV infections related to blood or plasma contamination became almost non-existent. Since 2015, nearly two decades after the initial HIV outbreak, no cases resulting from blood or plasma contamination have been reported (Wu et al. 2019, p. 460f.).

(6) Mother-to-Child Transmission (MTCT)

The HIV prevalence among pregnant women in China receiving antenatal care (ANC) is notably low, standing at less than 0.1%. Effectively managing the HIV epidemic in pregnant women and reducing the risk of mother-to-child transmission relies heavily on the reach and effectiveness of Prevention of Mother-to-Child Transmission (PMTCT) programmes. Statistics show that there has been significant progress in the coverage of HIV testing among pregnant women attending ANC and HIV-exposed infants at the age of 18 months. These rates have increased from 62.4% and 22.1% in 2003 to 90.3% and 82.8% in 2011, respectively.

According to national sentinel surveillance data, the prevalence of HIV infection among pregnant women was 19.8 per 100,000 in 2011. It subsequently saw a slight decrease to 9.1 per 100,000 in 2016. However, a recent study that screened 15 million pregnant women in China for HIV infection reported a higher overall prevalence of 34.0 per 100,000.

In 2005, China launched its first PMTCT programme in eight cities, and by 2015 it had expanded this effort into a nationwide Integrated Prevention of Mother-to-Child Transmission of HIV, Syphilis, and Hepatitis B programme (iPMTCT Programme). This expansion has led to significant improvements in access to care and treatment for HIV-positive mothers and their children. The uptake of antiretroviral therapy (ART) prophylaxis among HIV-infected pregnant women and their infants has seen substantial growth, rising from 35.2% and 26.9% in 2003 to 86.2% and 90.3% in 2011, respectively. Consequently, the rate of vertical transmission of HIV has notably decreased, plummeting from 31.8% before the commencement of PMTCT programmes to just 2.3% in 2011. The continued expansion of PMTCT programmes remains vitally important in the ongoing management of HIV among pregnant women and their children (Wu et al. 2019, p. 462f.).

Comorbidities

The 2019 Covid-19 pandemic has significantly impacted efforts related to HIV prevention, treatment, and healthcare services. In Wuhan, China, from 1st January to 16th April 2020, 35 out of 6,001 people living with HIV (PLWH) (0.58%) experienced Covid-19 and 197 (3.3%) had to discontinue ART, despite extensive support from both government and non-governmental organisations. In Jiangsu province, HIV testing rates saw a sharp decrease of 49.0% (919,938 tests) in the first three months of implementing Covid-19 measures. Out of an estimated 1,555 new HIV diagnoses expected during the same period, only 63.0% were actually recorded. Additionally, access to HIV healthcare services like CD4 testing and ART was severely affected (He 2021, p. 1022ff.).

To address these challenges during the Covid-19 pandemic, alternative methods of accessing HIV healthcare have been considered. For instance, research by Jiang and colleagues (2021, p. 2) indicated that more MSM self-tested for HIV (52.1% vs. 41.6%), but fewer used facility-based HIV testing (42.9% vs. 54.1%) during the time when Covid-19 measures were in place compared to before. Furthermore, compared to PLWH in other countries and the general population worldwide, PLWH in China expressed relatively low willingness to receive the Covid-19 vaccination. Among PLWH, perceptions towards the Covid-19 vaccine and willingness to receive it appear to be influenced by the internet, social media, and interpersonal communications, which has important implications for immunisation programmes targeting this population.

Between 2010 and 2018, the annual number of newly reported PLWH aged 60 years or older saw a substantial increase, surging by over five times from 5,946 to 31,541 in total. This increase was seen in both older men (from 4,751 to 24,465) and older women (from 1,195 to 7,076). Consequently, the proportion of newly reported PLWH aged 60 years or older rose from 9.27% in 2010 to 21.22% in 2018, according to statistics from the Chinese NCAIDS (Ding et al. 2019, p. 425). Most of these individuals were infected through heterosexual contacts, likely due to limited knowledge of HIV/AIDS and a low awareness of HIV risks among the older population in China. To summarise, the HIV epidemic has been increasingly affecting older people, particularly older men, over the past decade. These older PLWH also contend with chronic diseases such as cardiovascular diseases, diabetes mellitus, kidney disease, liver fibrosis, neurocognitive impairment, malignant tumours, and more. Those on HIV treatment continue to experience much higher rates of chronic kidney disease (CKD) compared to HIV-negative individuals, elevating their risks for cardiovascular diseases, end-stage renal disease, and premature mortality (He et al. 2019, p. 439ff.).

Aunon and colleagues (2020, p. 362ff.) found that while men undergoing HIV treatment did indeed report higher levels of depression and anxiety, their data did not align with their initial hypothesis, which was informed by the minority stress theory. The researchers had expected that MSM would display greater psychological distress compared to men who have sex with women (MSW). Surprisingly, their findings indicate that the sex of sexual partners was not significantly associated with increased levels of depression or anxiety symptoms. Instead, the research suggests that higher levels of depression were linked to maladaptive coping strategies and a lower physical quality of life. Moreover, younger, more educated men with poorer physical quality of life and more adaptive coping skills were more likely to report symptoms of anxiety. These findings offer a nuanced perspective on the factors that contribute to psychological distress among men receiving HIV treatment.

Regional spread of HIV

While the overall pattern of HIV infection in China is now primarily driven by sexual contact, particularly heterosexual contact, it is important to note that the distribution of HIV cases varies significantly across the country. Initially, the HIV epidemic was concentrated in rural areas of south-western and western China, as depicted in Figure 1a. Over time, it began to spread into cities and urban areas in all provinces.

According to sentinel surveillance data, in 1998 over 1,000 cases were identified in both Yunnan and Xinjiang provinces, while the remaining provinces reported significantly fewer cases. However, as discussed earlier, these new infections did not remain confined to south-western China. Instead, due to increased drug use and unsafe sexual behaviours, the epidemic started to spread, and by the following decade, it had reached all provinces across the nation. While the largest number of PLWH continued to be in southern and south-western China, there was also a growing number of cases identified in central China, as depicted in Figure 1b.

In 2008, Yunnan remained the epicentre of the HIV epidemic in China, with over 100,000 PLWH. Following Yunnan were Xinjiang, Sichuan, Guangxi, Guangdong, and Henan, each reporting more than 50,000 cases during that year. Along the eastern coast of China, there was a noticeable increase in new cases, with numerous provinces in this region reporting more than 10,000 cases (as shown in Figure 1b). This trend has persisted, and as of 2018, south-western China still reports the highest number of HIV cases.

In 2018, Yunnan and Sichuan had over 100,000 PLWH, followed by Guangxi, Guangdong, and Henan, each with more than 50,000 cases that year (as depicted in Figure 1c). The HIV epidemic has continued to expand in eastern and northern China, while regions such as Inner Mongolia, Qinghai, Hainan, and Tibet reported the lowest number of PLWH, each with fewer than 5,000 cases in 2018 (Wu et al. 2019, p. 458ff.).

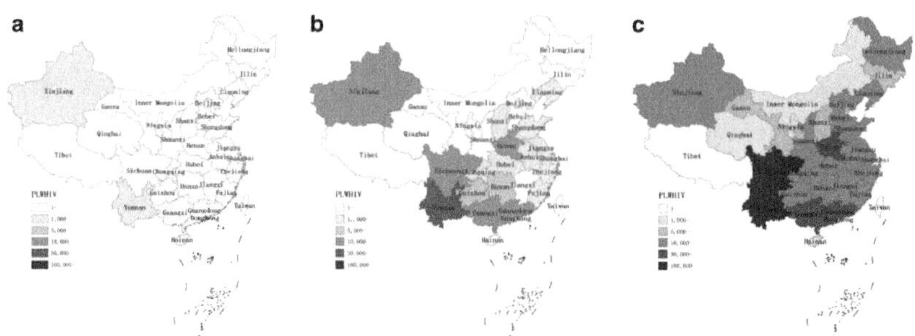

Figure 1a: Geographic distribution of PLWH in China in 1998
Figure 1b: Geographic distribution of PLWH in China in 2008
Figure 1c: Geographic distribution of PLWH in China in 2018

(Wu et al. 2019, p. 463)

The regions in south-western and south-central China, including provinces like Yunnan and Sichuan in the south-west, have historically been associated with drug abuse. Additionally, some of these regions are in close proximity to the 'Golden Triangle' and serve as trafficking routes for drugs to Hong Kong. The HIV epidemic initially emerged in the late 1980s to 1990s among drug users in these areas and has since become firmly established among FSWs (Zhang et al. 2020, p. 151ff.).

Zhang and colleagues (2020, p. 151ff.) conducted a thorough literature search and identified 51 publications that reported HIV prevalence rates among FSWs in Guangxi during the period from 2008 to 2018. These rates varied widely, ranging from 0.13% to 6.78%, with a median and interquartile range (IQR) of 1.08% (0.64%, 1.80%). Similarly, in Yunnan,

Zhang and colleagues identified 29 articles reporting HIV prevalence data among FSWs. These rates ranged from 0.13% to 10.12%, with a median of 1.50% (0.51%, 2.75%; as shown in Figure 2).

In regions with lower prevalence rates, there were fewer publications available. However, in economically developed eastern regions, encompassing seven provinces and municipalities, including Shanghai, the researchers found a substantial number of publications. These publications indicated extremely low HIV prevalence rates identified through sentinel surveillance. Nonetheless, it is worth noting that these studies did observe relatively high rates of syphilis among FSWs in these areas, with rates ranging from 0% to 10.12% (Zhang et al. 2020, p. 151ff.).

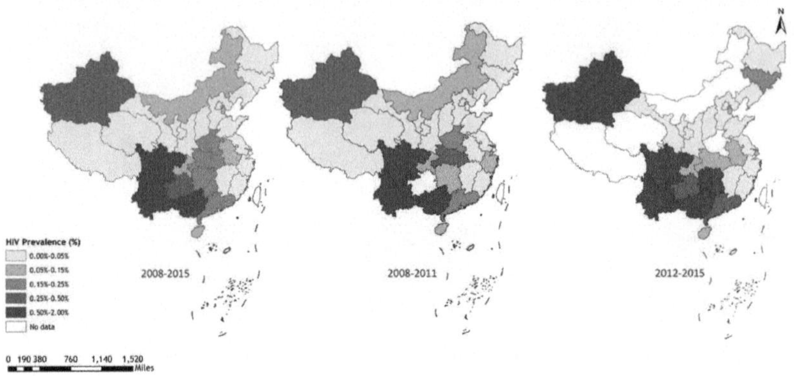

Figure 2: Median HIV prevalence among FSWs in China by province (Zhang et al. 2020, p. 158)

The prevalence of HIV among pregnant women was notably higher in southern China compared to northern China, with the highest prevalence observed in western China, reaching 93.5 cases per 100,000 individuals. Conversely, eastern Beijing had the lowest prevalence among pregnant women, with 8.6 cases per 100,000 individuals. This stark difference means that HIV prevalence in western China was approximately 11 times higher than in eastern China.

Among the 31 provinces, six had a prevalence rate exceeding 50.0 cases per 100,000 individuals. These provinces included Yunnan, Xinjiang, Sichuan, Guangxi, Guizhou, and Chongqing. Remarkably, even though these six provinces accounted for only 21% of all pregnant women in the country, they represented a staggering 76% of all HIV cases diagnosed among pregnant women in mainland China. Further analysis revealed that 30 cities reported an HIV prevalence rate among pregnant women exceeding 100.0 cases per 100,000 individuals, with 28 of these cities located in the south-west of China (Wu et al. 2019, p. 462f.).

Data availability

Data were collected from various sources, including survey reports, national publications, journal articles, and other less widely distributed literature. The scarcity of available data has significant implications for HIV prevention efforts and has the potential to impede a globally effective response to the epidemic. It is of utmost importance to closely monitor recent HIV infections in order to gain a comprehensive understanding of the epidemic's trajectory and effectively allocate resources. Urgent attention is required to establish robust surveillance systems that regularly track new infections using validated methodologies to estimate incidence rates. Ideally, these systems should also have the capacity to collect information about the risk factors associated with recent infections. Identifying the specific locations and demographics of new infections, as well as how these factors evolve over time, is crucial for guiding our response to the HIV epidemic and making optimal use of increasingly scarce resources (Dokubo et al. 2013, p. 67ff.).

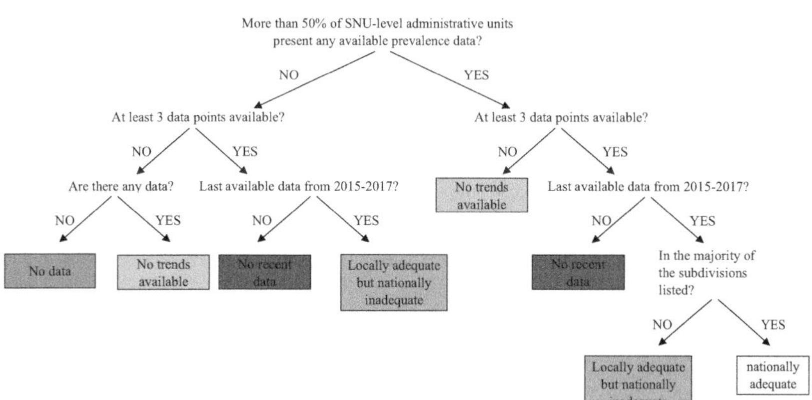

Figure 3: Decision tree depicting the categorisation of the subnational HIV prevalence data by key population (Arias Garcia et al. 2020, p. 4)

Access to treatment

Over the past two decades, China has invested substantial efforts in expanding access to ART regimens through the gradual expansion of the National Free Antiretroviral Treatment Program (NFATP). The country has also been dedicated to evaluating and optimising these regimens specifically for Chinese patients. Several domestic multicentre studies have consistently demonstrated the effectiveness and tolerability of available antiretrovirals in Chinese patients. They have also identified variations in the toxicity profiles of certain agents, proposed innovative strategies to reduce the occurrence of known adverse events, and identified cost-effective regimens suitable for low-resource settings, especially when patients are not suitable candidates for first-line regimens.

These achievements have led to a significant reduction in HIV/AIDS-related mortality in China. The number of patients receiving long-term ART has now surpassed 800,000. Nonetheless, challenges persist, particularly concerning late diagnosis and linkage to care. Additionally, long-term non-AIDS comorbidities have emerged as a new area of concern in HIV care. In response to these challenges, there have been proposals for the establishment of comprehensive 'all-in-one' HIV care centres. These centres would aim not only to physically integrate diagnosis and treatment but also to involve a trained, multidisciplinary team of healthcare professionals in the provision of HIV care.

Looking ahead, future priorities include the ongoing surveillance of drug resistance patterns, particularly acquired drug resistance (ADR), within China. Furthermore, research into innovative therapies to reduce chronic immune activation associated with HIV will be a key focus in the evolving landscape of HIV care in the country (Cao et al. 2020, p. 26ff.).

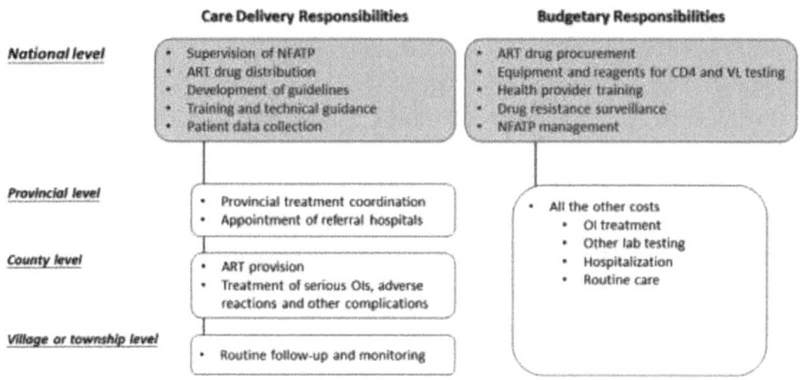

Figure 4: The structure of care delivery and budgetary responsibilities at different administrative levels of the National Free Antiretroviral Therapy Program (NFATP; Cao et al. 2020, p. 30)

2. HIV Policy in China

Legal Regulations

In 1998, China took a significant step towards halting the transmission of HIV via contaminated blood products by implementing its first blood safety law. Under this law, blood donation was allowed only if it was voluntary and repeated commercial donations were prohibited. Recognising the potential reluctance of individuals most likely infected with HIV to undergo testing, especially considering the absence of available treatment in China at that time, government officials took action. This was a period marked by severe stigma and limited awareness of HIV/AIDS within Chinese society. In response, the Chinese government introduced the 'Four Frees and One Care' AIDS policies as a comprehensive strategy to address the HIV/AIDS crisis (Wu et al. 2019, p. 460).

Main State Institutions Responsible for HIV

The introduction of MMT for PWID took place in early 2004, beginning in provinces such as Sichuan, Zhejiang, Guangxi, Yunnan, and Guizhou. By 2005, this pilot programme had expanded to include more than 30 MMT clinics spread across eleven provinces. The success and insights gained from this pilot initiative played a crucial role in shaping national policies related to NSP and MMT in China.

In 2019, there were over 760 MMT clinics catering to approximately 150,000 clients, along with 700 NSP sites serving around 40,000 PWID annually. The implementation of MMT and NSP programmes has become a cornerstone of China's response to HIV/AIDS, significantly curbing the spread of the virus among drug users. Studies have demonstrated a reduction in needle-sharing behaviours among PWID since the introduction of these programmes. However, a persistent challenge remains in ensuring that PWID continue to engage with and benefit from these programmes, as their retention poses an ongoing challenge for effectively controlling the HIV epidemic (Wu et al. 2019, p. 461).

HIV policy in China

In 2003, the Chinese government introduced the 'Four Frees and One Care' initiative. This programme included offering free ART to all PLWH, providing free voluntary counselling and testing, delivering free services to prevent mother-to-child transmission (PMTCT), granting free education to children who had lost parents to HIV or AIDS, and extending economic support to households affected by PLWH. This policy has notably alleviated the health and financial challenges associated with HIV, leading to increased HIV screening, better access to medical care, and enhanced well-being for those living with the virus (Wu et al. 2019, p. 458).

In response to the challenge of preventing ongoing HIV transmission among MSM, the government has taken proactive measures. They have developed national guidelines aimed at controlling HIV within this high-risk group. China is also collaborating with community-based organisations (CBOs) to introduce innovative strategies for HIV testing among MSM. These efforts include exploring the feasibility and acceptability of HIV self-testing, making testing kits available in vending machines on college campuses, and utilising social networking applications for HIV counselling and testing services. Innovative initiatives, in partnership with public health agencies and CBOs, leverage the internet and WeChat to enhance care efforts. Moreover, there is a strong emphasis on scaling up condom promotion campaigns and outreach services using novel techniques like social networking applications to combat rising HIV prevalence among MSM.

Despite these endeavours, the need for additional interventions, such as the potential rollout of pre-exposure prophylaxis (PrEP) for this group, is under consideration (Wu et al. 2019, p. 462).

Despite having supportive policies in place since 1998, there was a notable absence of former plasma or blood donors seeking HIV screening. As a result, no cases of HIV infection linked to plasma donation or blood transfusion were reported. It became evident that without HIV testing, no infections could be identified or documented. Consequently, the Ministry of Health initiated a nationwide HIV testing campaign during 2004 and 2005, specifically targeting individuals who had previously been involved in commercial plasma donation in the mid-1990s. Each province actively sought out these former donors and encouraged them to undergo HIV screening. Additionally, each province had the choice to extend testing to other key populations, such as PWID, MSM, sex workers, and patients attending sexually transmitted diseases (STD) clinics. This comprehensive HIV testing campaign was conducted throughout China from July 2004 to June 2005. Over the course of this twelve-month period, nearly one million former plasma donors were tested for HIV, resulting in approximately 23,000 diagnoses. The prevalence of HIV infection among former commercial plasma donors was found to be 2.3% (Wu et al. 2019, p. 462).

Major Changes or Reforms in HIV Policy

Over the past two decades, China has made remarkable strides in the battle against HIV/AIDS. According to a progress report by the NCAIDS of the China CDC, as of the end of 2017, a total of 610,000 individuals living with HIV were receiving ART in China, representing 80.4% of all reported cases. Impressively, more than 90% of those on ART had successfully achieved virologic control. The mortality rate among HIV/AIDS patients in China has seen a significant decline, dropping from 22.6 per 100 person years in 2003 to 3.1 per 100 person years in 2014. Moreover, the increasing availability of data from research networks like the China HIV/AIDS Clinical Trial Network (CACT) has directly informed the development of treatment guidelines tailored to the unique biology of Chinese HIV patients and the healthcare landscape in China. The 2018 Chinese National Guidelines for HIV/AIDS Diagnosis and Treatment marked the third update of these guidelines within a decade. Despite these tremendous achievements, it's important to acknowledge that potential challenges and risks still persist in the ongoing fight against HIV/AIDS (Cao et al. 2020, p. 30).

(1) Late Presenters and Delayed Diagnosis

Regularly monitoring key populations is a vital aspect of the national strategy for detecting HIV/AIDS cases. However, the issue of delayed diagnosis remains significant, especially in regions with limited healthcare access. The period between HIV acquisition and the onset of AIDS can be lengthy, and initial symptoms are often non-specific, posing challenges to early diagnosis without routine screening programmes. To effectively address this challenge, it's imperative to increase awareness about HIV infection and its varied clinical presentations among healthcare providers across different medical fields. At the same time, there's an equal need to enhance education and awareness among high-risk populations, particularly in areas with a high prevalence of HIV. This multi-faceted approach is essential for improving early diagnosis and ensuring that those affected by HIV/AIDS have access to appropriate care (Cao et al. 2020, p. 31).

(2) Drug Resistance

The emergence of HIV drug resistance poses a significant challenge to the effectiveness of ART. China has traditionally been considered a country with a low prevalence of transmitted drug resistance (TDR), also known as primary drug resistance, in comparison to some industrialised nations. TDR refers to a situation in which a person becomes infected with a strain of a virus, such as HIV or Hepatitis, that is already resistant to certain antiretroviral or antiviral drugs. This resistance can potentially limit the effectiveness of standard treatments from the outset. TDR is a concern in the management of infectious diseases, requiring continuous monitoring and adaptation of treatment strategies. Additionally, these rates have remained relatively stable over time. To address this issue, it is crucial to prioritise enhanced education and monitoring, particularly regarding treatment adherence. Moreover, maintaining adequate intervals for viral surveillance, especially during the initial year of treatment, is essential for controlling ADR. Furthermore, a key strategy in managing HIV drug resistance involves expanding access to antiretroviral drugs that target various virus–host interaction sites. This diversified approach will continue to be instrumental in combating the development of drug resistance and ensuring the efficacy of ART (Cao et al. 2020, p. 31f.).

(3) Novel Strategies for Unresolved Immune Activation

Despite the remarkable successes achieved with modern ART, completely eradicating HIV remains a challenging objective for researchers worldwide. Even after years of suppressive treatment, there are lingering levels of viral replication, along with unresolved low-grade immune activation. This creates a problematic cycle leading to incomplete immune recovery and an elevated risk of non-AIDS-related health issues. *Tripterygium wilfordii Hook F* (TwHF) is a well-documented immune-modulating agent approved by the China Food and Drug Administration (CFDA). It has been widely employed in China for treating autoimmune diseases like rheumatoid arthritis, showing effectiveness in controlling inflammation. Building on insights from the field of rheumatology, researchers have been exploring the hypothesis that TwHF may have a role in reducing residual immune activation in individuals with HIV infection (Cao et al. 2020, p. 32).

Cooperation of State Institutions with International Organisations (UNAIDS, Global Fund, Private Donors, etc.)

UNAIDS has established ambitious treatment targets to be met by 2030, crucial for the global elimination of HIV. These objectives entail diagnosing 95% of people with HIV (PHIV), providing treatment to 95% of those diagnosed, and achieving viral suppression in 95% of those under treatment. However, in a study featured in the AIDS journal, Shen and colleagues (2023, p. 1137ff.) analyse the transmission dynamics of the HIV epidemic in China, where the actual achievement of these targets stands at 71%, 80%, and 65%, respectively. Their study emphasises that a substantial rate of attrition poses a significant obstacle to achieving these goals. The authors of the study forecast the repercussions of attrition, particularly when expanding treatment, on various aspects, including HIV transmission, the risk of developing drug-resistant strains (acquired resistance), the transmission of drug-resistant strains (transmitted resistance), and HIV-related mortality. These insights shed light on the complex dynamics surrounding HIV control and management in the Chinese context (Blower et al. 2023, p. 1175f.).

Enhanced HIV detection can be achieved using various approaches. These include implementing more comprehensive testing programmes that specifically target high-risk groups, engaging in partner notification and testing initiatives, and providing increased education to primary care providers regarding the significance of routine HIV testing within primary care settings to identify undiagnosed individuals. Both primary care and specialised care providers play a pivotal role in improving patient follow-up. This involves tasks such as ordering and interpreting results of HIV RNA viral load tests and assessing immune surrogate markers like CD4 cell counts. Viral load levels continue to be the most reliable indicator of medication efficacy, and an effective treatment regimen is likely to boost adherence and reduce attrition rates among patients. These combined efforts contribute to more effective HIV management and care (Blower et al. 2023, p. 1175f.).

3. NGOs Working in the Field of HIV in China

Services for People Living with HIV, Provided by NGOs

Non-governmental organisations (NGOs) have played an invaluable and irreplaceable role in HIV/AIDS prevention and control efforts in China. These organisations serve as essential service providers and are actively engaged in various aspects of HIV/AIDS initiatives, including education, service delivery, and the provision of other critical services. Their contributions are instrumental in complementing government efforts and ensuring a holistic approach to addressing the HIV/AIDS epidemic in the country (Wang et al. 2016, p. 418).

Community Organisations (as a Special Type of NGOs)

In China, there are two main types of NGOs: actual NGOs and 'government-organised' NGOs (GONGOs). Actual NGOs are organisations that originate at the grassroots level and often have limited size, capacity, and access to political and financial resources. They are typically more independent from government influence. GONGOs are NGOs that receive government sponsorship and support. They are generally larger in size, have staff who have undergone extensive professional training, and often adopt a bureaucratic structure. Examples of GONGOs in China include organisations like the Family Planning Associations, Women's Federation, Red Cross, Youth League, trade unions, and various academic associations. These distinctions reflect the diverse landscape of NGOs in China, with varying levels of independence and resources based on their origin and relationship with the government (Wang et al. 2016, p. 418f.).

Advocacy by NGOs

NGOs have been acknowledged as a crucial social force in driving health initiatives, and their role in the response to AIDS has become increasingly vital. Their adaptability and popularity among HIV/AIDS patients have positioned them as more accessible providers of HIV/AIDS services. This has effectively supported the Chinese government in addressing the needs and demands of individuals affected by HIV/AIDS. NGOs play a significant role in complementing government efforts and ensuring a comprehensive response to the HIV/AIDS epidemic in China (Wang et al. 2016, p. 419).

Participation of NGOs in International and Regional Networks

The concept of civil society, known as '*minjian shehui*' in Chinese, was not traditionally a part of the political system in pre-modern China. The emergence of a relatively independent civil society is a product of modern China. This transformation was driven by changing socio-economic relations, largely influenced by the 'Open Door Policy', which resulted in the recognition and growth of civil society for the first time in Chinese history. However, the Chinese government's perspective on civil society underwent a significant shift after the 1999 *Falun Gong* incident. This event highlighted, in the eyes of the government, the potentially destructive power of civil society and raised concerns that a robust, well-organised, and uncontrollable civil society could threaten the ruling position of the Chinese Communist Party (CCP).

Simultaneously, authorities recognised that NGOs could play a supplementary role in policy implementation. To address this dilemma, the Chinese government adopted a 'state-led' approach to managing civil society in China. This approach, based on Frolic's concept of 'state-led civil society', views civil society as being created by and belonging to the state. As a result, the independence and autonomy of civil society are always constrained by the state's influence. The state legitimises social organisations and expects a disciplined partnership. In this authoritarian regime, any form of antagonism inherent in the Western concept of civil society is not permitted in state–society relations. Any alternative force that challenges the state is viewed as an attempt to undermine its political legitimacy and authority. This approach underscores the complex and controlled nature of civil society in contemporary China (Lo 2018, p. 4f.).

The Chinese state apparatus has implemented various legislative measures to manage and control the growth of both international and grassroots NGOs. These measures allow NGOs to operate openly but also aim to restrict their expansion. For international non-governmental organisations (INGOs), their operations in China are regulated by the 1989 Interim Procedures on Foreign Chambers of Commerce (*waiguo shanghui guanli zhanhang guiding*). According to this law, INGOs are limited to establishing only one branch office in China. This restriction effectively confines the geographic scope of INGOs' activities within the country, which, in turn, limits their potential political or social influence.

Additionally, to regulate the rapid influx of foreign funding into China, particularly in the field of HIV/AIDS interventions, the State Council introduced the Regulations on the Management of Foundations (*jijin guanli tiaoli*) in 2004 (Lo 2018, p. 5). These regulations are designed to oversee and control the activities of foundations and organisations that receive foreign endowments, including NGOs involved in HIV/AIDS work. These legislative measures reflect the Chinese government's dual approach of permitting NGO activities while simultaneously keeping a tight rein on their growth and influence, especially when it comes to foreign-funded NGOs and their potential impact on Chinese society and politics.

Indeed, when contrasted with grassroots NGOs, the Chinese authorities had historically granted relatively more autonomy to INGOs operating within its borders. This approach allowed the government to tap into international expertise and access foreign funding to address emerging social issues in China. However, the situation changed significantly with the introduction of the Foreign NGOs Management Law (*jingwai fei zhengfu zuzhi guanli fa*) in April 2016. Under this law, INGOs operating in China are required to register with public security officials and are prohibited from engaging in political or religious activities that could be perceived as damaging 'China's national interests' or 'ethnic unity'. The implementation of this law was perceived by the international community and Western governments as a reinforcement of restrictions on the numbers and scope of foreign entities operating within China's authoritarian regime (Lo 2018, p. 5). It marked a shift in the government's stance towards INGOs, bringing them under tighter scrutiny and control. This change in policy has raised concerns about the ability of INGOs to continue their work in China and has implications for their autonomy and the nature of their activities within the country.

Grassroots NGOs in China are subject to regulation under the Regulation on Registration and Administration of Social Organizations (*shehui tuanti dengji guanli tiaoli*). According to the 1998 regulation (amended in February 2016), in order to register with the Ministry of Civil Affairs (MOCA), a grassroots NGO must meet specific requirements, including having a minimum asset of 100,000 yuan and establishing a 'professional management unit' (*zhuguan danwei*) to serve as a supervisory body for the organisation.

Meeting these two requirements can be quite challenging for grassroots NGOs, as many of them face financial difficulties due to limited sources of funding. The majority of grassroots NGOs receive limited financial support from the government, especially if they lack political connections. Additionally, these organisations often struggle to secure donations from local communities for two main reasons: first, newly established NGOs may not have a track record that instils trust among the local population, and second, donors may not receive tax benefits for their contributions to unregistered NGOs (Lo 2018, p. 5). These financial challenges pose significant obstacles for grassroots NGOs in China, affecting their ability to operate effectively and sustainably.

Many government departments in China tend to reject the registration applications of grassroots NGOs out of concern for the potential consequences and responsibilities associated with officially recognising and supporting these organisations. Consequently, numerous grassroots NGOs either remain unregistered or register as business entities with the Ministry of Industry and Commerce (MOIC) to navigate these challenges. Furthermore, the Regulation on Registration and Administration of Social Organizations imposes restrictions by prohibiting the coexistence of 'similar organisations' at various administrative levels. This provision facilitates government management and control over the legal status of grassroots NGOs in China. Official registration is vitally important for the survival of these organisations. Legal status grants NGOs official recognition and the eligibility to receive legal and financial support from the government. By contrast, unregistered NGOs are viewed as illegal entities and are subject to potential prosecution and coercion by the state apparatus (Lo 2018, p. 5). This legal status distinction underscores the challenges faced by grassroots NGOs in China and the potential risks associated with their work.

Given the restrictive environment for grassroots NGOs in China, early responses to HIV/AIDS at the societal level were primarily carried out by GONGOs. Notable GONGOs involved in HIV/AIDS efforts included The Chinese Association of STD and AIDS Prevention and the Chinese Preventive Medicine Association. However, a limited number of NGOs focused on HIV/AIDS began to emerge in response to the growing number of infections in China during the 1990s. One such organisation was AIDS Action (*aizixing*), founded in 1994 by Dr. Wan Yanhai. Based in Beijing, AIDS Action became one of the earliest and most prominent NGOs dedicated to addressing HIV/AIDS-related issues in China (Lo 2018, p. 5). Despite the challenging environment for NGOs in the country, these organisations played a crucial role in raising awareness and providing support for individuals affected by HIV/AIDS in China.

However, there has been a notable surge in the quantity of HIV/AIDS-focused NGOs in China since 2003. According to data from the 2009/2010 China HIV/AIDS NGO Directory (*zhongguo aizibing shehuizuzhi minglu*), the number of both registered and unregistered NGOs dedicated to HIV/AIDS matters in China grew significantly, rising from 52 before 2003 to over 600 by 2010. Given the relatively low priority of health policies in the context of economic reforms, the restrictions on 'third sector' activities allowed in China's authoritarian system, and the political sensitivity surrounding the HIV/AIDS issue in the country, it is intriguing to delve into the underlying factors contributing to the expansion of HIV/AIDS-focused NGOs in China since 2003 (Lo 2018, p. 5).

Cooperation of NGOs with State Institutions

Many countries in Asia have established formal local networks for HIV/AIDS-related NGOs or civil society groups; however, such a coordination mechanism among non-state actors is largely absent in China. During interview sessions, it was observed that the HIV/AIDS NGO community in China is fragmented. Among the interviewees, the majority of NGO respondents believed that cooperation had significantly increased between the government and NGOs working on HIV/AIDS, particularly in the areas of treatment, care, and prevention. Only a few interviewees mentioned that communication and coordination among NGOs in policy implementation were lacking. A nationwide NGO respondent stated, 'We rarely collaborate with other NGOs or INGOs; we have our own teams to handle the work' (national NGO-3). Some grassroots NGO respondents in Shanghai and Kunming expressed their reluctance to cooperate with what they referred to as 'unauthentic' NGOs or NGOs with a 'government background' (Lo 2018, p. 11).

Cooperation of NGOs with International Organisations

Considering the emerging HIV/AIDS epidemic in China, the Chinese government readily embraced the international securitisation of HIV/AIDS in 2000. China was among the 189 signatories to the 2001 Declaration of Commitment on HIV/AIDS, demonstrating its dedication to aligning with the global consensus framework in response to the HIV/AIDS challenges. Significantly, the 2001 Declaration outlined a series of goals that national governments pledged to accomplish within specified timeframes, with most targets set to be achieved by either 2003 or 2005.

Table 1: Global Fund Grant Portfolio for HIV/AIDS in China (Lo 2018, p. 8)

Table 1 Global Fund Grant Portfolio for HIV/AIDS in China

Round	Grant title	Requested amount (in USD)	Lifespan
3	China CARES (China Comprehensive Aids Response): A Community- Based HIV Treatment, Care and Prevention Program in Central China	97,888,170	2004–2009
4	Reducing HIV transmission among and from vulnerable groups and alleviating its impact in seven provinces in China	63,742,277	2005–2010
5	Preventing a new wave of HIV Infections in China	28,902,073	2006–2011
6	Mobilizing Civil Society to Scale Up HIV/AIDS Control Efforts in China	14,395,715	2007–2012
8	Reaching vulnerable migrants with HIV/AIDS prevention and care services in seven provinces in China	61,413,199	2009–2014
RCC[a]	China Global Fund AIDS Program	509,000,000	2010–2015

[a]RCC stands for Rolling Continuation Channel Program

The role of NGOs in China's national HIV/AIDS programmes gained significant prominence during Round 6 of the Global Fund. This was particularly evident in the grant proposal submitted by the CCM, which directly emphasised the development of civil society groups (as indicated in Table 1). During interviews, a director of an NGO based in Hong Kong underscored the profound impact of Round 6 on NGO development, stating, 'Round 6 of the Global Fund serves as a catalyst for the government to engage more grassroots NGOs in HIV/AIDS interventions' (national

NGO-1). This perspective aligns with Kaufman's argument that Round 6, in particular, was widely perceived as a mechanism to further institutionalise the roles of HIV/AIDS NGOs in China's response to HIV/AIDS (Lo 2018, p. 8f.).

The Role of Social Work in Dealing with the HIV Epidemic

Social work courses impart essential skills encompassing psychosocial diagnostics, counselling, crisis intervention, intervention planning, case management, motivational interviewing, social group work, and street work. Social workers primarily engage in addressing mental health disorders and substance abuse, and play a pivotal role in HIV prevention and guidance. Moreover, social work is a profession that facilitates discussions at a local level to ensure the provision of adequate healthcare and social services for individuals living with HIV. This includes access to and support for adherence to antiretroviral therapy, housing initiatives, qualifications, and occupational opportunities. These achievements hinge on collaborative efforts involving diverse disciplines, professions, and policymakers.

In the context of both mental health and HIV/AIDS prevention, social work has contributed significantly to containing the HIV/AIDS epidemic. The profession has established a framework for harm reduction services, empowering individuals who use drugs to safeguard against viral transmission. Key interventions include ensuring clean needles for those with HIV, providing psychosocial support, and offering assistance to individuals living with HIV, including gay men and other populations (Henrickson et al. 2017, p. 106f.).

4. Epidemiology of HCV in China

Development of the HCV Epidemic in China

Chronic hepatitis C presents a significant global medical challenge, with China being home to one of the world's largest populations affected by this condition. In China, approximately 200,000 new cases of hepatitis C arise annually, resulting in 360,000 liver cancer-related deaths. Hepatitis C is responsible for 37.48% of liver cancer cases in China, contributing to at least 133,000 fatalities each year (Mei/Lu 2021, p. 270).

Earlier research indicated that the reported cases of hepatitis C in China exhibited a gradual increase from 1997 to 2003, with an annual growth rate of 27.89%. Subsequently, from 2004 to 2011, there was a substantial and rapid increase, averaging 48.79% annually. According to the Chinese Center for Disease Control and Prevention, one study showed a significant rise in cases from 52,927 in 2005 to 201,622 in 2012, with a more stable trend observed from 2012 to 2017. These findings are consistent with previous studies. Additionally, it was noted that the number of new cases displayed seasonality, with a peak in March each year, and a similar pattern was observed in the incidence rate. The data on deaths caused by hepatitis C showed fluctuations, with an average of ten deaths reported monthly. In a 2006 epidemiological survey of serum specimen testing in China, the prevalence of HCV infection in the total population was found to be 0.43%. However, the actual reporting rate for that year was only 5.41 per 100,000, suggesting that only one out of ten individuals potentially harbouring an HCV infection might be identified and officially reported (Zhao et al. 2022, p. 2).

Vulnerable Groups

The age distribution of reported HCV incidence displays variability. A prominent characteristic is that HCV incidence tends to affect younger individuals, while the prevalence remains elevated in older adults, particularly those aged 60 and above. In 2004, the prevalence was higher in people aged 25–44 and those aged 55 or older. However, by 2017, the prevalence was more evenly distributed across all age groups above 25. The incidence of HCV infection in infants (0–1-year-olds) showed a pattern of increase and subsequent decline, peaking in 2012 (11.71 cases per 100,000) during the period from 2004 to 2017. Mother-to-infant transmission became the most common route of hepatitis C virus infection. Risk factors for this transmission included the titre of HCV RNA, IgM positivity, high viral load, active drug use, and HIV coinfection in the mother. There was a notable upward trend in prevalence between 2004 and 2012, with a smoother trend in prevalence observed among people aged 85 and older after 2012. Starting in 2012, the incidence of hepatitis C experienced a clear upward trend among people aged 50–55, reaching its highest incidence rate (37.061 cases per 100,000) in 2017. Moreover, previous studies have consistently shown that the prevalence of hepatitis C generally increases with age, with seropositivity being strongly correlated with higher age, particularly in individuals aged 60 and older (Zhao et al. 2022, p. 4).

A study conducted in Liaoning province revealed that the seropositivity for hepatitis C was significantly higher in men than in women. Detection rates ranged from 0.18% to 2.40% for men and from 0.20% to 2.07% for women. Another study reported a prevalence ratio of 1.6:1 between men and women. This gender difference is closely associated with risk behaviours, including unprotected sex among MSM, syringe sharing, and tattooing (Zhao et al. 2022, p. 4).

Hepatitis C is found across various occupational groups in China, with retirees, farmers, and workers representing the largest proportion. Among female sex workers, the prevalence ranged from 0.32% to 1.14%, and it was even higher among those with lower socio-economic status. For male truck drivers and passengers, the prevalence was in the range of 0.3% to 0.5%, while it was 0.2% for pregnant women and young students (Zhao et al. 2022, p. 4).

The use of infected syringes is currently one of the primary modes of HCV transmission in China. The prevalence of HCV was 66.97% among IDUs and 18.30% among non-injecting drug users. Research has underscored a substantial disease burden of HCV infection among IDUs in China, with a high seropositivity rate of 71.6% (95% CI: 65.7%–77.6%; confidence interval [CI] is a statistical concept used to quantify the uncertainty or precision associated with a particular estimate). Another study reported a prevalence of 60.1% (95% CI: 52.8%–67.0%) among outpatients on methadone maintenance treatment. Importantly, the prevalence of HCV infection among IDUs in China surpasses that of general drug users. This discrepancy is primarily attributed to the sharing of needles, syringes, or other drug-related equipment, resulting in cross-contamination. Consequently, effective interventions are imperative for the prevention and control of HCV infection among IDUs (Zhao et al. 2022, p. 4f.).

Blood transmission represents another significant route of HCV infection in China, with a prevalence of 166.56 per 100,000 among first-time blood donors and 15.21 per 100,000 among regular blood donors. Hepatitis C prevalence in haemodialysis patients stood at approximately 10%, exceeding that of the general population. China's economic transformation and the introduction of the National New Urbanization Plan (2014–2020) have encouraged the orderly growth of the agricultural transfer population. Consequently, the scale of domestic migration in China has continued to expand. Rural workers have been migrating to urban areas in pursuit of better job opportunities, often engaging in 3D (dirty, dangerous, and difficult) occupations. Migrants, as a socially vulnerable group, face elevated health risks. One study indicated that the prevalence of hepatitis C among Chinese internal migrants reached 0.45%, which is 3.8 times higher than in the general population (Zhao et al. 2022, p. 5).

Among various high-risk groups for HCV infection, MSM exhibit a notably higher prevalence, ranging from 0.7% to 1.2%, compared to the general population. Additionally, HCV prevalence among clandestine sex workers falls within the range of 0.7% to 0.9%, while it ranges from 0.8% to 0.9% among men attending STD clinics (Zhao et al. 2022, p. 5).

Comorbidities

Both HIV and HCV share the same modes of transmission and common risk factors. Immunocompromised individuals are particularly vulnerable to HCV infection, and high active antiretroviral therapy (HAART) is associated with hepatotoxicity, making HIV/HCV co-infection common. A prior study discovered a 24.7% HCV prevalence among HIV-infected individuals. As of October 2020, a cohort study of HIV patients in Guangxi Zhuang Autonomous Region, China, revealed that 8.1% of these patients were co-infected with HCV. In a cross-sectional survey conducted in Yunnan province, 6.5% of a total of 5,922 HIV/AIDS cases were found to be infected with HCV. With the number of people living with HIV in China reaching 1.14 million as of October 2021 and continuing to increase, it suggests that there might be between 74,100 and 281,580 cases of HIV/HCV co-infection in China (Zhao et al. 2022, p. 5).

Data Availability

Data on hepatitis C infection is accessible through the national surveillance system as well as investigator-driven studies, and these resources are available in both Chinese and English languages.

Access to Treatment

In 2021, the Chinese Medical Association introduced the 'Process of In-Hospital Screening for Hepatitis C in China'. This process includes recommendations for the establishment of a multidisciplinary team (MDT) and suggests that clinical departments, laboratory services, and infection control at healthcare facilities should strengthen their efforts in referring and treating patients who test positive for anti-HCV antibodies. Furthermore, it encourages the screening, diagnosis, and antiviral treatment of patients with chronic hepatitis C (Mei/Lu 2021, p. 273).

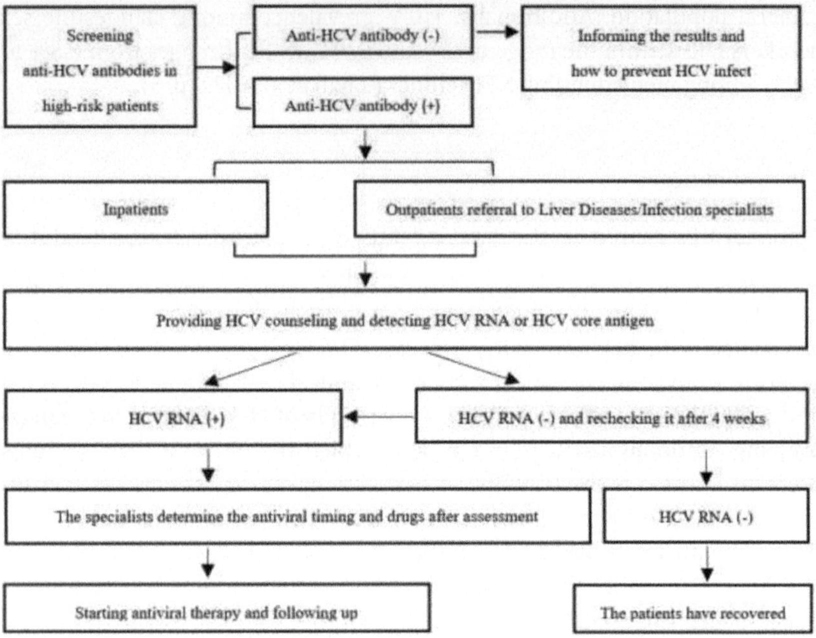

Figure 5: Flow chart for the process of in-hospital screening for hepatitis C in China. Abbreviations: HCV, hepatitis C virus; (+), positive; (-), negative (Mei/Lu 2021, p. 273)

5. HCV Policy in China

Legal Regulations

In 2019, the Chinese Medical Association updated its hepatitis C guidelines to align with international standards. The government is making concerted efforts to fully implement a range of comprehensive prevention and control measures. These include extensive health promotion and education, reinforced comprehensive intervention for key populations, standardised implementation of measures such as epidemic monitoring and response, hospital infection prevention and control, and supervision and inspection. Moreover, there's a comprehensive drive to implement clinical hepatitis C virus nucleic acid testing, ensure safe injections in medical institutions, consistently enhance patient detection, and establish standardised treatment protocols. The authorities are also actively exploring community management for chronic Hepatitis patients and working towards the inclusion of hepatitis C treatment drugs in the list of medications covered by medical insurance in China (Mei/Lu 2021, p. 272).

Main State Institutions Responsible

In China, the extensive promotion of HCV-infected patient screening and management has been facilitated through the establishment of several information technology platforms. Notable examples include the HCV community-self-management system for liver disease patients and the HCV Screening and Management Information Platform at Shengjing Hospital of China Medical University. The HCV Screening and Management Information Platform is designed to integrate screening, alerting, reporting, and management intervention functions. These platforms are closely linked with hospital information systems, enabling regulatory tracking of HCV-infected patients and significantly enhancing management efficiency (Zhao et al. 2022, p. 7).

HCV Policy in China

China has implemented proactive strategies to bolster the prevention and control of HCV infection. The goal of HCV infection elimination has been integrated into the 'Healthy China 2030' plan, as outlined by the State Council of the People's Republic of China in 2016. In 2017, China established the HCV Infection Elimination Alliance and initiated pilot programmes to offer free HCV screening in high-incidence counties, as reported by People's Daily Online in 2017. Furthermore, the government issued guidelines for HCV infection prevention and treatment in 2019. These comprehensive policies underline the determination and commitment to eliminating HCV infection in China (Zhao et al. 2022, p. 7).

Major Changes or Reforms in HCV Policy

In 1993, the Chinese government implemented a policy to screen all blood donors and enacted corresponding laws to test them for anti-HCV antibodies. Beginning in 2015, China expanded its screening procedures to include HCV RNA testing for blood donors who initially tested negative for anti-HCV antibodies. Moreover, the methods of recruiting blood donors have evolved over time. In addition to these measures, China has developed and enforced standards for disinfection, nosocomial infection control, and hepatitis C prevention and control guidelines to enhance safety and reduce HCV transmission (Mei/Lu 2021, p. 271).

Before 2017, the primary treatment for hepatitis C in China involved interferon and ribavirin (PEG/RBV) for durations of 24 or 48 weeks, depending on the genotype. However, since 2017, China's health authorities have made significant advancements in the prevention and treatment of hepatitis C. Multiple direct-acting antivirals (DAAs) have received approval for use in the Chinese market. These DAAs, administered orally for 8–16 weeks, have demonstrated a sustained virological response (SVR) in over 90% of patients infected with any HCV genotype. Additionally, adverse reactions are rare, and patients exhibit improved tolerance and compliance with these newer treatments (Mei/Lu 2021, p. 272).

Lately, China has started to employ AI and information technology to identify patients through their medical data, which represents a significant step in managing HCV. However, challenges persist, including low general awareness of hepatitis C, low screening rates, and insufficient connections to medical care. In the future, it's essential to further refine the existing prevention and control strategies and strengthen coordination among public health departments, centres for disease control, and tertiary medical facilities. Promoting more cost-effective screening and treatment for HCV within the population could pave the way for the successful elimination of Hepatitis C in China by 2030. Efforts in this direction are crucial to address the remaining issues in the management of HCV and achieve the goal of eliminating the disease (Mei/Lu 2021, p. 273).

Cooperation of State Institutions with International Organisations

In 2016, the World Health Organization (WHO) unveiled its initial global strategy aimed at eliminating viral hepatitis as a public health threat by

2030. This strategy's definition of elimination entails an 80% reduction in HCV incidence and a 65% decrease in mortality compared to 2015. It also established targets for diagnosing 90% of HCV patients and treating 80% of those eligible for treatment. This prompted international efforts to identify gaps in the existing research landscape and to create country-specific strategies to achieve this objective. However, as of 2016, it was estimated that only 18% of the HCV-infected population in China had been diagnosed. Even though 25% of the ten million patients with chronic hepatitis C required urgent treatment, fewer than 1.3% had actually received treatment, highlighting the need for substantial progress in diagnosis and treatment to meet the WHO's elimination targets (Li et al. 2019, p. 763).

Drawing from international experiences and acknowledging the distinctive demographic and socio-economic factors in China, a micro-elimination approach appears to be a more practical path towards achieving the WHO targets. This strategy could involve the prioritisation of high-risk populations, including PWIDs, haemodialysis patients, individuals co-infected with HIV and HCV, and women of child-bearing age or pregnant women (Li et al. 2019, p. 770). By focusing on these specific at-risk groups, China can take targeted measures to combat HCV transmission more effectively and improve access to diagnosis and treatment, ultimately working towards the goal of hepatitis C elimination.

6. NGOs Working in the Field of HCV in China

Services for People Living with HIV

The Center for Liver Health of The Chinese University of Hong Kong (CUHK) is one of the largest centres in Hong Kong dedicated to combatting hepatitis, including HCV. The centre offers the public up-to-date knowledge and information on liver diseases, along with a variety of tests to detect viral hepatitis and its associated complications. Caritas Lok Heep Club is another esteemed organisation in Hong Kong that caters to the needs of drug abusers. With shared objectives, CUHK and Caritas Lok Heep Club launched the New Life New Liver programme in 2009. This programme is specifically aimed at ex-intravenous drug users (IVDU), who represent a population at the highest risk of HCV infection. The programme's primary focus is on preventing the transmission of hepatitis, preserving liver function through early screening, and offering counselling and referrals to specialist clinics for prompt treatment (Lai et al. 2021, p. 283).

Community Organisations and Advocacy

Through the dedicated efforts of these two pioneering centres, the programme has gradually transformed into a collaboration between CUHK and numerous other NGOs that support the rehabilitation of ex-IVDUs. These NGOs offer a range of services, including substance abuse counselling and various rehabilitation treatment programmes. Examples of such organisations include Operation Dawn, The Society of Rehabilitation and Crime Prevention in Hong Kong, The Society for the Aid and Rehabilitation of Drug Abusers, Rehabilitation Centers of the Christian Zheng Sheng Association, Evangelical Lutheran Church Social Service, Ling Oi Centre, Pui Hong Self-Help Association, Barnabas Charitable Service Association Limited, St. Stephen's Society, DACARS Limited, and Glorious Praise Fellowship (Hong Kong) Limited. Some of these NGOs also provide religious guidance and support in addition to the services mentioned above (Lai et al. 2021, p. 284).

New Life New Liver programme

The New Life New Liver programme is a specialised initiative that focuses on individuals who were previously PWID in Hong Kong. This programme was launched in 2009, initially as a collaborative effort between Caritas Lok Heep Club and the CUHK. Over time, it has expanded into a collaborative endeavour involving CUHK and numerous other NGOs dedicated to the rehabilitation of ex-PWID. This programme is designed as a targeted screening and assessment programme for ex-PWID. It accepts referrals from social workers and requires confirmation of abstinence from intravenous drug use for at least one year. The programme includes educational talks and utilises point-of-care anti-HCV testing, employing the HCV Rapid Card from Bio Focus Company in Ui-Wang, Korea. The objectives of this programme are outlined in Table 2 (Lai et al. 2021, p. 284).

Table 2: Objectives of New Life New Liver Programme (Lai et al. 2021, p. 284)

Icon	Objective
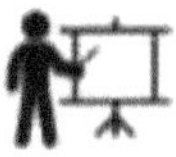	Provide education on HCV infection and its complications.
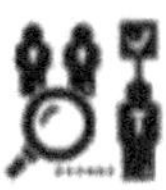	Screen for HCV infection and other liver diseases (*e.g.* HBV, HIV).
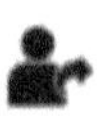	Refer for antiviral treatment for those who are HCV infected.
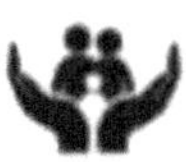	Support the social and psychological aspects of patients before, during and after antiviral treatment.
	Promote the avoidance of drug abuse to the public.

HBV, hepatitis B virus; HCV, hepatitis C virus; HIV, human immunodeficiency virus.

In the New Life New Liver programme, a diverse group of professionals collaborates within a multidisciplinary team to care for patients. This team includes hepatologists, psychiatrists, psychologists, social workers, project coordinators, and laboratory technicians. The programme has three main components. First, educational talks about HCV infection, its complications, and available treatments are provided to PWID and their family members. Adequate time is allocated for participants to ask questions following the presentation. Many PWID express concerns, particularly about the side effects of treatment. This was especially the case during the era when peginterferon-alpha and ribavirin were the only reimbursed antiviral treatments. The second phase entails a risk assessment for HCV infection, which involves blood tests and transient elastography examinations to measure liver stiffness. These assessments are typically scheduled within three months of the educational session. Due to the referral policy of the

Hospital Authority in Hong Kong, HCV patients are referred to their respective regional hospitals based on their residential address for long-term follow-up and social worker support provided by the relevant NGOs (Lai et al. 2021, p. 284).

7. Conclusions

The HIV/AIDS epidemic in China has undergone significant transformations over the past 35 years. China has implemented a multitude of laws, policies, and guidelines to support the response to HIV/AIDS, demonstrating a strong commitment both politically and economically in the battle against HIV/AIDS. Domestic multicentre studies conducted over the years have confirmed the effectiveness and tolerability of available antiretroviral treatments in Chinese patients. These studies have also revealed variations in toxicity profiles for certain medications, proposed innovative strategies to minimise known adverse events, and identified cost-effective regimens suitable for low-resource settings when patients are not eligible for first-line treatments. These achievements have led to a remarkable reduction in mortality from HIV/AIDS over the past two decades, and the number of patients on long-term ART now exceeds 800,000. Nevertheless, challenges such as late diagnosis and linkage to care continue to be significant barriers, and the emergence of non-AIDS comorbidities represents a new area of concern in HIV care. This has spurred the concept of comprehensive 'all-in-one' HIV care centres, which would not only streamline the diagnosis and treatment process but also involve a trained, multidisciplinary team of healthcare professionals providing comprehensive HIV care. Looking ahead, future priorities include the ongoing monitoring of drug resistance patterns, particularly ADR, within China. Additionally, research into innovative therapies to mitigate HIV-related chronic immune activation is on the agenda to further advance the field of HIV care (Cao et al. 2020, p. 32).

The most significant challenge in eliminating HIV in China lies in identifying currently undiagnosed infections and ensuring that infected individuals are rapidly linked to treatment. Approximately 30% of HIV infections in China go undetected. Since 2003, China has offered free HIV counselling and testing, along with free antiretroviral therapy for those meeting specific eligibility criteria based on CD4 cell count. In 2016, these criteria were aligned with the WHO's policy of treating all PHIV. However, at present, many high-risk individuals do not seek testing, and among those who do, a substantial number do not follow up on their diagnosis. Multiple strategies can be employed to enhance HIV detection, such as implementing more intensive testing programmes that target high-risk groups, partner notification and testing, and providing greater education for primary care providers on the importance of routine testing in the primary care setting to identify undiagnosed individuals. Both primary care and specialised care providers play a crucial role in improving patient follow-up, which includes ordering and interpreting results of HIV RNA viral load and immune surrogate markers like CD4 cells. Viral load levels continue to be the most effective indicator of medication efficacy; an effective regimen is likely to promote adherence and reduce attrition. Consequently, the most plausible scenario is that by 2030, treatment coverage will have significantly increased, HIV transmission rates will have decreased, drug resistance will remain at low levels, and China will be on the verge of realising UNAIDS' second and third treatment targets. However, the foremost challenge will likely revolve around achieving UNAIDS' first treatment target by 2030 (Blower et al. 2023, p. 1175f.).

The primary challenge in HCV management in China is a complex issue that involves identifying HCV-infected patients, ensuring their access to treatment options, and making these treatments affordable. Furthermore, patient adherence and physician guidance could introduce additional variability in the eventual therapeutic outcomes. The absence of a comprehensive epidemiological monitoring system in China also presents additional hurdles in enhancing HCV management at a national level (Li et al. 2019, p. 770).

Enormous progress has been made in the management of HCV in China over the past five years. Healthcare communities and governmental bodies in the country have been actively working towards increasing public awareness, enhancing access to healthcare, and providing more extensive training for healthcare professionals. Despite these recent efforts, the challenge of achieving the WHO's 2030 goals for HCV elimination in China remains formidable due to the extensive scale, complexity, and cost of implementation. Given that China is the most populous country globally, there may be significant variations between different Chinese cities and even counties concerning factors like the epidemiology, transmission routes, and the composition of HCV-infected patient groups. Variabilities may also arise in the availability of healthcare resources, reimbursement policies, and the financial capabilities of municipal governments, impacting the provision of HCV care (Li et al. 2019, p. 770).

In early 2018, the 'Seek and Cure Hepatitis C' patient assistance programme, launched by the China Primary Health Care Foundation, was introduced on a national scale. This initiative aims to offer free DAA drugs to patients who live on the minimum subsistence level and provide a half-course of medication free of charge to individuals with low incomes. Such endeavours represent a positive step forward, contributing to the enhancement of the accessibility of HCV management (Li et al. 2019, p. 770).

To bring it all together, China has undoubtedly made substantial strides in HCV management, but there is still a significant journey ahead. Over the next five years, it is anticipated that both the healthcare community and governmental stakeholders will place growing emphasis on the accessibility and affordability of HCV medications, specifically DAAs. Furthermore, more patients are expected to benefit as DAAs become the established standard of care within an enhanced HCV management framework that relies on micro-elimination strategies. With any luck, a well-informed HCV management coalition will allocate essential funds and resources to areas with the most pressing needs, thus accelerating the nation's progress towards achieving the WHO's HCV elimination goal (Li et al. 2019, p. 770).

Bibliography

Arias Garcia, Sonia/Chen, Jia/Garcia Calleja, Jesus/Sabin, Keith/Ogbuanu, Chinelo/Lowrance, David/Zhao, Jinkou (2020): Availability and Quality of Surveillance and Survey Data on HIV Prevalence Among Sex Workers, Men Who Have Sex With Men, People Who Inject Drugs, and Transgender Women in Low- and Middle-Income Countries: Review of Available Data (2001-2017). In: JMIR Public Health and Surveillance 6, No. 4, pp. 1–12. DOI: 10.2196/21688.

Aunon, Frances M./Simoni, Jane M./Yang, Joyce P./Shiu, Chengshi/Chen, Wei-Ti/Edmunds, Sarah R./Ramaiya, Megan et al. (2020): Depression and anxiety among HIV-positive men who have sex with men and men who have sex with women in China. In: AIDS Care 32, No. 3, pp. 362–369. DOI: 10.1080/09540121.2019.1683803.

Blower, Sally/Okano, Justin T./Kahn, James S. (2023): Modeling UNAIDS treatment targets for China. In: AIDS 37, No. 7, pp. 1175–1176. DOI: 10.1097/QAD.0000000000003571.

Cao, Wei/Hsieh, Evelyn/Li, Taisheng (2020): Optimizing Treatment for Adults with HIV/AIDS in China: Successes over Two Decades and Remaining Challenges. In: Current HIV/AIDS Reports 17, No. 1, pp. 26–34. DOI: 10.1007/s11904-019-00478-x.

Cui, Yan/Guo, Wei/Li, Dongmin/Wang, Liyan/Shi, Cynthia X./Brookmeyer, Ron/Detels, Roger et al. (2016): Estimating HIV incidence among key affected populations in China from serial cross-sectional surveys in 2010-2014. In: Journal of the International AIDS Society 19, No. 1, pp. 1–8. DOI: 10.7448/IAS.19.1.20609.

Ding, Yingying/Ma, Zhonghui/He, Jiayu/Xu, Xiaoyi/Qiao, Shijie/Xu, Lulu/Shi, Ruizi et al. (2019): Evolving HIV Epidemiology in Mainland China: 2009–2018. In: Current HIV/AIDS Reports 16, pp. 423–430. DOI: 10.1007/s11904-019-00468-z.

Dokubo, E. Kainne/Kim, Andrea A./Le, Linh-Vi/Nadol, Patrick J./Prybylski, Dimitri/Wolfe, Mitchell I. (2013): HIV Incidence in Asia: A Review of Available Data and Addessment of the Epidemic. In: AIDS Reviews 15, No. 2, pp. 67–76.

He, Na (2021): Research Progress in the Epidemiology of HIV/AIDS in China. In: China CDC Weekly 3, No. 48, pp. 1022–1030. DOI: 10.46234/ccdcw2021.249.

He, Na/Ding, Yingying/Li, Jing/Yuan, Shiying/Xu, Lulu/Qiao, Shijie et al. (2019): HIV and Aging in Mainland China: Implications for Control and Prevention Research. In: Current HIV/AIDS Reports 16, No. 6, pp. 439–447. DOI: 10.1007/s11904-019-00473-2.

Henrickson, Mark/Chipanta, David/Lynch, Vincent/Muñoz Sanchez, Hernando/Nadkarni, Vimla/Semigina, Tetyana/Sewpaul, Vishanthie (eds.) (2017): Getting to Zero: Global Social Work Responds to HIV. Auckland: Massey University Press.

Jiang, Hongbo/Xie, Yewei/Xiong, Yuan/Zhou, Yi/Lin, Kaihao/Yan, Yao et al. (2021): HIV self-testing partially filled the HIV testing gap among men who have sex with men in China during the COVID-19 pandemic: results from an online survey. In: Journal of the International AIDS Society 24, No. 5, pp. 1–6. DOI: 10.1002/jia2.25737.

Lai, Jimmy Che-To/Ho, Agnes Hiu-Yan/Wu, Claudia Wang-Kwan/Wong, Grace Lai-Hung (2021): HCV elimination in Hong Kong – Non-government organization (NGO) activities. In: Global Health & Medicine 3, No. 5, pp. 283–287. DOI: 10.35772/ghm.2021.01049.

Li, Mingyang/Zhuang, Hui/Wei, Lai (2019): How would China achieve WHO's target of eliminating HCV by 2030? In: Expert Review of Anti-infective Therapy 17, No. 10, pp. 763–773. DOI: 10.1080/14787210.2019.1675509.

Lo, Catherine Yuk-ping (2018): Securitizing HIV/AIDS: a game changer in state-societal relations in China? In: Globalization and Health 14, No. 50, pp. 1–14. DOI: 10.1186/s12992-018-0364-7.

Mei, Xue/Lu, Hongzhou (2021): Prevalence, diagnosis, and treatment of hepatitis C in Mainland China. In: Global Health & Medicine 3, No. 5, pp. 270–275. DOI: 10.35772/ghm.2021.01080.

Shen, Mingwang/Xiao, Yanni/Rong, Libin/Zhuang, Guihua/Song, Chang/Zhao, Quanbi et al. (2023): The impact of attrition on the transmission of HIV and drug resistance: a mathematical modelling study. In: AIDS 37, No. 7, pp. 1137–1145. DOI: 10.1097/QAD.0000000000003528.

Wang, Danni/Mei, Guangliang/Xu, Xiaoru/Zhao, Ran/Ma, Ying/Chen, Ren et al. (2016): Chinese non-governmental organizations involved in HIV/AIDS prevention and control: Intra-organizational social capital as a new analytical perspective. In: BioScience Trends 10, No. 5, pp. 418–423. DOI: 10.5582/bst.2016.01134.

Wang, Lu/Tang, Weiming/Wang, Lan/Qian, Shasha/Li, Yin-ge/Xing, Jiannan et al. (2014): The HIV, Syphilis, and HCV Epidemics Among Female Sex Workers in China: Results From a Serial Cross-Sectional Study Between 2008 and 2012. In: Clinical Infectious Diseases 59, No. 1, pp. 1–9. DOI: 10.1093/cid/ciu245.

Wu, Zunyou/Chen, Junfang/Scott, Sarah Robbins/McGoogan, Jennifer M. (2019): History of the HIV Epidemic in China. In: Current HIV/AIDS Reports 16, pp. 458–466. DOI: 10.1007/s11904-019-00471-4.

Xu, Jun-Jie/Han, Meng-Jie/Jiang, Yong-Jun/Ding, Hai-Bo/Li, Xi/Han, Xiao-Xu et al. (2021): Prevention and control of HIV/AIDS in China: lessons from the past three decades. In: Chinese Medical Journal 134, No. 23, pp. 2799–2809. DOI: 10.1097/CM9.0000000000001842.

Zhang, Hanxi/Hsieh, Evelyn/Wang, Lu/Liao, Susu (2020): HIV/AIDS Among Female Sex Workers in China: Epidemiology and Recent Prevention Strategies. In: HIV/AIDS Reports 17, No. 2, pp. 151–160. DOI: 10.1007/s11904-019-00477-y.

Zhao, Zeyu/Chu, Meijie/Guo, Yichao/Yang, Shiting/Abudurusuli, Guzainuer/Frutos, Roger/Chen, Tianmu (2022): Feasibility of Hepatitis C Elimination in China: From Epidemiology, Natural History, and Intervention Perspectives. In: Frontiers in Microbiology 13, pp. 1–11. DOI: 10.3389/fmicb.2022.884598.

3. HIV and Hepatitis C in Kazakhstan

Dinara Yessimova, Mariya Prilutskaya, Dalida Mukasheva, Medet Kudabekov, Sandugash Ismagulova

Introduction

The issue of HIV infection in Kazakhstan remains a public health priority. A step-by-step reform of the nation's health policies guarantees that the country's population will receive a timely diagnosis of HIV infection and the earliest possible prescription of the necessary therapy, in accordance with the UNAIDS '90-90-90' recommendations. Kazakhstan has managed to keep the spread of HIV infection at a concentrated stage, with infections remaining concentrated in key populations. Meanwhile, coverage of HIV-focused services for key populations, including harm reduction interventions, remains limited due to a range of barriers and challenges. The aim of this chapter is to systematise information on the history of the spread of HIV infection in the country and the phased roll-out of HIV policies. The statistical data presented here show the epidemiological situation as regards HIV among both the general population and key populations. The chapter describes the context for establishing HIV services for key populations, emphasising the role of NGOs in these endeavours. In addition, the chapter provides information on the spread of viral hepatitis C (HCV) in Kazakhstan, which is on the verge of implementing comprehensive HCV screening among the general population. While the chapter sheds light on the country's achievements in rolling out free direct-acting antiviral therapy for those living with HCV, it underlines the gap in the involvement of NGOs in HCV preventive initiatives for key populations.

HIV in Kazakhstan: Epidemiology, Key Populations and Services

In the era of global modernization and economic intensification, the issue of public health stays on the international agenda as one of the most concerning topics of political discussions and social science debates. The COV-ID pandemic has shown the vulnerability of the global space to infectious threats and forced the world to take a new look at systemic measures to limit the spread of pathogenic microorganisms and viruses. HIV continues to pose a significant worldwide public health challenge, having caused the loss of approximately 40.4 million lives (with an estimated range of 32.9 million to 51.3 million) up to this point. The virus persists in all countries across the globe, and in certain nations, there are reports of rising rates of new infections, despite earlier declines (World Health Organization [WHO] 2023b). Worldwide, approximately 58 million individuals are living with a chronic hepatitis C infection, and roughly 1.5 million new infections emerge annually. An estimated 3.2 million adolescents and children are affected by chronic hepatitis C infection (WHO 2023a).

According to the World Health Organization's (WHO) report, every region has made progress in their own way and, at the same time, has to deal with specific gaps in their anti-HIV and HCV strategies. Central Asia, as a large and unique WHO European subregion, demonstrates its uniqueness in terms of its political structures, socio-economic characteristics, and health indicators. According to the latest United Nations' (UN) estimates, the current population of Central Asia is more than 75 million people – about 1% of the global population. Over the past ten years, the population of Central Asia has increased annually by an average of more than one million people (Tukumov 2023). This territory is characterised by intense migration, uneven access to medical care, and differences in preventive and harm reduction approaches (Renton et al. 2006). In parallel, since the beginning of the 1990s, Central Asian countries have been facing drug challenges (including illicit drug traffic and high prevalence of people who inject drugs [PWID]) in parallel with severe criminalisation and penalisation of those who are involved in drug use. All of these factors drive the growth of HIV and HCV in the country. Over the past ten years, the regions of Eastern Europe and Central Asia (EECA) have consistently recorded the highest rates of new HIV cases. In 2019, there were 100,000 new HIV infections in these regions alone, as reported by the Joint United Nations Programme on HIV and AIDS (UNAIDS) in 2019. What is particularly concerning is that in Eastern Europe and Central Asia, a staggering 95% of all new HIV infections are attributed to specific high-risk groups, including people who inject drugs, commercial sex workers, men who have sex with men, individuals in prison, and their sexual partners, as indicated by UNAIDS in 2019 (Davlidova et al. 2021).

Within the region of Central Asia, Kazakhstan was the first country exposed to HIV. Information about the first patients in Kazakhstan already appeared in 1987, when the country was part of the Soviet Union (USSR). HIV infection was diagnosed in six foreign students who were subjected to immediate deportation from the Soviet Union. At that time, the Soviet authorities imparted an unambiguous message about the extreme danger of the HIV epidemic and associated it with the Western lifestyle, which was stigmatised as depraved and vicious. The agenda was widely supported by the national and local press. Headlines at the time compared HIV to the plague. Only few doctors had the courage to speak openly about the need for prevention services, increased healthcare capacity, and staff training before the first cases were registered among residents (Romashkina 2021). But even then, health experts argued that the threat of HIV spread lay not only in the behaviour of key population groups but also in insufficient anti-epidemic measures in hospitals. The insufficient supply of disposable medical instruments for clinics exacerbated the situation. For example, one Ministry of Health employee confided that the Kazakh Soviet Republic received only 21 million syringes from the Central Soviet Government in 1990, which covered only 10% of its real demand. At the same time, there was a hepatitis B epidemic in the country, with thousands of cases recorded. In parallel, the incidence of syphilis increased. For instance, in 1990, 13,000 new cases of syphilis were registered. Syphilis rose from the level of 1.4 cases per 100,000 population at the beginning of the 1990s to 640 cases per 100,000 at the beginning of the 2000s (Zhusupov 2000).

At the end of 1990, the Republican AIDS Center was established, followed by the networks of regional centres across Kazakhstan. The first HIV case among the Kazakhstan population was diagnosed in Almaty in 1990. By 1st December 1991, up to twenty HIV-positive patients were registered, nine of whom were foreign students. At the same time, at the dawn of its independence, Kazakhstan was facing a severe economic crisis, increased levels of crime, and drug trafficking. The first case of HIV among PWID was registered in 1996. The man was never registered at a drug treatment centre but was diagnosed with HIV and substance use disorders (SUD) in prison. Unlike with the homosexual HIV cases, the index case resulted in an instant outbreak of the epidemic, initially limited to Temirtau, a small town in the Karaganda region. From 1996 to 1997, specialists have faced exponential growth in the number of infections (from 30 cases in 1996 to 300 cases in 1997). It was in the city of Temirtau that the work of non-governmental organisations focusing on providing HIV services began. These NGOs were launched by active patients and community members in collaboration with the local AIDS centre. The first HIV preventive services included the distribution of informational leaflets and the opening of syringe exchange points in Temirtau (Sukhorukov 2023). At the time, this was a rather exceptional example of a progressive approach towards HIV services; by comparison, the main policy approaches were repressive and included forced HIV testing, police raids, and severe stigmatisation. Newspapers of the time wrote about mass cases of acquired immune deficiency syndrome (AIDS) panic, with parents refusing to vaccinate their children out of fear that they would be infected with HIV. People with HIV often had to relocate, due to the harassment they faced and the threats made to their lives when others discovered their HIV status. The media fuelled this general AIDS phobia. By 1999, the number of registered HIV patients comprised 1,000 persons, the significant majority of whom were infected through injecting drug use. At the same time, experts believe that the real number of HIV cases exceeded the aforementioned figure at least tenfold. The year 2000 witnessed a growth in the number of HIV infection cases in other cities, namely Shymkent in Southern Kazakhstan and Pavlodar in Northern Kazakhstan. Kazakh authorities reported that in 2001 alone the number of HIV infections rose by about 240% (Human Rights Watch 2003). As of 1st June 2001 in the Republic of Kazakhstan, the total number of people diagnosed with HIV infection since the first case was registered in 1987 was 1,799. 37 people living with HIV (PLWH) have gone on to develop AIDS, and 31 of them have died to date. The rate of first-identified HIV prevalence in 2000 was 35 per 100,000 persons surveyed. In the first five months of 2001, the HIV prevalence was 99 per 100,000 people surveyed, five times higher than in the same period in 2000.

Several factors have contributed to the rapid growth of HIV infection in Kazakhstan. Firstly, the population had little information or awareness about HIV. That was especially true for young people. According to the Kazakhstan Demographic and Health Surveillance Report, 16.9% of men and 33% of women aged 15–19 did not know how to prevent an HIV infection (Institute of legislation and legal information of the Republic of Kazakhstan of the Ministry of Justice of the Republic of Kazakhstan 2001). As many as 27.4% of men and 65% of women had experience of unprotected sexual intercourse with a non-regular partner. The young age was an additional risk factor associated with an increased likelihood of getting an HIV infection (a 2.5-fold increased risk) (Institute of legislation and legal information of the Republic of Kazakhstan of the Ministry of Justice of the Republic of Kazakhstan 2001). According to reports on the drug use situation in five regions of Kazakhstan, about one third of university students reported personal experience of drug use. It was also of considerable concern that the proportion of people using drugs at that time was extremely high (the estimated number was up to 250,000) (Institute of legislation and legal information of the Republic of Kazakhstan of the Ministry of Justice of the Republic of Kazakhstan 2001). As of 2012, only 15%–20% of drug users engaged in behaviours that are safe in terms of HIV transmission. At that time, the most common types of drugs in Kazakhstan were cannabinoids (500–750 tons consumed per year) and opioids (29.3 tons consumed per year), in addition to other drugs (14.4 tons consumed per year) (Katkov 2013).

Considering the high prevalence of parenteral HIV transmission, drug use and heroin addiction have been the key drivers of HIV epidemics all across Kazakhstan for more than two decades. The growth of the prison population in the country has also been a significant driver in terms of the spread of HIV. Surveys conducted among anonymous visitors of injection drug use drop-in centres in Almaty and Shymkent indicated that drug-dependent individuals accounted for up to 30% of people in penitentiary institutions, where, despite the measures taken, drugs remained available. Injecting equipment was not sterilised and was used until it was completely unusable. The results of epidemiological surveillance conducted in 2001 in penitentiary institutions of the Karaganda region showed 42% seroprevalence of HCV among inmates (Institute of legislation and legal information of the Republic of Kazakhstan of the Ministry of Justice of the Republic of Kazakhstan 2001).

Since 2005, additional vulnerability to HIV has been registered among the female population. According to official state statistics, women accounted for 19% of newly registered HIV cases in 2001, increasing to 28% by 2005. One of the causal factors here was the steady increase in the proportion of HIV cases that were transmitted through sexual activity, which accounted for 5% of newly registered cases in 2001, compared to 25% in 2005 (Institute of legislation and legal information of the Republic of Kazakhstan of the Ministry of Justice of the Republic of Kazakhstan 2006). The groups of people with unsafe injecting and sexual behaviours, among whom HIV infection is currently concentrated, are predominantly drawn from the least socially protected segments of the population. Their vulnerability to HIV infection is determined by their lack of access to information and education programmes and their inability to use any knowledge they do have to protect themselves from HIV. The issue was also aggravated by poor knowledge about HIV among medical specialists and insufficient anti-epidemic standards in clinics. The first requirements for mandatory HIV screening among blood donors and arriving foreigners were adopted in the early 1990s. However, these requirements were not sufficiently fulfilled, given the low material resources of the clinics. In 2006 an outbreak of nosocomial HIV transmission was registered in Kazakhstan. The tragedy was that 150 children were infected at one time in the city of Shymkent. The children were infected due to the repeated use of disposable instruments during blood transfusions. Overall, 21 doctors were brought to criminal liability (Kommersant 2007). The repercussions of these mass HIV infection cases included not only the punishment of doctors but also the worsening of stigmatisation issues in Kazakhstan. The victims of the tragedy confessed that discrimination and stigma was a key part of their daily lives (Akulova 2023).

Stigma in its various forms has proved to be one of the key problems associated with HIV epidemics. It is obvious that HIV stigma hinders preventive and treatment approaches. At the same time, stigma has its direct impacts on those who are beyond the scope of the HIV problem being a key factor in the epidemic's spread (Li et al. 2017). Stigma refers to the societal devaluation and disapproval linked to specific attributes, actions, medical conditions, and social positions (Stringer et al. 2019). In the context of HIV, stigma is made worse by issues such as contempt for drug addiction, the criminalisation of and punishment for risky behaviour (such as drug use, commercial sex, and belonging to a sexual minority), and a lack of evidence-based information about the infection. Stigma can manifest through isolation, criticism, verbal harassment, aggression, threats, penalisation, denial of care and testing, poorer treatment provision, and administrative barriers. According to the Stigma Index Report in 2016, one in three (39.3%) of people living with HIV who was interviewed was afraid of being gossiped about because of his/her positive HIV status or feared sexual rejection (37.5%).

One in five people living with HIV (21.3%) experienced the fear of being verbally affronted, harassed, and/or threatened. Every tenth person feared physical harassment, threats, or being physically assaulted. People living with HIV in Kazakhstan reported that they had been gossiped about (44.6%), had been verbally affronted, harassed, and/or threatened (23.2%), had experienced sexual rejection (15.8%) or psychological pressure and manipulation by their partner (13.0%), or that members of their household had been discriminated against (12.3%). 8.8% of people interviewed reported having been physically harassed and/or threatened, and 8.2% had been physically assaulted. In Kazakhstan, individuals with HIV frequently encounter discrimination, primarily from healthcare providers (with 6.0% reporting strong discrimination and 12.4% indicating signs of discrimination) and government employees (with 4.0% experiencing strong discrimination and another 4.0% reporting signs of discrimination) (Amanzholov et al. 2016). As many as 30%–40% of Kazakhstanis stated that they would not buy food from a person with HIV or allow their children to learn alongside HIV-infected peers (The Joint United Nations Programme on HIV/AIDS [UNAIDS] 2021). Additionally, one of the significant drivers of HIV stigma are service providers who exhibit stigmatising behaviour in narcology dispensaries, tuberculosis (TB) clinics, and places that provide reproductive and maternal healthcare services. Taking unnecessary precautions, such as using masks, actively denying care, and segregating clients who were living with HIV, were signs of widespread stigmatisation and were hardly perceived by health workers as devaluating (Stringer et al. 2019).

All these events showed that Kazakhstan had to reconsider its HIV policy. Since the early 2000s, the country has started to change its HIV policy in terms of treatment, prevention, and surveillance of infection. The first preventive HIV programmes were already launched in the mid-1990s, but at that time their efficiency was limited by poor financial policy and a lack of international support. The first large-scale international collaboration started in 2003 when the Republican Aids Center received the Global Fund's grant for capacity building for the response to HIV/AIDS. Within the framework of the grant, Kazakhstan received money to cover the first antiretroviral therapy (ART) campaign for those patients who had already been diagnosed with AIDS. Since 2006, ART programmes have been fully covered by the state budgets. To date, in the era of health insurance, ART and all diagnostic procedures for HIV patients are provided free of charge, regardless of the individual's insurance status, within the guarantee package of free medical care.

However, in 2017, Kazakhstan adopted clinical protocols on the principle of early ART initiation. According to WHO recommendations, HIV patients receive ART regardless of their CD4+ count. But, according to the Almaty Centre for AIDS Prevention and Control's recent survey conducted in Kazakhstan, it was estimated that as of 2017, 75% of PLWH were aware of their HIV status, of which only 59% received ART (Denebayeva et al. 2020). In 2003, Kazakhstan introduced the first sentinel surveillance procedures in pilot mode in one of the regions with the highest HIV prevalence in the country (Karaganda). In the following years, sentinel surveillance spread nationally. It helped to monitor the spread of HIV infection among vulnerable population groups, to determine estimated national rates of HIV infection among adults, and to evaluate the HIV response and plan further prevention and treatment programmes (Kazakh Research Centre of Dermatology and Infectious Diseases 2012). The following sentinel groups have been included in the surveillance since 2003: PWID, sex workers, men who have sex with men (MSM), pregnant women, people with sexual diseases, and prisoners. The first sentinel surveillance among MSM was carried out in 2003 in Karaganda alone. In 2005, it was expanded to four sites, and then during 2008 to 2010 to eight sites. Sentinel surveillance among pregnant women was carried out from 2003 to 2007. Since 2008, Kazakhstan has carried out mandatory double (in the first and third trimesters) HIV testing of pregnant women upon obtaining informed consent. In this regard, surveillance among pregnant women was cancelled. HIV surveillance among people with sexually transmitted infection (STI) symptoms was stopped in 2011.

The last two decades, Kazakhstan has experienced a concentrated stage of HIV epidemics with a prevalence in 2022 of 0.3% in the general population, compared to the 0.6% worldwide rate. As reported by the Minister of Healthcare Azhar Giniyat, for the last ten years, the morbidity rate in the country has doubled, while the mortality rate of AIDS has decreased 1.7 times (Figure 1) (Official Information Source of the Prime Minister of the Republic of Kazakhstan 2023). According to statistical prognosis, morbidity prevalence is on the rise and will potentially reach the level of 0.47%–0.60% by 2030 (Mussina/Kadyrov et al. 2023).

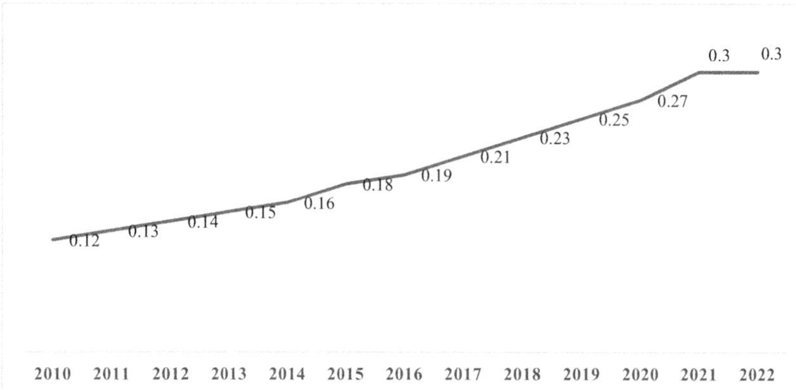

Figure 1: Prevalence of HIV in the general population of Kazakhstan (%) (Official Information Source of the Prime Minister of the Republic of Kazakhstan 2023)

When it comes to discussing epidemiological data on HIV in Kazakhstan, the majority of research publications underline the poor quality of statistical data in the field. In most cases, that refers to the underreporting of statistical indicators. Among the reasons for this underreporting, Thorne and her co-authors listed stigma and discrimination, over-centralisation of the surveillance systems, insufficient linkages between services, and insufficient involvement of civil sectors in data gathering and distribution. Additionally, the authors mentioned universal technical and methodological challenges while estimating epidemics concentrated in stigmatised, vulnerable population groups (Thorne et al. 2010).

In 2022, the absolute number of people living with HIV in Kazakhstan was 30,558, with 3,877 new cases registered that year. In terms of gender, there are significantly more cases among men (67.2% of all cases). Currently, sexual transmission is the most prevalent way for HIV to spread (74.7%), and parenteral is as high as 20.3%. Overall, 82.6% of people living with HIV are of working age. According to Mussina et al. (2023), the rate of HIV infection in Kazakhstan varies considerably depending on the data source used. In practice, for 2020, UNAIDS reported 3,600 newly diagnosed HIV cases in the country, while official governmental bodies confirmed just 93% of that indicator. Likewise, data on mortality is also sparse and fragmental. For instance, the Ministry of Healthcare reported a 1.7% decrease in the AIDS mortality rate (Official Information Source of the Prime Minister of the Republic of Kazakhstan 2023), while Mussina et al. (2023) revealed a sharp escalation in the mortality rate (248%) in the cohort of PLWH hospitalised due to various somatic diseases in the period of 2014–2019. According to the study of Mussina and her co-authors, people with TB comorbidity and an older age had lower survival chances. Stigmatisation, poor social support, and barriers to medical health utilisation were listed as the main drivers of increased mortality risks for inpatients with a positive HIV status (Mussina/Abbay et al. 2023). The HIV prevalence in key population groups is presented in Table 1 (Petrenko 2023).

Table 1: HIV prevalence in key populations in Kazakhstan (Petrenko 2023)

Key groups	**2019/ 2020**	**2021/ 2022**
PWID	8.3%	7.6%
Sex workers	1.4%	1.3%
MSM	6.5%	6.9%
Inmates	4.2%	4.1%

While the HIV prevalence in sex workers and inmates has remained stable, the rate of HIV in MSM is on the rise. HIV incidence among MSM has increased sevenfold since 2009. Specialists face significant difficulties in estimating the prevalence among MSM, which is related to the fact that official data often give lower figures than studies among MSM (Semchuk 2018). The reason could lie in stigmatisation, the segregation of this closed community, and the low attractiveness of the services offered in state medical and preventive organisations. Recent surveys indicate that as many as 70% of individuals in Kazakhstan maintain prejudiced attitudes towards people living with HIV (UNAIDS 2019).

In 2017, the estimated number of MSM in Kazakhstan was 154,000 individuals. National research indicates that HIV testing rates among MSM in Kazakhstan are below 50%, and as a result, up to 50% of those living with HIV may not be aware of their HIV-positive status. Furthermore, in this context, MSM seem to have lower testing rates than other demographic groups in Kazakhstan (Wu et al. 2017). The low rate of HIV test uptake is associated with poor community connectedness with sexual and gender communities (Paine et al. 2021). According to the data of Berry et al. (2012), unprotected receptive anal sex raised the risk of HIV infection twofold. In turn, unprotected sex among MSM living in Almaty was associated with low access to lubricants, transactional sex, STI symptoms, and non-injection drug use (Berry et al. 2012).

Given these statistics, the government has set a course to change prevention approaches among the LGBT community. For example, a pre-exposure prophylaxis programme for HIV was introduced in 2020. More than 3,000 people currently receive free, regular pre-exposure prophylaxis funded by the state budget. This programme's most frequent clients are MSM. In financial terms, the price of one course of the drug for pre-exposure prophylaxis does not exceed five dollars, which is undoubtedly one of the most efficient and low-cost HIV prevention approaches available in Kazakhstan (Institute of legislation and legal information of the Republic of Kazakhstan of the Ministry of Justice of the Republic of Kazakhstan 2020a).

Another equally important facilitator of the HIV response among MSM is the work carried out in the community by NGOs. Currently, NGOs in Almaty, Astana, Karaganda, Shymkent, and Pavlodar conduct informational campaigns, work to minimise stigma, and provide support to overcome discrimination and increase tolerance towards LGBT people (such as AFEW Kazakhstan, Community Friends, Human Health). Unfortunately, the number of condoms and lubricants provided by state organisations is quite low (no more than 150 per person who injects drugs annually) (Institute of legislation and legal information of the Republic of Kazakhstan of the Ministry of Justice of the Republic of Kazakhstan 2020a). The decision to increase the number of preventive products issued (up to 300 units annually) is currently under consideration by the government. Given the low coverage of diagnostic testing among key populations (including MSM), the issues of distribution of rapid HIV tests through NGOs remain relevant (Alibayeva et al. 2019). At present, programmes for distributing rapid tests through trust points have been introduced across Kazakhstan. As additional options, international projects have supported the implementation of distribution saliva test systems through pharmacies, including online ordering and home delivery options.

A successful example is the HIV Flagship project funded by the United States Agency for International Development (USAID), which raised the capacity of NGO testing through teams of peer test navigators. They have extended HIV testing to nearly 10,000 individuals in the Pavlodar and East Kazakhstan regions by utilising rapid test kits. This effort led to almost 600 individuals receiving their first positive HIV test result through community-level testing, with over 500 of them subsequently becoming clients of community case management. Moreover, more than 400 people initiated ART as a result of this initiative. Overall, the case management programme welcomed 1,347 former clients, and approximately half of them commenced ART (USAID 2020). In 2019, HIV testing was conducted by 23 stationary laboratories in all regions of the country. There are no mobile laboratories in the Republic of Kazakhstan; instead, there are 23 mobile trust points that travel to the points with the highest concentration of key group representatives and conduct rapid testing, among other services. In 2019, 1,224 self-test kits (saliva) were distributed, with 4,856 MSM getting tested in 2019 (Prilutskaya 2020).

In addition to MSM, people who use drugs are also at significant risk of HIV infection. As illustrated in research conducted by Strathdee et al. (2010), as well as Krüsi et al. (2010), various behavioural elements contribute to the spread of HIV among PWID. These factors encompass challenges such as limited access to clean needles and syringes, concerns about facing discrimination, arrest, or imprisonment, and encountering obstacles that hinder their ability to access HIV testing and drug addiction treatment services (Krüsi 2010; Strathdee et al. 2010). In 2017, the Republican AIDS Center of Kazakhstan estimated that the nation had 11,207 PWID living with HIV. Among them, 9,072 individuals (80.9%) were aware of their HIV-positive status. Nevertheless, less than half of these individuals, specifically 4,340 (38.7%) of them, were receiving ART, and only 2,318 (20.6%) of them had achieved viral suppression below 1,000 copies/mL (McCrimmon et al. 2019).

Despite the fact that a decrease in HIV prevalence among PWID has been registered in the last five years, the coverage of prevention programmes does not reach the target values. For example, in 2019, the direct coverage of three preventive services (syringes, condoms, and informational leaflets) was no higher than 52%. Systematic coverage of PWID with three preventive services (at least once a month during 2019) only amounted to 27% (Prilutskaya 2020). The quality and coverage of preventive programmes continue to be relevant for PWID. According to the study of El-Bassel et al. (2013), no more than 10% of PWID living in Almaty visited needle-exchange points (NEP). Overall, 25% has never been tested for HIV. Furthermore, another concerning fact was the high risk of bridge transmission of HIV in the non-drug-using injection partners of PWID. El-Bassel et al. (2013) found that HIV prevalence among non-PWID partners of PWID was as high as 10.4%. In this regard, the relevance of systemic preventive campaigns among discordant couples is on the rise.

An example of successful intervention for couples is Project Renaissance funded by the National Institute on Drug Abuse (NIDA), which showed positive results in the Almaty region with a reduction in the injection rate and an increase in condom use, achieved by implementing couple's counselling (Gilbert et al. 2010). The Project Renaissance showed that social enablers play an extremely significant role in curtailing the barriers to accessing HIV services among PWID, such as differentiated service delivery, decriminalisation, and destigmatisation, which was underlined by several regional HIV-policy experts (Deryabina/El-Sadr 2019).

The estimated number of PWID is currently decreasing due to the changing drug scene in the country. Official government estimates have stated that there were approximately 122,850 injection drug users (IDUs) in Kazakhstan in 2011, while that rate was just above 85,000 in 2020. In terms of ways of transmitting HIV, injecting has been overtaken by sexual transmission, including through increased unsafe sexual practices among synthetic stimulant users. The official data on HIV prevalence in users of new psychoactive drugs is lacking, although the scope of the problem can be observed through sporadic studies in the field. According to Prilutskaya et al. (2020), up to 10% of all hospital-based admissions for SUD were associated with problematic use of new psychoactive substances (NPS).

Selected research assessments in the country indicate that there are special needs for HIV prevention among people who use synthetic stimulants (Prilutskaya 2020). Sexual arousal following polydrug use and a binge mode of drug consumption are additional drivers of raised HIV transmission risks, even without drug injections (Su et al. 2018). International research data states the higher risks of HIV transmission among people who use synthetic stimulants, due to the lack of evidence-based information, rare use of condoms, higher likelihood of chemsex practices and commercial sex, and higher risk of stigmatisation, even among people who use traditional drugs. In parallel with HIV, stimulant use is associated with a higher prevalence of STIs (e.g. syphilis) (Chen et al. 2014; Sun et al. 2018). In Kazakhstan, HIV spread in NPS-using people can be accelerated by the lack of tailored HIV services for those subgroups of key populations. It should be noted that people who use stimulants in a form other than injections are not covered by regular preventive HIV services, being beyond the scope of three key groups (PWID, MSM, and sex workers).

The pilot study by Prilutskaya (2020) showed poor knowledge about HIV risks while using NPS, even among outreach peer-to-peer counsellors and NGO representatives. By 2019, no NGOs in Kazakhstan offered any NPS-tailored services to communities. The multinational qualitative study, in which both Kazakhstan providers and patients participated, revealed that harm reduction should encompass the following range of new approaches and services: providing support and tools for non-injecting users of NPS, offering a wider array of supplies for those who do inject, delivering targeted education about NPS usage and the associated hazards, implementing peer-driven initiatives, providing drug-testing services, and offering training to healthcare professionals and harm reduction workers on NPS-related matters (Kurcevič/Lines 2020).

To date, the first steps have been taken towards web outreach harm reduction initiatives, supported by the United Nations Office on Drugs and Crime (UNODC 2023a) and the Global Fund (Kazakh Research Centre of Dermatology and Infectious Diseases 2022b). In 2019, the first harm reduction channel was launched in Kazakhstan through the Telegram platform. To date, six channels in four Kazakhstan regions have provided harm reduction counselling. Overall, eleven web-outreach specialists were trained and are now working successfully in this field. The current phase of the web-outreach project focuses on establishing the distribution of harm reduction kits for people who use NPS in three regions of Kazakhstan: Almaty, Karaganda, and Oskemen (Figure 2).

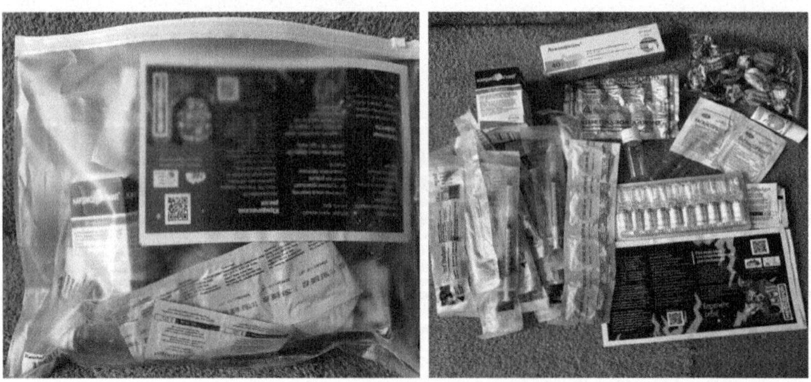

Figure 2: Harm reduction packages (kits) distributed among people who use synthetic stimulants (Valentina Mankieva, representative of the Kazakhstan Forum of people who use drugs)

According to a piece of expert information, in 2023, six online trainings were provided for NGOs, 217 consultations were provided online for

PWID, and 138 persons were tested, with one positive HIV case identified. Developing a relatively new direction in harm reduction, experts noted the need for systemic funding, capacity building for human resources, and security for web-based outreach in the context of severe criminalisation of all NPS distribution in Kazakhstan. Another important issue is the pressing need to establish an NPS early warning system with data triangulation to monitor the harms and risks of NPS, considering the best practices of the European Monitoring Centre for Drugs and Drug Addiction (EMCDDA 2023) and the United Nations Office on Drugs and Crime (UNODC 2023b). That requires the systemic modernisation of legal acts and operational standards, including those related to HIV monitoring (such as a national sentinel surveillance system).

The key role of NGOs in HIV prevention and treatment was acknowledged over three decades ago by the whole international community. Building the partnership between the governmental and non-governmental sectors is a critical step for the dissemination and implementation of state-of-art approaches and for transparency and equality in the distribution of services, especially in the context of the vulnerability of key population groups. NGOs provide critical support and care services to PLWH and key populations by offering counselling services to help PLWH and individuals at risk of HIV infection cope with the emotional and psychological challenges associated with HIV; by facilitating access to healthcare services, including ART and essential medical treatments; by ensuring that PLWH receive the care they need; and by employing peer educators and support workers who have personal experience with HIV or harm reduction. These peers build trust and provide practical guidance, making it easier for individuals to navigate the challenges of living with or preventing HIV.

To date, Kazakhstan has seen a rapid development of the civil sector in various aspects of social welfare service. HIV programmes are not an exception to this trend. Capacity building and increased representation of NGOs in the healthcare sector (including HIV prevention initiatives) are both on the agenda of current state policies. The main support is supposed to be provided through the local budgets of 20 Kazakhstani regions. In practice, the regional capacities of NGOs are not equal as they depend on the regional budgets and readiness of state bodies to invest in and prioritise civil actions at a regional level. The government has reported a decrease in the number of NGOs financed by state budgets, from 21 NGOs in 2019 to seven NGOs in 2023 (International news agency "Kazinform" 2023). In 2019, the share of state funding costs for NGOs did not exceed 0.2%

of the total HIV budget. In this regard, international grants play a key role in the sustainable development of the civil sector when it comes to providing transparent and timely HIV services for various representatives of key population groups in the country.

NGOs often collaborate with the Global Fund to access funding, technical expertise, and best practices. Kazakhstan's NGOs actively engage with UNAIDS to align their strategies with international standards and to access data, research, and policy guidance (UNAIDS 2023). The UNODC has been a vital partner in Kazakhstan's efforts to combat HIV/AIDS, particularly in addressing the intersection of drug use, harm reduction, and HIV prevention (UNODC 2020). On a national level, NGOs in Kazakhstan are active participants in regional networks that facilitate cooperation, advocacy, and resource sharing through several key stakeholders. These NGOs are as follows: the Central Asian Network of PLWH, the Eurasian Harm Reduction Network, and the Central Asia Program for AIDS Control and Prevention. NGOs in Kazakhstan have also played an active role in advocating for policies that prioritise HIV prevention and harm reduction. Their advocacy efforts include policy development, resource mobilisation, and community empowerment. Moreover, NGOs provide critical support and care services to PLWH and key populations through counselling, facilitating access to healthcare services, and peer-to-peer education.

The Role of Social Work in the Prevention and Treatment of HIV/AIDS

People living with HIV still face a number of challenges around the world. The role of social work is critically important in improving the quality of life of people living with HIV and their families.

Social work, as a relatively new profession, is going through a period of institutionalisation in Central Asian countries. At present, social work in the prevention and treatment of HIV is gradually developing in Kazakhstan. However, in most cases, the work is carried out with a focus on medical care, without due attention being paid to family factors or social and psychological needs. Today, professional social work in the field of HIV prevention is largely carried out by non-profit organisations (NPOs), which train outreach workers to provide targeted social work and carry out work with communities. Also, elements of social work for people living with HIV can be found in the primary healthcare system.

The results of the international research project InBeAIDS by the Frankfurt University of Applied Sciences (Frankfurt am Main, Germany 2018), entitled 'Prevention of Infectious Diseases and Treatment of HIV/AIDS and Hepatitis among Injecting Drug Users in Central Asia and the Contribution of Social Work to Serving Drug Addicts', show that the state of professional social work in the field of HIV prevention is unsatisfactory in terms of its state institutionalisation, if we talk about the state system of providing social services, as well as the development of education in the field of social work at the level of training qualified social workers (Bachelor of Social Sciences, 'pre-service' level) (InBeAIDS 2020).

Kazakhstan became the first country in the Commonwealth of Independent States (CIS) to introduce standards of psychosocial support for children and adolescents living with HIV. These standards were put into practice after a joint meeting of the United Nations Children's Fund (UNICEF), the Ministry of Health, and the Kazakh Scientific Center for Dermatology and Infectious Diseases in 2019. In 2020, in accordance with the action plan of the 2019–2021 grant of UNICEF in Kazakhstan, the Ministry of Labor and Social Protection of the Population of the Republic of Kazakhstan, experts from UNICEF, the National Alliance of Professional Social Workers, the Research Group on Social Work of the L.N. Gumilyov Eurasian National University conducted research into the needs of families with children and teenagers living with HIV. The purpose of this study was to monitor and supervise the implementation of the 'needs assessment' tool among families with children and adolescents living with HIV according to the methodology of the Standard of Psychosocial Support for Families with Children Living with HIV.

The study involved the Centers for the Prevention and Control of AIDS, the Centers for Primary Medical and Social Care, and the Departments for the Coordination of Employment and Social Programs of the East Kazakhstan, Almaty, and Turkestan regions and the cities of Shymkent and Almaty.

As this study shows, the functions of social workers are most often performed by quasi- professionals, i.e. employees with medical education, which significantly reduces the quality of services for the integrated management of family cases. This situation is due to the insufficient level of educational support from the state at both the bachelor's and master's levels. For example, in 2019, the Ministry of Education allocated just 80 educational grants for undergraduate programmes throughout the country

(Ministry of Labor and Social Protection of Population of the Republic of Kazakhstan 2020).

In general, it has been over the past two decades that the professional training of social work specialists has been carried out in Kazakhstan. In the country, one of the key roles in solving the problem of undertraining of social workers is played by the National Alliance of Professional Social Workers (NAPSW), which was established in 2019 and in 2022 initiated the creation and registration of the Association of Schools of Social Work (ASSOR) in Kazakhstan to promote and strengthen education in the field of social work. In December 2022, the NAPSW of Kazakhstan joined the International Federation of Social Workers.

Over the years, the Alliance has carried out work in several areas, such as improving the quality of education in the field of social work (for example, providing advanced training of social work specialists in various fields, including the social workers of AIDS centres and NGOs providing social support to people living with HIV; developing a curriculum for bachelor's and master's programmes in the fields of social work and social work in healthcare; and implementing advanced training programmes for social workers in social protection and healthcare), developing and maintaining the institution of supervision in the field of healthcare (since 2016, the Alliance experts have been conducting supportive monitoring of specialists of primary health care organisations and AIDS centres), and training trainers in social work technologies and case management.

In order to increase the role of social work and its impact on providing support and assistance to people living with HIV, it is recommended to develop training programmes at the bachelor's level in the field of social work with HIV, addiction, etc., at the postgraduate level (for students who already hold a bachelor's degree), and for paraspecialists who carry out the tasks of a social worker in NPOs. It is also necessary to conduct trainings for case management professionals that include information on assessment, intervention design, and how to evaluate social work practice, as well as specific courses for people living with HIV, with a focus on future outreach work (InBeAIDS 2020).

Legal Regulations and State Guarantees for PLWH

Compared to other Central Asian countries, Kazakhstan demonstrates the highest economic growth and intensification of modernisation processes that embrace digitalisation, the decentralisation of administrative processes, and focusing on social policies. In this regard, economic growth is measured not only by the growth rate of financial well-being but also by the strengthening of socially oriented approaches and the expansion of institutions that provide social support for the population. The Constitution of the Republic of Kazakhstan (1995) states that 'citizens of the Republic of Kazakhstan have the right to health protection and are entitled to receive the guaranteed volume of medical care established by law free of charge' (Article 29). In addition, concealment of facts and circumstances threatening the life and health of people is punishable by law (Article 31). During the years of Kazakhstan's independence, from 1993 to the present day, about 2,000 normative legal acts were issued concerning policy issues on the reduction and treatment of HIV/AIDS morbidity, 848 of which are still in place today and regulate current standards in the field of HIV-related issues (Figure 3).

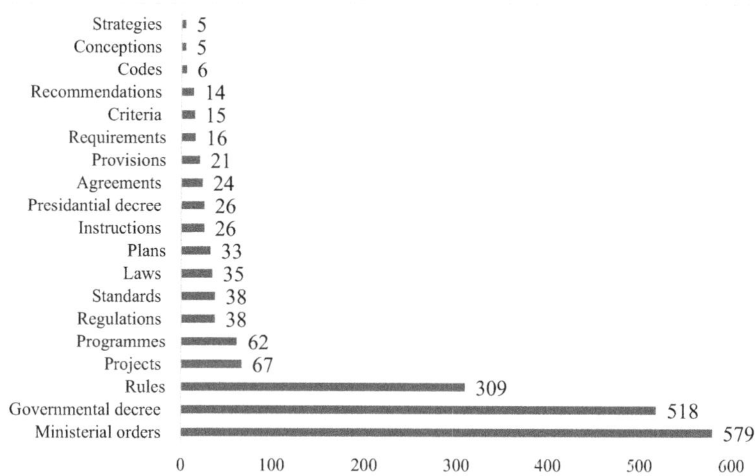

Figure 3: Legal documents regulating HIV-related issues in Kazakhstan (authors' compilation)

According to the Eurasian Harm Reduction Association (EHRA 2021), Kazakhstan has not yet adopted a comprehensive national HIV strategy. Instead, issues to improve HIV policy are presented at three levels: (i) the long-term state strategy 'Kazakhstan-2050', (ii) documents on the strategic economic development of the country and regions, and (iii) operational documents on the implementation of the aforementioned strategies (EHRA 2021).

Legislation on HIV infection was established in Kazakhstan for the first time in 1994. The first edition of the law established legal definitions of a range of terms, including 'HIV', 'HIV-infected person', and 'HIV diagnostics'. It listed the responsibilities of state authorities to prevent HIV spread in Kazakhstan. Ten years later, the law was amended and articles about rights and guarantees for PLWH were introduced. Guarantees for the social security of medical workers in case of HIV infection were also enshrined (Institute of legislation and legal information of the Republic of Kazakhstan of the Ministry of Justice of the Republic of Kazakhstan 1994). Since 2007, social guarantees have been extended to other persons infected with HIV, especially education guarantees for minors living with HIV. Since 2000, issues relating to HIV prevention and response have become part of the state concept. The main principles of the state anti-HIV policy include the consolidation of the forces of the state and society as regards AIDS prevention; broad cooperation with international and public organisations; ensuring respect for human rights in the implementation of AIDS prevention programmes; encouraging healthy lifestyles; education and awareness-raising; and guaranteeing that vulnerable population groups receive basic healthcare at the same level as the rest of the population. The state concept named the following groups as the priority population groups when it comes to HIV prevention: people who use drugs, sex workers, and youth. This document underlined the need for NGOs in the field, as well as the importance of coverage with ART and preventive measures (Institute of legislation and legal information of the Republic of Kazakhstan of the Ministry of Justice of the Republic of Kazakhstan 2000). In 2005, the Governmental Decree established the Country Coordinating Committee as the main governmental body responsible for regulating the Global Fund projects in Kazakhstan, modernising legal regulations, and controlling the implementation of national prevention and treatment policies. A significant political achievement and innovation for that time was the inclusion of representatives of non-governmental organisations in the Committee, which in essence provided an opportunity for a transparent dialogue platform for the government, civil society, and international organisations (Institute of legislation and legal information of the Republic of Kazakhstan of the Ministry of Justice of the Republic of Kazakhstan 2004). The next step in the area of health safeguards for HIV was the adoption of the Health Code in 2009. Four articles of the Code were dedicated to regulations and state guarantees for HIV prevention, testing, and social insurance for PLWH (Institute of legislation and legal information of the Republic of Kazakhstan of the Ministry of Justice of the Republic of Kazakhstan 2009). The current version of the Health Code provides more advanced steps and guarantees in terms of HIV prevention and health promotion, not only for the general population but also for vulnerable key groups. Monitoring campaigns (epidemiological surveillance) have been introduced as a mandatory biennial procedure of the national HIV policy. The principles of peer-to-peer counselling and universal ART coverage (test and treat) are also declared by the current Code of the Republic of Kazakhstan (Institute of legislation and legal information of the Republic of Kazakhstan of the Ministry of Justice of the Republic of Kazakhstan 2020).

As of 1st January 2021, Kazakhstan had 17 state medical organisations in the field of HIV prevention, one republican umbrella organisation, and 29 so-called 'friendly clinics' (*druzhestvennye kliniki*) to provide preventive and therapeutic-diagnostic assistance to HIV-positive patients and key populations. Overall, 139 drop-in centres provided syringe exchange services and 485 outreach workers practised peer counselling (329 of them funded by local budgets and 156 funded by donors). In total, 39 HIV-service NGOs were registered in the country, of which nine NGOs received state social contracts. Preventive services that are spread across Kazakhstan, guaranteed and controlled by the government, are as follows: HIV awareness in all medical organisations, ensuring infectious safety as concerns organ donation and transplantation; the integration of HIV education into the education system and at the workplace; the surveillance of HIV prevalence among the population, including key groups; treatment and prevention services for key populations in drop-in centres and friendly offices on the principle of confidentiality and voluntariness; funding of NGOs through state social grants; the prevention of mother-to-child transmission of HIV; pre- and post-contact prophylaxis; and ART (EHRA 2021). In 2014, Kazakhstan adopted new initiatives presented by the WHO and the UNAIDS, such as '90-90-90'. In 2021, Kazakhstan ratified new '95-95-95' targets of the UNAIDS fast-track approach (Kazakh Research Centre of Dermatology and Infectious Diseases 2022a). According to the recent data (2021–2022), this indicator has reached the level of '87-84-87', which is significantly lower than the UN target of '95-95-95'. Reaching these targets will involve systemic reforms in HIV prevention and treatment, changing a significant number of policy approaches and funding.

A phased increase in funding for HIV treatment and prevention is an important component of government policy in this area. In 2017, expenditure on HIV services in Kazakhstan totalled USD 34,816,918 (UNAIDS 2018). Budgets and the amount of funding allocated are key, as the Global Fund estimates that funding has the potential to directly impact population losses from HIV. By 2030, through a more efficient allocation of resources, it should be possible to prevent an extra 52,000 disability-adjusted life years (DALYs) (Optima Consortium for Decision Science 2020). HIV/AIDS services are covered by a guaranteed finance package, with free provision for all citizens across all regions of Kazakhstan. For medical and social assistance and HIV/AIDS prevention services, the financial coefficient is calculated per person infected with HIV and is supposed to cover specialised medical care in outpatient settings, medical and social assistance for persons infected with HIV, and preventive measures to reduce the risk of HIV transmission from mother to foetus and child. An additional budget is allocated to preventive services provided in friendly offices and trust points, which is directly dependent on the type of service and the likelihood of receiving it. In 2019, according to the data obtained from in-depth interviews with experts of the Kazakh Scientific Center of Dermatology and Infectious Diseases, USD 3.5 million were spent on the prevention and treatment of HIV infection, which amounted to 9.3% of the state expenditure on healthcare in general (the total public health budget of Kazakhstan in 2019 was approximately USD 33.5 million). The share of the expenditure allocated to financing NGOs working in the field of HIV/AIDS amounted to 0.2% (approximately USD 70,000) of the expenditure on prevention and treatment. According to estimations from the Global Fund, in order to meet the '95-95-95' targets, it will be necessary to increase the HIV programme budget for 2019 to 2030 to 160% of the most recent reported budget level, requiring an extra USD 13 million each year. This increase should be carefully directed towards enhancing and prioritising ART, as well as focusing on HIV testing and prevention initiatives for PWID, HIV testing and prevention programmes aimed at MSM, and broad-scale HIV testing for the general population (Optima Consortium for Decision Science 2020).

In 2019, more than USD 35 million was spent on the HIV response in the Republic of Kazakhstan. More than USD 30 million was covered by the state budget (95%), while the remaining 5% were funds from international partners. The international assistance provided to the Republic of Kazakhstan includes funds allocated by the US government (USAID/PEPFAR, CDC/PEPFAR), the Global Fund to Fight AIDS, Tuberculosis and Malaria, UN agencies, and other partners. International cooperation between Kazakhstan and donor organisations has made a significant contribution to improving national policy over three decades of HIV epidemics. Kazakhstan became the first country in the post-Soviet region to receive stable funding from the Global Fund. From 2003 to 2014, the Global Fund committed five grants to the Republic of Kazakhstan, with USD 89.5 million for the first decade and USD 111.8 million later (The Global Fund. Office of Inspector General 2015). The share of Global Fund investments allocated to the HIV response from 2016 to 2020 amounted to about 51.1% of the total amount of international donor funding (UNAIDS 2021). It was with the support of the Global Fund that the procurement of ART became possible in 2006. After achieving upper-middle-income country status in 2006, Kazakhstan has recently experienced a decrease in HIV funding from international donors (EHRA 2021). However, the donors continue to show their support in terms of advocacy, anti-stigma campaigns, capacity-building programmes, and research initiatives that explore new factors as regards the spread of HIV epidemics. According to the estimations of the Global Fund, if the HIV support programme had not been put into action between 2015 and 2017, by 2018, there could have been nearly 170% more new HIV infections (almost 8,300 more cases) and over 220% more fatalities related to HIV (roughly 2,800 more deaths) during that time frame (Optima Consortium for Decision Science 2020). To date, Kazakhstan has the resources to cover its own ART needs for all citizens. According to Aktayeva (2021), ART coverage increased fifteenfold between 2010 and 2020 (going from 1,336 PWLH in 2010 to 20,177 PWLH in 2020).

Thus, the above data shows the progress Kazakhstan has made in the field of HIV response and the full range of results achieved. However, an analysis of the situation among key populations would not be complete without taking into account the parallel spread of viral hepatitis C and the challenges that require solutions in this field.

HCV in Kazakhstan: Epidemiology, Policies, and Services

According to WHO statistics from 2019, approximately 58 million individuals are afflicted by persistent hepatitis C infection, leading to approximately 400,000 fatalities annually (WHO 2023d). The Ministry of Health's official figures show a population-wide prevalence of hepatitis C of up to 3.1%. In 2022, there were 27,835 patients registered as having hepatitis B and 30,862 patients registered as having hepatitis C (WHO 2023c). According to an independent NGO assessment, just above 8,000 new HCV cases were identified in 2022, whereby the prevalence was higher among women (53.2% of new cases) than men (46.8% of new cases) (Biryukov/Rastokina 2023). According to national experts, epidemiological data on viral hepatitis in Kazakhstan is scattered and inconsistent (Ashimkhanova et al. 2022). In most cases, the data were obtained either from several research projects among PWID or from several different transplant clinics. Notably, the HCV seroprevalence among PWID fluctuated between 14% and 90%, depending on the research methodology and the region of Kazakhstan where the fieldwork was focused (Davlidova et al. 2021). The study by Mukhatayeva et al. (2021) identified the coinfection of HIV and HCV in 43% of the 500 PWLH who took part. According to official statistics, in 2018, among PL-WH in Kazakhstan, 62% and 63% were found coinfected with, respectively, HBV and HCV funding (UNAIDS 2021). In the study by Mukhatayeva et al. (2021), the significant factors of HIV and HCV coinfections were described: male gender, age group of 30–49, a more than ten-year duration of HIV infection, and residence in the Kostanay region.

WHO's global hepatitis strategy, endorsed by WHO Member States, aims to reduce new hepatitis infections by 90% and deaths by 65% between 2016 and 2030. As a country that supports the WHO 2022 international strategy, Kazakhstan is aiming to develop new strategies for HCV screenings among the general population, including rolling out the HCV test campaigns piloted in Astana city. To date, free HIV screenings are available for medics who provide invasive procedures, patients who need surgical procedures, patients in haemodialysis, oncology, transplantology, or oncology departments, pregnant women, and a population of key groups. The latter receives all HCV services through an HIV-service organisation. The other groups can be tested for HCV at general hospitals or primary healthcare units. Since 2011, Kazakhstan has covered all its treatment needs with the state budget within the framework of the guaranteed package of free medical help. Since 2018, internationally acknowledged direct-acting antiviral (DAA) treatment regimens, consisting of a combination of sofosbuvir, daclatasvir, and ribavirin, have been available under the state insurance programme (Figure 4). The cost of a single course of DAA therapy ranges from USD 450 to USD 1,200 (Public Foundation "AGEP'C" 2023). In 2022, 6,590 patients received DAA therapy with an effectiveness rate of 96.5%.

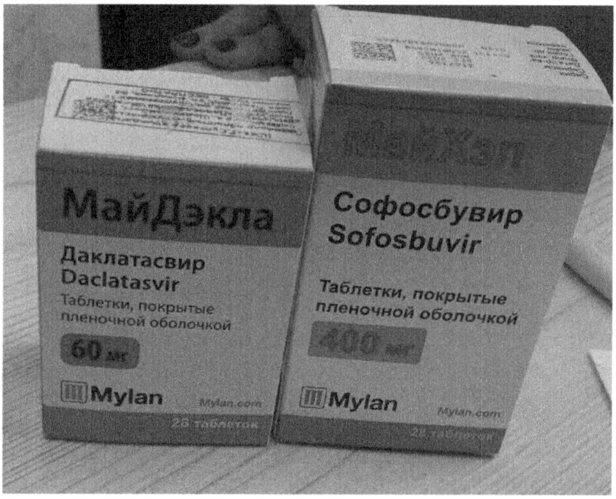

Figure 4: Antiviral medications used for HCV treatment in Kazakhstan (authors' compilation)

However, in practice, all the testing procedures to identify and officially diagnose HCV and qualify someone for free antiviral treatment are available only for those citizens who are insured. This is a significant issue, given the fact that many individuals with HCV are from vulnerable population groups that are underinsured. Another major practical barrier is limited treatment options for people who continue to use drugs. Based on an expert interview undertaken to gather information for this chapter, it appears to be normal practice for hepatologists to request special notification about stable remission from a psychiatrist for those patients who have experienced any drug use. According to expert opinions shared in the interviews, the reason for this is that hepatitis therapy becomes unsafe for the patient when active drug use is present.

These barriers to accessing HCV treatment are not unique to Kazakhstan, but can be observed in many countries of the world (Rodríguez Torres 2006). Most of them are related to social factors such as poverty, homelessness, infrequent contact with healthcare providers, and unreliable follow-up treatment. These barriers and pitfalls cannot be overcome without multidisciplinary efforts, including harm reduction interventions implemented by NGOs, HIV-service organisations, and social work specialists. Our investigation for this chapter revealed the paucity of information about NGO activity in combating HCV. To the best of our knowledge, there is only one NGO that focuses its work on issues of viral hepatitis and facilitates the implementation of patient-oriented approaches in general populations. Their activities include also key populations but only tangentially, in collaboration with HIV-service NGOs. 'AGEP'C' projects aim to distribute evidence-based information and consultations about free treatment options for HCV. Other than that, in 2020, only four NGOs implemented harm reduction projects with HCV information campaigns as an element of their initiatives (Public Foundation "AGEP'C" 2023).

Conclusions

This analysis of the situation regarding HIV and HCV in Kazakhstan has revealed the gradually shifting trends in parenteral infections over the thirty years of Kazakhstan's independence. The policy focus on infection prevention in the general population and key populations remains on the agenda. The standards of treatment and approach to preventing infections are in line with international protocols and recommendations. A significant achievement is the possibility for all citizens of the country to receive these services free of charge.

ART and DAA regimens are implemented throughout the country. However, the '95-95-95' indicators have not yet been achieved in Kazakhstan. There is a need to expand systemic measures for multidisciplinary efforts that address various barriers for vulnerable populations. The key element of HIV and HCV prevention policies should lie in the decriminalisation of drug use and in focusing on a public health approach in the field, while promoting equity and fairness in the provision of care. This is desirable in order to expand the range of services available by coordinating the efforts of state organisations and the civil sector, where social work can be a powerful bridge. The principle of equity in the services received should not only address the transfer of prison health issues to the general healthcare system but also aim to improve access to treatment, prevention, and harm reduction for other key populations. This need is particularly strong in the area of access to HCV testing and treatment among people who use drugs.

Given the changing drug markets in Kazakhstan, it is increasingly important to monitor the epidemiological situation of hepatitis and HIV in the context of NPSs It is also crucial to continue efforts to introduce bundled services for the prevention and treatment of parenteral infections, tailored to the needs of key populations. For example, there is no experience in the country of providing opioid substitution treatment (OST) concurrently with hepatitis C therapy. The approach of providing ART together with OST has not been implemented as a publicly available service. The state's approach to harm reduction policy remains ambiguous. Although some measures are enshrined in legislation, they cannot be assessed as systemic. Meanwhile, sufficient scientific material has been accumulated to demonstrate the importance of all eight harm reduction principles for Kazakhstan (National Harm Reduction Coalition 2021).

It is important to continue to build the capacity of NGOs as key actors in reducing stigma and discrimination and changing public attitudes towards HIV and viral hepatitis. Transparent communication and advocacy of community efforts should be the key to policy change at the level of standards and laws as a bottom-up principle. In a top-down manner, funding opportunities for civil society should be expanded. HIV and hepatitis policies should not only focus directly on public safety issues but also become more comprehensive, whereby common access to services among vulnerable populations should be promoted under a single umbrella. At the same time, a promising step towards achieving the UN Sustainable Development goals could be to more actively support social work institutes in countries like Kazakhstan, where social work is still a developing profession.

One of the recommendations from the external assessment of eight AIDS centres in Kazakhstan carried out by local UNICEF initiatives was the recommendation to establish new positions for social worker in multidisciplinary teams that currently do not include social workers. Furthermore, social work tools can be improved in HIV prevention, folloing theUNAIDS strategy. Another area for further smart interventions relates to the question of professionalisation of outreach workers who provide the majority of harm reduction services in fields of HIV. If the next decades are more supportive of professional social work in Kazakhstan, in terms of achieving the UN Sustainable Development goals, then Kazakhstan will be able to make progress in HIV prevention and treatment.

Bibliography

Akulova, Oksana (2023): "Behind the wall". Stigma: People living with HIV. www.vlast.kz/obsshestvo/51328-za-stenoj-stigma-ludi-zivusie-s-vic.html, 30.10.2023.

Alibayeva, K./Saparbekov, M./Baiserkin, B./Abishev, A./Tazhibaeva, G./Kasymbekova, S. (2019): Study of the possibility of introduction of Kazakhstan NGO-based rapid HIV testing procedures. In: HIV/AIDS – Research and Palliative Care 11, pp. 219–227. DOI: 10.2147/HIV.S212718.

Amanzholov, Nurali/Yakovleva, Anna/Kamaldinov, Denis (2016): The people living with HIV. Stigma index. Analytical report. www.caapl.org/wp-content/uploads/2020/11/kazakhstah_stigma_index_report_eng_17_05_2017.pdf, 30.10.2023.

Ashimkhanova, Aiymkul/Syssoyev, Dmitriy/Gusmanov, Arnus/Yesmembetov, Kakharman/Yespotayeva, Arina/Abbay, Anara et al. (2022): Epidemiological Characteristics of Chronic Viral Hepatitis in Kazakhstan: Data from Unified Nationwide Electronic Healthcare System 2014–2019. In: Infection and Drug Resistance 15, pp. 3333–3346. DOI: 10.2147/IDR.S363609.

Berry, Mark/Wirtz, Andrea L./Janayeva, Assel/Ragoza, Valentina/Terlikbayeva, Assel/Amirov, Bauyrzhan et al. (2012): Risk factors for HIV and unprotected anal intercourse among men who have sex with men (MSM) in Almaty, Kazakhstan. In: PloS One 7, No. 8, p. e43071. DOI: 10.1371/journal.pone.0043071.

Biryukov, Sergey/Rastokina, Elena (2023): Report on the study of procurement of antiretroviral drugs for the treatment of HIV and drugs for the treatment of viral hepatitis C in the Republic of Kazakhstan in 2022. www.itpc-eeca.org/wp-content/uploads/2023/08/pdf-dokument.pdf, 30.10.2023.

Chen, Huai L./Zhang, Jian X./Xu, Qi/Dai, Ying X./Huang, Yu L. (2014): Synthetic Drug Boom: Potential Threat to HIV/AIDS Transmission in China. In: Sexually Transmitted Diseases 41, No. 10, p. 618. DOI: 10.1097/OLQ.0000000000000184.

Davlidova, Salima/Haley-Johnson, Zoë/Nyhan, Kate/Farooq, Ayesha/Vermund, Sten H./Ali, Syed (2021): Prevalence of HIV, HCV and HBV in Central Asia and the Caucasus: A systematic review. In: International Journal of Infectious Diseases 104, pp. 510–525. DOI: 10.1016/j.ijid.2020.12.068.

Denebayeva, Alfiya/Abrahamyan, Arpine/Sargsyan, Aelita/Kentenyants, Karine/Zhandybayeva, Ainur/Nugmanova, Zhamilya et al. (2020): Antiretroviral therapy among patients with HIV in Almaty, Kazakhstan: The implication for HIV-associated tuberculosis control. In: Journal of Infection in Developing Countries 14, No. 11.1, pp. 128S–132S. DOI: 10.3855/jidc.11924.

Deryabina, Anna P./El-Sadr, Wafaa M. (2019): Optimizing HIV prevention and treatment outcomes for persons with substance use in Central Asia: What will it take? In: Current Opinion in HIV and AIDS 14, No. 5, pp. 374–380. DOI: 10.1097/COH.0000000000000565.

El-Bassel, Nabila/Gilbert, Louisa/Terlikbayeva, Assel/Wu, Elwin/Beyrer, Chris/Shaw, Stacey et al. (2013): HIV among injection drug users and their intimate partners in Almaty, Kazakhstan. In: AIDS and Behavior 17, No. 7, pp. 2490–2500. DOI: 10.1007/s10461-013-0484-2.

Eurasian Harm Reduction Association (EHRA) (2021): A brief overview of the results of the sustainability assessment of the HIV response among Key Populations in nine countries of the EECA region in the context of transition from Global Fund support to domestic funding. Vilnius: EHRA.

European Monitoring Centre for Drugs and Drug Addiction (EMCDDA) (2023): The EU Early Warning System on new psychoactive substances (NPS). www.emcdda.europa.eu/publications/topic-overviews/eu-early-warning-system_en, 30.10.2023.

Gilbert, Louisa/El-Bassel, Nabila/Terlikbayeva, Assel/Rozental, Yelena/Chang, Mingway/Brisson, Anne et al. (2010): Couple-based HIV prevention for injecting drug users in Kazakhstan: A pilot intervention study. In: Journal of Prevention & Intervention in the Community 38, No. 2, pp. 162–176. DOI: 10.1080/10852351003640914.

Human Rights Watch (2003): Fanning the Flames: How Human Rights Abuses are Fueling the AIDS Epidemic in Kazakhstan. www.refworld.org/docid/3f4f595711.html, 09.01.2024.

InBeAIDS (2020): Prevention of infectious diseases and treatment of HIV / AIDS and hepatitis among injecting drug users in Central Asia and the contribution of social work to the services for drug using people (InBeAIDS). Frankfurt am Main: Frankfurt University of Applied Sciences. DOI: 10.13140/RG.2.2.24808.62727.

Institute of legislation and legal information of the Republic of Kazakhstan of the Ministry of Justice of the Republic of Kazakhstan (1994): On the prevention and treatment of HIV infection and AIDS. Law of the Republic of Kazakhstan [05 October 1994]. www.adilet.zan.kz/rus/docs/Z940006000, 30.10.2023.

Institute of legislation and legal information of the Republic of Kazakhstan of the Ministry of Justice of the Republic of Kazakhstan (2000): About the Concept of State Policy to Counter the Epidemic. Decree of the Government of the Republic of Kazakhstan [No. 41, 29 January 2011]. www.adilet.zan.kz/rus/docs/P000001808_#z0, 30.10.2023.

Institute of legislation and legal information of the Republic of Kazakhstan of the Ministry of Justice of the Republic of Kazakhstan (2001): On approval of the Program to combat the AIDS epidemic in the Republic of Kazakhstan for 2001-2005. Decree of the Government of the Republic of Kazakhstan [No. N 1207, 14 September 2001]. www.adilet.zan.kz/rus/docs/P010001207, 30.10.2023.

Institute of legislation and legal information of the Republic of Kazakhstan of the Ministry of Justice of the Republic of Kazakhstan (2004): About the Coordination Council for the Prevention and Control of AIDS and Tuberculosis. Decree of the Government of the Republic of Kazakhstan [No. N 922, 01 September 2004]. www.adilet.zan.kz/rus/docs/P040000922, 30.10.2023.

Institute of legislation and legal information of the Republic of Kazakhstan of the Ministry of Justice of the Republic of Kazakhstan (2006): On approval of the Program to combat the AIDS epidemic in the Republic of Kazakhstan for 2006-2010. Decree of the Government of the Republic of Kazakhstan [No. N 1216, 15 December 2006]. www.adilet.zan.kz/rus/docs/P060001216, 30.10.2023.

Institute of legislation and legal information of the Republic of Kazakhstan of the Ministry of Justice of the Republic of Kazakhstan (2009): Code of the Republic of Kazakhstan: On public health and healthcare system [No. 193-IV, 18 September 2009]. www.adilet.zan.kz/rus/docs/K090000193, 30.10.2023.

Institute of legislation and legal information of the Republic of Kazakhstan of the Ministry of Justice of the Republic of Kazakhstan (2020): Code of the Republic of Kazakhstan: On public health and healthcare system [No. 360-VI, 07 July 2020]. www.adilet.zan.kz/eng/docs/K090000193, 29.02.2024.

Institute of legislation and legal information of the Republic of Kazakhstan of the Ministry of Justice of the Republic of Kazakhstan (2020a): On approval of the rules for carrying out activities to prevent HIV infection. Order of the Minister of Health of the Republic of Kazakhstan [No. KR DSM-137/2020, 19 October 2020]. www.adilet.zan.kz/rus/docs/V2000021467, 30.10.2023.

International news agency "Kazinform" (2023): Head of the Ministry of Health: Kazakhstan does not use the potential of NGOs to combat HIV. www.inform.kz/ru/glava-minzdrava-v-kazahstane-ne-ispol-zuetsya-potencial-npo-dlya-bor-by-s-vich_a4072990, 30.10.2023.

Katkov, Alexander (2013): Destructive Social Epidemics: New Conceptual and Organizational Approaches of Effective Response. DOI: 10.2139/ssrn.2370633

Kazakh Research Centre of Dermatology and Infectious Diseases (2012): Sentinel epidemiological surveillance (SES) in the Republic of Kazakhstan. www.kncdiz.kz/ru/sentinel_surveillance/, 30.10.2023.

Kazakh Research Centre of Dermatology and Infectious Diseases (2022a): Towards achieving UNAIDS goals 95-95-95. www.kncdiz.kz/ru/news/item/7023/, 30.10.2023.

Kazakh Research Centre of Dermatology and Infectious Diseases (2022b): Training for outreach workers and web consultants. www.kncdiz.kz/en/news/item/7083/, 30.10.2023.

Kommersant (2007): Kazakh doctors were convicted of mass infection of children with HIV. www.kommersant.ru/doc/778412, 30.10.2023.

Krüsi, Andrea/Wood, Evan/Montaner, Julio/Kerr, Thomas (2010): Social and structural determinants of HAART access and adherence among injection drug users. In: International Journal of Drug Policy 21, No. 1, pp. 4–9. DOI: 10.1016/j.drugpo.2009.08.003.

Kurcevič, Eliza/Lines, Rick (2020): New psychoactive substances in Eurasia: A qualitative study of people who use drugs and harm reduction services in six countries. In: Harm Reduction Journal 17, No. 94. DOI: 10.1186/s12954-020-00448-2.

Li, Xin/Yuan, Lili/Li, Xiaoxia/Shi, Jingli/Jiang, Liying/Zhang, Chundi et al. (2017): Factors associated with stigma attitude towards people living with HIV among general individuals in Heilongjiang, Northeast China. In: BMC Infectious Diseases 17, No. 154. DOI: 10.1186/s12879-017-2216-0.

McCrimmon, Tara/Gilbert, Louise/Hunt, Timothy/Terlikbayeva, Assel/Wu, Elwin/Darisheva, Meruyert et al. (2019): Improving HIV service delivery for people who inject drugs in Kazakhstan: Study protocol for the Bridge stepped-wedge trial. In: Implementation Science 14, No. 62. DOI: 10.1186/s13012-019-0909-z.

Ministry of Labor and Social Protection of Population of the Republic of Kazakhstan (2020): Report on the study of the needs of families with children and adolescents living with HIV. Nur-Sultan [unpublished report].

Mukhatayeva, Ainur/Mustafa, Aidana/Dzissyuk, Natalya/Issanov, Alpamys/Bayserkin, Bauyrzhan/Vermund, Sten H. et al. (2021): Hepatitis B, Hepatitis C, tuberculosis and sexually-transmitted infections among HIV positive patients in Kazakhstan. In: Scientific Reports 11, No. 13542. DOI: 10.1038/s41598-021-92688-w.

Mussina, Kamilla/Abbay, Anara/Sakko, Yesbolat/Syssoyev, Dmitriy/Gusmanov, Arnur/Abdrakhmanova, Ainur et al. (2023): Dynamics of hospital admissions and all-cause mortality of HIV infected patients in Kazakhstan: Data from unified nationwide electronic healthcare system 2014-2019. In: Frontiers in Public Health 11, No. 1138604. DOI: 10.3389/fpubh.2023.1138604.

Mussina, Kamilla/Kadyrov, Shirali/Kashkynbayev, Ardak/Yerdessov, Sauran/Zhakhina, Gulnur/Sakko, Yesbolat et al. (2023): Prevalence of HIV in Kazakhstan 2010-2020 and Its Forecasting for the Next 10 Years. In: HIV/AIDS – Research and Palliative Care 15, pp. 387–397. DOI: 10.2147/HIV.S413876.

National Harm Reduction Coalition (2021): Harm Reduction Principles. www.harmreduction.org/about-us/principles-of-harm-reduction/, 29.02.2024.

Official Information Source of the Prime Minister of the Republic of Kazakhstan (2023): Strict control of infection safety in medical services and other procedures is necessary – Alikhan Smailov on HIV prevention. www.primeminister.kz/en/news/strict-control-of-infection-safety-in-medical-services-and-other-procedures-is-necessary-alikhan-smailov-on-hiv-prevention-24284, 30.10.2023.

Optima Consortium for Decision Science (2020): Resource optimization to maximize the HIV response in Kazakhstan. www.optimamodel.com/pubs/Kazakhstan_2020.pdf, 30.10.2023.

Paine, Emily A./Lee, Yong G./Vinogradov, Vitaliy/Zhakupova, Gulnara/Hunt, Timothy/Primbetova, Sholpan (2021): HIV Stigma, Homophobia, Sexual and Gender Minority Community Connectedness and HIV Testing Among Gay, Bisexual, and Other Men and Transgender People Who Have Sex with Men in Kazakhstan. In: AIDS and Behavior 25, No. 8, pp. 2568–2577. DOI: 10.1007/s10461-021-03217-9.

Petrenko, Irina I. (2023): Epidemiological situation in the Republic of Kazakhstan. Prospects and problems in the implementation of prevention programmes. www.ccmkz.kz/meeting, 10.01.2024.

Prilutskaya, Mariya (2020): Pilot study to assess the needs and availability of HIV prevention and treatment services for people using new psychoactive substances/stimulants in the Republic of Kazakhstan. Vienna: United Nations Office on Drugs and Crime (UNODC) [unpublished report].

Prilutskaya, Mariya/Yussopov, Oleg/Negay, Nikolay/Altynbekov, Kuanysh/Tokayeva, Makpal (2020): Prevalence of new psychoactive substances addiction: A hospital-based cross-sectional study. In: Journal of Clinical Medicine of Kazakhstan 1, No. 55, pp. 11–16. DOI: 10.23950/1812-2892-JCMK-00730.

Public Foundation "AGEP'C" (2023): Information for Kazakhstanis infected and living with hepatitis C virus. www.hepatit.kz/, 30.10.2023.

Renton, Adrian/Gzirishvilli, David/Gotsadze, George/Godinho, Joana (2006): Epidemics of HIV and sexually transmitted infections in Central Asia: Trends, drivers and priorities for control. In: International Journal of Drug Policy 17, No. 6, pp. 494–503. DOI: 10.1016/j.drugpo.2006.09.003.

Rodríguez Torres, Maribel (2006): Treatment of hepatitis C virus infection in drug addicts. In: Annals of Hepatology 5, No. 1, pp. S60–S62. DOI: 10.1016/S1665-2681(19)31976-3.

Romashkina, Svetlana (2021): "We had to send her to Moscow, to save from persecution". What Kazakh newspapers wrote about HIV/AIDS in the 80s and 90s. www.vlast.kz/obsshestvo/47641-prislos-ee-otpravit-v-moskvu-daby-spasti-ot-presledovanij.html, 30.10.2023.

Semchuk, Nadiya (2018): Brief information about HIV among MSM in Kazakhstan 2018. www.ecom.ngo/resource/files/2021/05/brief-on-hiv-among-msm-in-kazakhstan.pdf, 29.02.2024.

Strathdee, Steffanie A./Hallett, Timothy B./Bobrova, Natalia/Rhodes, Tim/Booth, Robert/Abdool, Reychad et al. (2010): HIV and risk environment for injecting drug users: The past, present, and future. In: The Lancet 376, No. 9737, pp. 268–284. DOI: 10.1016/S0140-6736(10)60743-X.

Stringer, Kristi L./Mukherjee, Trena/McCrimmon, Tara/Terlikbayeva, Assel/Primbetovac, Sholpan/Darisheva, Meruyert et al. (2019): Attitudes towards people living with HIV and people who inject drugs: A mixed method study of stigmas within harm reduction programs in Kazakhstan. In: International Journal of Drug Policy 68, pp. 27–36. DOI: 10.1016/j.drugpo.2019.02.007.

Su, Su/Mao, Limin/Zhao, Jinxian/Chen, Liang/Jing, Jun/Cheng, Feng et al. (2018): Epidemics of HIV, HCV and syphilis infection among synthetic drugs only users, heroin-only users and poly-drug users in Southwest China. In: Scientific Reports 8, No. 1. DOI: 10.1038/s41598-018-25038-y.

Sukhorukov, Ivan (2023): Patient zero. How HIV was first discovered in Kazakhstan in the 90s. www.tengrinews.kz/article/nulevoy-patsient-v-90-e-kazahstane-vpervyie-obnarujili-vich-2048/, 30.10.2023.

Sun, Yyanming/Guo, Wei/Li, Guiying/He, Shufang/Lu, Hongyan (2018): Increased synthetic drug abuse and trends in HIV and syphilis prevalence among female drug users from 2010–2014 from Beijing, China. In: International Journal of STD & AIDS 29, No. 1, pp. 30–37. DOI: 10.1177/0956462417715174.

The Global Fund. Office of Inspector General (2015): Report on the results of the investigation Global Fund grants in the Republic of Kazakhstan. Violations of procurement rules by suppliers and principal recipients. www.theglobalfund.org/media/2795/oig_gf-oig-15-002_report_ru.pdf, 30.10.2023.

The Joint United Nations Programme on HIV/AIDS (UNAIDS) (2018): Miles to Go. The Response to HIV in Eastern Europe and Central Asia. www.unaids.org/sites/default/files/media_asset/miles-to-go_eastern-europe-and-central-asia_en.pdf, 30.10.2023.

The Joint United Nations Programme on HIV/AIDS (UNAIDS) (2019): Community at the Centre. Defending Rights. Breaking Barriers. Reaching People with HIV Services. www.unaids.org/en/resources/documents/2019/2019-global-AIDS-update, 30.10.2023.

The Joint United Nations Programme on HIV/AIDS (UNAIDS) (2021): Country Progress Report – Kazakhstan. Global AIDS Epidemic Monitoring 2020. www.unaids.org/sites/default/files/country/documents/KAZ_2020_countryreport.pdf, 30.10.2023.

The Joint United Nations Programme on HIV/AIDS (UNAIDS) (2023): Young activists fight HIV stigma in Central Asia. www.unaids.org/ru/keywords/kazakhstan, 30.10.2023.

Thorne, Claire/Ferencic, Nina/Malyuta, Ruslan/Mimica, Jadranka/Niemiec, Tomasz (2010): Central Asia: Hotspot in the worldwide HIV epidemic. In: The Lancet. Infectious Diseases 10, No. 7, pp. 479–488. DOI: 10.1016/S1473-3099(10)70118-3.

Tukumov, Erkin (2023): "The region is entering a new phase". The expert named 3 scenarios for Central Asia. www.tengrinews.kz/article/region-vstupaet-novuyu-fazu-ekspert-nazval-3-stsenariya-1939/, 30.10.2023.

United Nations Office on Drugs and Crime (UNODC) (2020): About UNODC in Central Asia. www.unodc.org/centralasia/ru/unodc-in-central-asia.html, 30.10.2023.

United Nations Office on Drugs and Crime (UNODC) (2023a): Webinar Series – "Web-outreach as a Harm Reduction tool". www.unodc.org/centralasia/en/news/webinar-series---web-outreach-as-a-harm-reduction-tool.html, 30.10.2023.

United Nations Office on Drugs and Crime (UNODC) (2023b): Early Warning Advisory. www.unodc.org/unodc/en/scientists/ewa.html, 30.10.2023.

United States Agency for International Development (USAID) (2020): Central Asia Factsheet: HIV Flagship Activity. www.reliefweb.int/report/kazakhstan/usaid-central-asia-factsheet-hiv-flagship-activity, 30.10.2023.

World Health Organization (WHO) (2023a): Hepatitis C. Key Facts. www.who.int/news-room/fact-sheets/detail/hepatitis-c, 30.10.2023.

World Health Organization (WHO) (2023b): HIV and AIDS. Key Facts. www.who.int/news-room/fact-sheets/detail/hiv-aids, 30.10.2023.

World Health Organization (WHO) (2023c): Kazakhstan is leading light for free hepatitis testing and treatment in Central Asia. www.who.int/news-room/feature-stories/detail/kazakhstan-is-leading-light-for-free-hepatitis-testing-and-treatment-in-central-asia, 30.10.2023.

World Health Organization (WHO) (2023d): WHO publishes updated guidance on hepatitis C infection – with new recommendations on treatment of adolescents and children, simplified service delivery and diagnostics. www.who.int/news/item/24-06-2022-WHO-publishes-updated-guidance-on-hepatitis-C-infection, 30.10.2023.

Wu, Elwin/Terlikbayeva, Assel/Hunt, Timothy/Primbetova, Sholpan/Gun Lee, Yong/Berry, Mark (2017): Preliminary Population Size Estimation of Men Who Have Sex with Men in Kazakhstan: Implications for HIV Testing and Surveillance. In: LGBT Health 4, No. 2, pp. 164–167. DOI: 10.1089/lgbt.2015.0152.

Zhusupov, Baurzhan (2000): Women, Youth and HIV/AIDS in Kazakhstan. Public Opinion Research Centre. Kazakhstan. www.un.org/womenwatch/daw/csw/hivaids/Zhusupov.html, 30.10.2023.

4. HIV and Hepatitis C in Kyrgyzstan

Jarkyn Shadymanova, Nurgul Musaeva

Introduction

The epidemiological situation in the Kyrgyz Republic regarding HIV and hepatitis C infections presents a complex problem. There is an intensification of HIV and hepatitis C transmission pathways not only among vulnerable groups with risky behaviours but also among the general population, leading to an increase in the number of people living with these infections. The specifics of sexual behaviour and strategies for protection against unintended pregnancies and sexually transmitted infections play a significant role in the development of HIV/AIDS and hepatitis C epidemics in the country. In this chapter, we provide a comprehensive examination of the epidemiological conditions surrounding HIV/AIDS and hepatitis C in Kyrgyzstan. This includes a presentation of statistical data and a critical discussion of the response of the governmental healthcare system as well as international organisations and non-governmental organisations (NGOs). We also discuss the prevention programmes addressing HIV/AIDS and hepatitis C in Kyrgyzstan. In our discussion, we pay attention to the issue of stigmatisation and discrimination against vulnerable groups affected by HIV and hepatitis C.

HIV/AIDS and hepatitis C are medical and social issues with far-reaching consequences. The high level of stigma and discrimination against people living with HIV (PLWH) and those infected with hepatitis C, as well as the stigma against key population groups, complicates the response to the two diseases. This makes it more difficult to achieve key prevention objectives, such as reducing the incidence and mortality rates and preventing the further spread of HIV and hepatitis C in the country due to the inaccessibility of key population groups and their refusal to participate in testing, prevention, and treatment programs. The increase in the number of cases of HIV and hepatitis C transmitted through sexual contact indicates the duration of the latent stage of the development of these epidemics among injection drug users and the initiation of infection transmission within the general population. Therefore, preventive programmes, including harm reduction programmes, remain a vital component of comprehensive measures to combat these epidemics in Kyrgyzstan.

The epidemiological situation in the Kyrgyz Republic regarding HIV and hepatitis C infections presents a complex problem. There is an intensification of HIV and hepatitis C transmission pathways not only among vulnerable groups with risky behaviours but also among the general population, leading to an increase in the number of people living with these infections. The specifics of sexual behaviour and strategies for protection against unintended pregnancies and sexually transmitted infections play a significant role in the development of HIV/AIDS and hepatitis C epidemics in the country. In this chapter, we provide a comprehensive examination of the epidemiological conditions surrounding HIV/AIDS and hepatitis C in Kyrgyzstan. This includes a presentation of statistical data and a critical discussion of the response of the governmental healthcare system as well as international organisations and NGOs. We also discuss the prevention programmes addressing HIV/AIDS and hepatitis C in Kyrgyzstan. In our discussion, we pay attention to the issue of stigmatisation and discrimination against vulnerable groups affected by HIV and hepatitis C.

HIV and hepatitis C are spread unevenly within Kyrgyzstan. The highest prevalence of HIV and hepatitis C are found in the Chui and Osh regions, as well as in the cities of Bishkek and Osh. The central parts of these regions are better covered by HIV and hepatitis C testing services. However, in other regions, the intensity of infection transmission is lower as these regions were impacted by the epidemic at a later stage. Additional research and strategies are needed to effectively combat these epidemics in Kyrgyzstan.

Hepatitis C, sometimes referred to as the 'silent killer' is a serious infectious disease that affects people's health and lifestyles. This disease, caused by the hepatitis C virus (HCV), primarily targets the liver and can lead to chronic impairments in the organ's function, including cirrhosis and liver cancer. Hepatitis C has a global presence and represents a significant threat to public health in various countries. HCV transmission occurs through contact with infected blood, which means there is a risk of infection through the use of contaminated injection needles, improper use of medical equipment, and blood transfusions. It is worth noting that many infected individuals are unaware of their status since the disease often progresses without noticeable symptoms. A deep understanding of HIV and hepatitis C is becoming increasingly important in the context of global healthcare, requiring collaborative efforts from healthcare professionals, researchers, and society to combat and control these serious diseases.

Development of the HIV Epidemic in Kyrgyzstan

In the Kyrgyz Republic, the first case of HIV infection was recorded in 1987, involving a foreign citizen who was a student at the military school. According to the World Health Organisation (WHO) data, until 1996 Kyrgyzstan remained the only country in the Central Asian region without reported cases of HIV infection.

Between 1996 and 2000, 14 cases of HIV infection were registered among Kyrgyz citizens, most of them resulting from sexual transmission. After that, sporadic cases of HIV infection were observed, primarily among vulnerable groups. In most cases, infections occurred among Kyrgyz seasonal migrant workers who were infected while out of the country.

From 1987 to 2000, a total of 53 cases were registered, including 14 among citizens. However, significant growth in HIV infections began in 2000 (Sultanalieva et al. 2018).

From 2001 to 2006, the beginning of the HIV epidemic was observed in major regions of the country, including large cities such as Bishkek, Osh, and the regions of Osh and Chui. This epidemic primarily affected male injecting drug users (IDUs) aged 20 to 39.

Starting in 2001, there was a sharp increase in the spread of HIV infection in the country, with 149 cases among Kyrgyz citizens in 2001. The number of new infections that year was significantly higher than the total number of cases in the entire previous period of the epidemic. This increase was associated with an outbreak of HIV infection among IDUs, constituting 95.5% of the people living with HIV registered in 2001 (Mamadzhanov 2021).

From 2007, the HIV epidemic in Kyrgyzstan developed rapidly, affecting various social groups and transmission routes. The epidemic spread to the other six regions of the country, with an increase in HIV registration among women, particularly women of reproductive age. Cases of HIV infection in children, both through vertical transmission and parenteral transmission, were also identified. There was also increase in HIV transmission through sexual contact.

In the following years, there was a continuous increase in the registration of new cases, and the cumulative number of HIV infection grew annually.

The epidemic continued to affect various social groups and transmission routes. There were more cases of HIV infection in children. The transmission of HIV through sexual contact also increased.

The development of the HIV/AIDS epidemic started at the end of the 1990s.

In 2001, 9.5% of PLWH were women, but by 2010 this had increased to 30%.

In the last ten years, the number of women living with HIV increased by 77 times. However, in the last three years, it increased only 2.4 times, in January 2011. For the same reason, the number of cases of vertical transmission of HIV increased from 0% in 2005 to 2.4% of the registered cases of PLWH in 2010. The increase in the number of HIV-positive women and children indicated the transition of the epidemic from people who inject drugs (PWID) to the general population (Government of the Kyrgyz Republic 2012).

From 2011 to 2016, the total number of officially registered cases of HIV infection in the country more than doubled (from 3,270 cases in 2011 to 7,108 in 2016). According to WHO/UNAIDS estimates, in 2016 there were 8,307 PLWH in the country, which is 1.6 times higher than the official data (5,158). The number of women with HIV increased by 2.8 times (from 802 in 2011 to 2,313 in 2016 cumulatively). In 2011, approximately 30.7% of newly registered HIV cases were among women, while in 2016, this proportion increased to 41.8%, indicating a rise in the percentage of women living with HIV during that time period (Kyrgyz Republic Ministry of Justice 2017a, No. 852).

The changing nature of the HIV epidemic in Kyrgyzstan is reflected in the increasing number of infected women, leading to a change in the ratio of HIV-infected men and women and an increase in the proportion of women in the structure of HIV-infected people (Mamadzhanov 2020).

The existing infrastructure allowed for the identification of 83% of the estimated number of PLWH. Over the years, there has been a consistent pattern of change in the distribution of the main modes of HIV transmission. The proportion of cases resulting from sexual transmission has steadily increased, climbing from 81% in 2018 to 90% in 2022, while the percentage of cases attributed to injection transmission has notably decreased, dropping from 19% in 2018 to merely 4% in 2022 (Republican Center for Control of Bloodborne Viral Hepatitis and Human Immunodeficiency Virus 2022).

The HIV epidemic in Kyrgyzstan continues to evolve among key groups, especially among men who have sex with men (MSM), who account for up to 10% of new cases each year. However, a larger proportion of the newly identified cases (around 80%) occurs among individuals who do not belong to key vulnerable groups (Kadyrkulova 2018).

What are the Drivers of the HIV Epidemic?

Kyrgyzstan is home to a concentrated HIV/AIDS epidemic, with a disproportionately high percentage of the infections found among vulnerable groups, including PWID and MSM. A population-based bio-behavioural survey (BBS) found that the prevalence of HIV ranged from 13.3% to 25.9% among PWID and from 5.3% to 16.2% among MSM in Bishkek, the country's largest city (Republican AIDS Center/Centers for Disease Control and Prevention [CDC]/Pepfar 2021). This BBS study also identified key areas of prevention needs within the framework of the global '95-95-95' HIV treatment cascade, highlighting significant disparities in the accessibility and provision of services for these population groups at high risk of HIV infection. Viral HCV is a key co-infection, with estimates indicating that 67% of PWID were previously infected and 39% are currently infected with HCV.

According to AIDS Center data, there are approximately 16,900 MSM, 25,000 PWID, and 7,100 sex workers (SW) living in Kyrgyzstan, with varying geographical distribution (Regional Expert Group on Migrant Health 2023). According to data from the United Nations Development Programme (UNDP) (the principal recipient of the Global Fund in Kyrgyzstan), the coverage of prevention programmes among vulnerable groups is as follows: 85% for MSM, 68% for PWID, and 65% for SW. However, these data should be treated with caution as the estimates of vulnerable group size were conducted some time ago (in 2013 and 2016). In the past five years, the coverage of preventive programmes among PWID has not exceeded 17,000 clients (AIDS Center 2022).

The findings from the 2021 BBS encompassed estimations of the population size of PWID at locations representing more than 60% of the total coverage for preventive services in various regions such as Bishkek, Osh, Chui, and Osh. The estimated median number for these sites was 6,638. Similarly, in the same year, a BBS indicated an estimated population of 6,126 MSM in Bishkek according to data from the AIDS Center (Republican AIDS Center/CDC/Pepfar 2021). Insufficient legal awareness and knowledge results in the denial of generally accepted legal norms, violations of established norms, and myths, prejudices, and stigmas that restrict access to prevention for populations at increased risk, leading to the hidden spread of HIV among these groups. The Law of the Kyrgyz Republic 'On HIV/AIDS in the Kyrgyz Republic' contains provisions for the protection against stigmatisation and discrimination. However, violations of rights and breaches of diagnosis confidentiality occur on a regular basis. The absence of documents, registration, and citizenship also hinders the realisation of the right to HIV prevention and treatment.

Stigma and discrimination against people living with HIV, which are prevalent in Kyrgyzstan, manifest in disrespectful treatment, disclosure of HIV status, and refusal to provide medical services. These are significant barriers to accessing HIV-related services. The refusal of representatives of vulnerable groups to undergo HIV testing and to participate in prevention and treatment programmes leads to the continued spread of HIV infection, delayed treatment seeking, and increased AIDS-related mortality. In 2015, for example, 15.2% of infections were discovered at an advanced stage of HIV infection (Kyrgyz Republic Ministry of Justice 2017a, No. 852). Some PLWH refuse antiretroviral treatment out of fear of disclosing their HIV status.

In order to reduce the level of stigma and discrimination to zero in government organisations providing HIV-related services to key groups of the population and PLWH, various studies have been conducted. Firstly, the Harm Reduction Network Association of Legal Entities conducted two national monitoring studies, 'The Index of stigma against PLWH', in 2018 and 2021 (Harm Reduction Network Association 2022). Secondly, the AIDS Centre and the Ministry of Health conducted two national studies (one basic and one monitoring study) on the level of stigma in relation to key groups, namely PWID, SR, MSM, TG (transgender people) and prisoners.

A strategic and communication plan was developed, aimed at reducing stigma and discrimination. In 2021, in partnership with NGOs (by agreement) and vulnerable groups, training on stigma and discrimination was provided to 50% of staff involved in HIV programmes, key ministries, and agencies. Efforts were also made to incorporate HIV-related disciplines into the curricula and postgraduate training programmes for pedagogical and other related programmes.

What are the Vulnerable Groups and Why?

Prevention initiatives, such as harm reduction programmes, continue to be essential elements in Kyrgyzstan's comprehensive approach to addressing the HIV epidemic among vulnerable populations. By 2022, there were 24 operational harm reduction sites across the country, including those run by NGOs and within the prison system. Fifteen NGOs offered services tailored to PWID, SW, MSM, and PLWH, complemented by two dedicated centres for PLWH and other vulnerable groups. Prevention programmes for vulnerable groups, including harm reduction programmes, remain one of the crucial components in the comprehensive efforts to combat the HIV epidemic in Kyrgyzstan. In 2022 there were 24 harm reduction sites across the country, as well as harm reduction programmes in NGOs and in the penitentiary system. Fifteen NGOs provided services for PWID, SW, MSM, and PLWH, and there were two centres for PLWH and other vulnerable groups. In 2022, more than 36,000 representatives of vulnerable groups were provided with HIV testing, harm reduction services, care, and support programmes. This activity was carried out with the support of the Global Fund, and since 2019, there has been a continued effort to provide care and support for PLWH through mechanisms of government social contracting.

The AIDS Center is developing an online (cloud) version of the electronic tracking system for HIV cases (AIDS Center 2023) and has also initiated the process of developing a unified information system for HIV prevention programmes that will integrate disparate databases and improve the accounting system and, accordingly, the ability to monitor the quantity and quality of services for PLWH, reduce duplication of medical services, and improve quality data (Republican AIDS Center/CDC/Pepfar 2021, p. 33).In 2022, the AIDS Center updated the clinical protocol for the pre-contact prevention of HIV infection (PREP). In 2021, the coverage of PREP totalled 68 cases, and by the end of 2022, this had increased to 266.

The southern regions of the Kyrgyz Republic are among the most affected areas in terms of HIV infection. Organisational and preventive measures to combat the HIV epidemic in these regions are insufficient and do not fully cover the primary drivers of the epidemic, which hinders the achievement of significant results in the fight against it. In these regions, the rate of HIV infection among the population is higher than the national indicator. The mortality and lethality rates of HIV-infected people in these regions are also 2.5 to 4.5 times higher than in the Republic (Mamadzhanov 2021, p. 7). The Osh region is characterised by a high population density with a multinational composition, population instability due to internal and external migration, and high unemployment among young people. The current situation undoubtedly has an impact on the spread of the HIV epidemic.

The prevalence of HIV, according to data from the Republican Centre for the Control of Hematogenous Viral Hepatitis and Human Immunodeficiency Virus of the Ministry of Health of the Kyrgyz Republic as of 1st January 2023, is as follows (Republican Center for Control of Bloodborne Viral Hepatitis and Human Immunodeficiency Virus 2023b):

Table 1: HIV Prevalence in Kyrgyzstan (own compilation, based on data of the AIDS Centre)

Cities and Regions	**Male**	**Female**	**Total**
Batken	156	136	292
Bishkek	1,883	1,009	2,892
Osh city	883	408	1,291
Jalal-Abad	715	600	1,315
Issyk-Kul	268	152	420
Naryn	162	85	247
Osh region	991	780	1,771
Talas	103	75	178
Chuy	2,088	1,033	3,121
Total	**7,249**	**4,278**	**11,527**

The highest prevalence of HIV is observed in the Chui and Osh regions, as well as in the cities of Bishkek and Osh. The central parts of these two regions are better covered by HIV testing services. Residents in peripheral and remote villages often have to travel to the nearest family medical centre or AIDS centre for testing. The highest concentration of private laboratories is found in Bishkek and Osh. According to the prevalence of HIV by regions in the country, 50% of the country's laboratory equipment is concentrated in Bishkek, Osh, the Osh region, and the Chui region (Association Partnership network 2020).

In other regions of the Republic, the intensity of HIV spread is lower as these regions were impacted by the epidemic at a later stage.

Mamadzhanov (2021) ranked the different regions in the country based on the degree of the population affected by HIV infection, with three categories identified: high, moderate, and low.

The first zone consists of regions with a high prevalence. The city of Osh and the Chui region can be classified as high-prevalence areas. In these regions, the HIV prevalence rate among the population is higher than the national average (which is 143.2±1.5 per 100,000 people) and stands at 382.3±11.3 and 291.5±5.6, respectively. HIV mortality and fatality rates in these regions are also 2.5 to 4.5 times higher than the national average in Kyrgyzstan. The analysis shows that Osh City and the Chui region are characterised by intensive migration processes (both internal and external), a high level of unemployment, widespread drug use, and commercial sexual services among youth.

The second zone consists of regions with moderate prevalence. The zone includes territories like Bishkek City (161.4) and the Osh region (112.3), with prevalence rates among pregnant women of 0.024 (Bishkek) and 0.05 (Osh region). HIV mortality and fatality rates are lower than the national level in these areas. These regions account for 37% of HIV cases in the country, with 36.8% of the country's population residing there.

The third zone consists of regions with low prevalence. This zone includes districts in the other four regions of the Republic. The epidemic process began to intensify in these regions starting in 2006 to 2007.

Comprehensive epidemiological studies of HIV infection, particularly the factors of diagnosis or spread in the context of regions or cities, have not been conducted in Kyrgyzstan. Consequently, there are no recommendations for improving the HIV surveillance and prevention system in specific regions of the country.

The steps taken by Kyrgyzstan allow for the containment of the epidemic in a concentrated stage, in which the spread of the infection is among groups considered the most vulnerable. However, due to objective and subjective factors, including changes in transmission routes, increased migration processes, religious intensification, and a decrease in donor funding, there is a threat of the epidemic transitioning to a generalised stage and the registration of HIV cases among the general population (The Joint United Nations Programme on HIV/AIDS [UNAIDS] 2020).

HIV Policy in Kyrgyzstan

The main government agencies responsible for HIV in the Kyrgyz Republic include state institutions, international organisations, and non-governmental (non-profit) organisations. Over the past 10 years, a close collaboration between the government and the non-governmental sector has allowed for an effective mutual integration of HIV service delivery. The results of this integration include specific action plans for each actor, common indicators of joint activities, and the incorporation of social services into state medical institutions.

One of the primary state institutions responsible for the detection, treatment, and prevention of HIV spread in the country is the Republican Centre for the Control of Hematogenous Viral Hepatitis and HIV of the Ministry of Health of the Kyrgyz Republic.

The governmental HIV/AIDS service system was established in 1989 and has been working at the national and local levels since then. It implements and adapts international experience, builds partnerships, and coordinates programmes for HIV treatment and prevention. It is currently named the Service for the Control of Hematogenous Viral Hepatitis and HIV. HIV treatment services are provided by the Republican Centre for the Control of Hematogenous Viral Hepatitis and HIV, which oversees eight regional and local centres that provide consulting, diagnostic, and treatment for PLWH throughout the country. The provision of antiretroviral therapy (ART) for PWLH has been delegated to healthcare organisations in primary healthcare (PHC).

The Kyrgyz governmental HIV/AIDS service system has been accumulating and analysing data on the current epidemiological situation for more than 30 years. Based on the information obtained, HIV prevention and treatment programmes have been developed. It shapes national HIV policy, establishes a legislative framework, mobilises human and technical resources, and contributes to effective dialogue with civil society leaders, government, and international organisations.

Moreover, the National Coordination Committee for Combating HIV/AIDS, Tuberculosis, and Malaria was formed under the Government of the Kyrgyz Republic (Kyrgyz Republic Ministry of Justice 2011). The Committee includes representatives from all institutions and organisations involved in the response to HIV/AIDS. In 2019, boards of trustees were established in each regional AIDS centre and other healthcare organisations. This measure helps ensure the efficiency and transparency of decisions made, improve the quality of services provided, and targets the use of funds.

Cooperation Between Government Institutions and International Organisations

Since 2004, Kyrgyzstan has received financial and technical assistance from the Global Fund to Fight AIDS, Tuberculosis, and Malaria in addressing various medical and social issues related to HIV infection. Despite a nearly twofold reduction in funding, the Global Fund remains the primary donor, covering 48% of the budget of the government programme on HIV for the period of 2017 to 2021 (Eurasian Harm Reduction Association [EACB] 2021).

The programme activities of the AIDS Centre have been implemented with the technical and financial support of various international organisations, including UNAIDS, UNICEF, USAID, CDC, WHO, ICAP, UNDP, AFEW, and AIDS Centre. The Central Asian Regional HIV/AIDS Programme (CARHAP), funded by DFID, supports harm reduction programmes for HIV. CARHAP financed 43 projects primarily in the Bishkek, Osh, Chui, Osh, Jalal-Abad, and Batken regions, as well as the penitentiary sector from 2006 to 2010 (Government of the Kyrgyz Republic 2012). The programme's activities ended in 2012.

In addition to the grant component, CARHAP provided technical assistance to the National Coordination Committee for Combating HIV/AIDS, Tuberculosis, and Malaria under the Government of the Kyrgyz Republic. It also supports advocacy activities for harm reduction programmes related to HIV, enhances the capacity to beneficiaries, and promotes the development of the monitoring and evaluation system for HIV prevention programmes, including financial monitoring.

The German KfW Development Bank has facilitated the purchasing of equipment for laboratory services for HIV diagnosis in healthcare institutions. Under the KfW grant, 34 laboratories in healthcare institutions were equipped with diagnostic equipment (Government of the Kyrgyz Republic 2012).

The German Technical Cooperation (GIZ) project (2010–2018) focused on two key areas: supporting medical organisations and educational programmes on health issues. A small aspect of the programme supports the civil sector.

USAID initiated a new five-year regional project called 'HIV and Tuberculosis Dialogue' in 2009. This project provided technical assistance and training to improve access to quality HIV and tuberculosis prevention services for populations at high risk of infection. In 2010, USAID also introduced the 'Quality Healthcare' project, in which HIV and tuberculosis prevention issues were key components.

The AIDS Foundation East-West (AFEW) has implemented a project to enhance the interaction between HIV/tuberculosis services in Central Asia and works with NGOs and correctional facilities. This project introduced social support programmes in the country for the first time.

The Joint United Nations Programme on HIV/AIDS (UNAIDS) addresses HIV issues at the policy level. UNAIDS supports legislative changes to create a favourable environment for promoting HIV prevention in collaboration with partners, especially with vulnerable groups. UNAIDS works on enhancing the capacity of both national partners and vulnerable groups. It supports partners in developing strategic documents and assists the country with strategic data.

The Main Legal Norms Related to HIV in Kyrgyzstan

In the Kyrgyz Republic, in accordance with international standards, specific legislative acts have been developed and are in effect to regulate the procedures for HIV medical examination and subsequent treatment.

The fundamental legal documents regulating the diagnosis and treatment of HIV in Kyrgyzstan are the 'Law on HIV/AIDS in the Kyrgyz Republic', as well as the 'Rules for Medical Examination for the Detection of the Human Immunodeficiency Virus, Medical Record Keeping, and Monitoring of Individuals with Positive or Suspicious HIV Test Results in the Kyrgyz Republic' (Kyrgyz Republic Ministry of Justice 2005); the 'List of Workers, Professions, Jobs, and Positions Subject to Mandatory Medical Examination', approved by the Government's Resolution No. 296 of 25th April 2006 (Kyrgyz Republic Ministry of Justice 2006); the 'Regulations on Psychosocial Counselling Related to HIV', approved by the Government's Resolution No. 683 of 20th October 2017 (Kyrgyz Republic Ministry of Justice 2017); the 'State Programme to Overcome HIV Infection for 2017–2021'; the 'Guidelines for Laboratory Diagnosis of HIV Infection in the Kyrgyz Republic' and the 'Methodological Guidance on Laboratory Diagnosis of HIV Infection'; the 'Standard Operating Procedures for Laboratory Diagnosis of HIV Infection' (Order of the Ministry of Health of the Kyrgyz Republic No. 637 dated 26th November 2014) (Ministry of Health of the Kyrgyz Republic 2014); and other orders of the Ministry of Health aimed at expanding testing, including the organisation of rapid testing.

As a result of representatives if civil society the implementation of state programmes to overcome HIV, the improvement of the legislative framework, the interaction of state structures, representatives of civil society, international organisations are getting stronger and it is possible to keep the spread of HIV infection in the country at a low level.

The Law on HIV/AIDS in the Kyrgyz Republic defines the legal framework for preventing the spread of HIV/AIDS within the territory of the Kyrgyz Republic, ensuring a system of measures to protect the rights of people living with HIV/AIDS, the safety of Kyrgyzstan's citizens, and national security in accordance with international law.

A new Government Programme to Overcome HIV has been adopted for the years 2022 to 2027. In this new programme project, under the first strategic direction focused on providing a comprehensive package of services for the diagnosis, treatment, care, and support of HIV, measures are outlined to ensure access to testing services, not only for vulnerable groups but also for migrants and their close contacts, people facing difficult life situations, and those living in remote regions of the country. Additionally, the programme highlights measures to improve the laboratory diagnostic structure as regards HIV, including equipping healthcare organisations and NGOs with appropriate equipment, technical support, and staff training, as well as the introduction of modern methods for the laboratory diagnosis of HIV. The fourth strategic direction, aimed at ensuring the sustainability of HIV programmes, involves implementing measures to procure expensive or unavailable medical devices through international organisations, optimising testing, diagnosis, and treatment schemes.

In accordance with the WHO recommendations, the clinical protocols for HIV treatment and testing approaches are regularly reviewed in Kyrgyzstan. On 25th September 2020, new clinical guidelines for the treatment of HIV and comorbid conditions was approved by the Kyrgyz Ministry of Health (Order No. 759, 2020). In 2021, additions to this guidance were submitted for approval. In addition to the new guidance, previously approved clinical protocols and instructions include: 'Guidance on the Evaluation of Laboratory Diagnosis of HIV Infection' and 'Instruction on the Laboratory Diagnosis of HIV Infection in the Kyrgyz Republic'.

The goal of these protocols was to expand testing by non-governmental organisations and testing based on epidemiological and clinical indications, as well as testing for citizens entering the country.

HIV rapid testing is actively carried out among vulnerable groups. Algorithms for the use of rapid tests in healthcare institutions and by NGOs were developed and approved for this purpose. Changes to clinical protocols, updates to laboratory diagnostic instructions, and the allocation of funds from the state budget for the procurement of ARV drugs and HIV diagnostic tools have allowed for the expansion of state purchasing of tests and reagents for HIV diagnosis.

As a result, the Republican Centre for AIDS fully funds the tests needed for routine testing among the general population, including blood services, maternity institutions, and the testing of sexual partners. Despite significant progress having been made in terms of ensuring the availability of HIV testing services, the sustainability of diagnostic measures among vulnerable groups is still at risk.

In 2020–2021, screening and rapid testing for these groups were carried out with funding from donor organisations. Recently, however, the funding from the Global Fund and other donors was decreased. This, in combination with the limitations of the country's budget, means that there is a substantial risk that the testing of vulnerable population groups will have to be reduced in scope.

Thanks to civil society's activism and the support of international donors, Kyrgyzstan became the first country in the Eastern Europe and Central Asia (EECA) region to legislatively establish all nine HIV prevention measures for people who inject drugs, including the introduction of prevention services in places of detention. Criminal and administrative legislation related to drug trafficking are being reformed.

It is important to note that in 2019, a revision of national protocols and guidelines for the diagnosis, treatment, care, and social support of PWLH was initiated. All necessary ARV drugs were included in the List of Vital Medicines and Medical Devices. The main aim of this list is to facilitate the registration of high-quality ARV drugs. A comprehensive campaign to revise the registration, reporting, and accounting procedures related to HIV is also underway. As part of this campaign, updated algorithms for the registration of HIV cases, deaths, and more, as well as unified or consistent accounting and reporting forms for all stakeholders at all levels, are being reviewed and developed.

Kyrgyzstan continues its efforts to increase access to medical and social services for vulnerable groups and PLWH. As part of the implementation of the WHO 'Test and Treat' strategy, HIV testing, treatment, and care are being introduced in all healthcare systems at the secondary and primary levels. Primary healthcare physicians conduct rapid testing, screening for HIV based on clinical indications, and other assessments, prescribe and distribute ARV medications, and treat opportunistic infections. Seminars and training sessions are held to educate primary healthcare doctors on HIV diagnosis and treatment. Additionally, healthcare aides are being integrated into healthcare organisations to facilitate the delivery of medical and social services to people living with HIV and vulnerable groups, and to encourage their participation in prevention programmes.

NGOs have played a significant role in Kyrgyzstan's response to the HIV epidemic. Often, they were the first to advocate for the need to implement prevention programmes, emphasising the importance of the epidemic at the political level. The rapid spread of the HIV/AIDS epidemic in Kyrgyzstan since 1992/1993 contributed to the emergence of new NGOs at the local and national levels.

Thanks to non-governmental organisations in Kyrgyzstan, it has become possible to gain access to hard-to-reach groups of the population, involve them in preventive work, take their needs into account, and test modern technologies and methods for preventing the spread of HIV/AIDS in the country.

During the period of 2006 to 2010, 16 clinics for anonymous services were established within NGOs and state structures. These clinics provide diagnostic and treatment services for sexually transmitted infections (STIs) to vulnerable groups. In 2009 to 2010, 9,606 people applied and received services at syringe exchange points. However, out of those who applied, only 85.4% underwent testing for sexually transmitted infections and subsequently received treatment.

Since 2017, Kyrgyzstan has implemented a new system of state financing for socially relevant projects. All NGOs working with PLWH can participate in the state grant competitions. In the years 2019 to 2021, six NGOs working with PLWH in seven regions of the country received state funding. The effectiveness of NGO activities was monitored during visits by conducting surveys of service recipients.

Kyrgyz NGOs working in the field of HIV/AIDS differ significantly in terms of programme direction, target audience, size, financial capability, and strategy. The most obvious distinction exists between NGOs operating at the national level and local-level NGOs. The largest and most well-known NGOs are based in the cities of Bishkek and Osh.

Currently, the majority of NGOs in Kyrgyzstan combine their work on human rights and social activities, providing a range of services. However, representatives of NGOs believe that the lack of state prevention programmes in Kyrgyzstan might soon become a problem of national scale. Since 1997, nearly all necessary measures in this direction have been implemented with the support of international donors. The government of Kyrgyzstan has contributed only 5% of all expenses during the entire period (1997–2023).

The implementation of activities within the framework of the state social order with the involvement of NGOs and the private sector will help achieve the set goals while making more efficient use of state resources.

The participation of NGOs in the national response to HIV is also provided for in departmental documents. Thus, according to the Order of the Ministry of Health 'On the introduction of HIV testing by rapid testing among vulnerable groups of the population' (Ministry of Health of the Kyrgyz Republic 2012), a number of NGOs were involved in rapid testing and consulting in various regions Kyrgyzstan. Later, the number of participating NGOs increased, with the adoption of the Ministry of Health's order on 'Expanding HIV Rapid Testing among Vulnerable Population Groups' (Ministry of Health of the Kyrgyz Republic 2014).

NGOs, collaborating with PLWH and MSM at sentinel sites, establish positive relationships with target groups and are familiar with the local context. This facilitates the conducting of bio-behavioural research. NGOs also participate in formative assessments of PWLH and MSM in Kyrgyzstan to plan methods for implementing integrated HIV programmes and actively disseminate research results. NGO staff provides access to social and medical services, referring or accompanying clients to specialists. They actively participate in the service delivery algorithm, including involving PWLH and their communities in HIV-related prevention, treatment, and support programmes.

In general, the NGOs are currently actively involved in organising and implementing social support for PWLH in the observation and treatment programme for HIV infection. Their focus includes the formation of adherence to treatment, social assistance, and support. The organisation provides advisory services on reproductive health, family planning, and the diagnosis and treatment of STIs. Additionally, they distribute condoms and other contraceptives to women living with HIV. One of the crucial tasks of NGOs is to conduct pre-test and post-test counselling and voluntary testing for HIV infection, as well as providing redirection and support in healthcare organisations. NGOs also carry out various initiatives, including the organisation of self-help groups, peer-to-peer counselling, and 'Patient School' to maintain adherence to ART in PWLH.

Some NGOs go beyond healthcare and provide psychological, social, and legal support to PWLH and children affected by the epidemic. They also play a significant role in research, participating in monitoring studies and conducting integrated bio-behavioural studies among key population groups (LUIN, CP, MSM, TG, prisoners). This includes assessing the number and gender composition of key population groups and monitoring the level of stigma and discrimination against people living with HIV and key population groups.

Thus, in the Kyrgyz sector, NGOs and organisations working in the field of HIV/AIDS perform various functions: they actively combat the HIV epidemic, provide healthcare services, and focus on HIV prevention (Stöver/Shadymanova 2022). They address the HIV epidemic, focus on healthcare, and emphasize HIV prevention. However, their work varies significantly depending on their target groups. Some NGOs primarily work in youth-oriented HIV prevention, while others specialise in serving vulnerable groups such as injection drug users, commercial sex workers, and MSM.

Epidemiological Situation of HCV in Kyrgyzstan

According to the WHO, around 58 million people worldwide suffer from chronic HCV, with approximately 1.5 million new infections occurring each year. This disease contributes significantly to mortality, primarily due to liver cirrhosis and hepatocellular carcinoma (primary liver cancer). Despite the existence of direct-acting antiviral drugs that can cure HCV in over 95% of cases, access to diagnosis and treatment remains inaccessible in many parts of the world (WHO 2023). Currently, there is no vaccine for hepatitis C, but the disease can be successfully treated with antiviral medications. Early detection and proper treatment help prevent serious liver damage and improve long-term health.

In 2021, a total of 2,090 cases of viral hepatitis were registered in Kyrgyzstan, compared to 4,805 cases in 2020, indicating a 2.3-fold decrease in hepatitis incidence. Of all the registered cases in 2021, hepatitis A, which can be transmitted through environmental factors such as water, food, 'unclean' hands, and everyday objects, accounted for 91.6%; hepatitis B constituted 5.7%; and hepatitis C made up 2.5% (Ministry of Health Department of Disease Prevention and State Sanitary 2022).

In Kyrgyzstan, there are 34 laboratories for HIV diagnosis that also now provide HCV diagnostic services for free. At the end of 2022, the government allocated 276 million Kyrgyz Som for laboratory diagnosis, vaccination, and treatment of viral hepatitis. Rapid tests and vaccines are available to all patients in need. In this regard, a free rapid testing programme was conducted between 15th September and 31st December 2022 in the cities of Bishkek and Osh, as well as in the Chui region. Since the beginning of 2023, rapid tests have been conducted before vaccination with 'Regevak B' (Republican Center for Health Promotion and Mass Communication 2023), and more than 31,000 people have undergone rapid testing for all types of hepatitis, identifying 830 new cases of hepatitis. These cases are confirmed using PCR and Iffar methods to determine viral load and subsequent treatment (Sputnik Radio Kyrgyzstan 2023).

The hepatitis C virus is a blood-borne virus. The main modes of transmission include the re-use or inadequate sterilisation of medical equipment, such as syringes and needles in healthcare facilities, transfusion of untested blood and blood products, and the sharing of injection equipment among drug users. This results in a higher prevalence of hepatitis C among people who inject drugs, three times higher than the prevalence of HIV (WHO 2017).

More than half of acute hepatitis C cases are linked to drug use, which is why this disease is often referred to as drug users and hepatitis in literature. Scientists attribute the peculiarities of hepatitis development in drug users to the toxic impact on the liver and changes in the immune system. Infection with hepatitis viruses occurs in the first year of drug use when the toxic impact on the liver is still minimal, and clinical symptoms are primarily caused by the viruses. Alcoholism, inadequate nutrition, and toxic impurities also contribute to liver damage in drug addiction (Global Commission on Drug Policy 2013).

Drug users become infected during the injection of narcotic substances, using the same needle, leading to a cycle of injection drug use. Over time, those who use psychotropic drugs experience impaired thinking and analysis and a weakened self-preservation instinct, leading to careless adherence to hygiene rules and the use of already-used syringes, ignoring the risk of infection transmission (Martínez-Pérez et al. 2021).

Over time, as the transmission of the hepatitis C virus through medical procedures has decreased, this virus has increasingly become associated with drug injection. This leads to reduced sympathy for individuals suffering from hepatitis C due to the widespread perception of drug addiction as a manifestation of weak character. In places where the 'war on drugs' is being waged, these beliefs are reinforced by the criminalisation and incarceration of drug users (Global Commission on Drug Policy 2013).

Hepatitis C is mainly transmitted through the injection of narcotic substances using shared needles, and limited access to sterile instruments is linked to drug policies and law enforcement actions. In Kyrgyzstan, according to the WHO, more than 100,000 people suffer from chronic hepatitis C infection, which constitutes a significant part of liver disease-related mortality. Even among those who are aware of their condition, at least 220,000 people are affected by hepatitis C (Zheenalieva 2022).

Based on the statistical data from the Republican Medical Information Centre, over a period of five years (2010–2015), 1,429 newly diagnosed cases of chronic hepatitis C were registered in Kyrgyzstan (Tobokalova et al. 2016). Unofficial estimations claimed that approximately 6%–10% of Kyrgyzstan's population was infected with the hepatitis C virus by the beginning of 2016 (Miroshnik 2015). According to the study by Botheju and colleagues (2019), the prevalence of HCV varied within different groups in Kyrgyzstan, ranging from 0.8% to 5.0% in the general population, with a median of 2.0%; from 0.0% to 35.0% in populations at intermediate risk, with a median of 7.0%; and from 4.0% to 33.3% in non-specific clinical populations, with a median of 8.0%. Among people who inject drugs, the HCV prevalence ranged from 17.0% to 60.4%, with a median of 46.4% (Botheju et al. 2019). The price for hepatitis C treatment in Kyrgyzstan ranged from 15,000 USD to 20,000 USD (Miroshnik 2015).

Co-infection of HIV and hepatitis C often occurs among injecting drug users. Co-infection is exacerbated by repressive drug policies that limit access to prevention programmes and alienate vulnerable groups from healthcare services, which also affects the treatment of both infections (Deryabina/El-Sadr 2017).

To improve the outcomes of HIV and HCV co-infection treatment, it is necessary to intensify the fight against HIV and hepatitis, such as by running informational campaigns and ensuring access to rapid testing.

HCV Testing

The WHO recommends that testing, medical care, and treatment for people with chronic hepatitis C be carried out by qualified doctors and nurses, even if they are not specialists in the field, using a simplified service delivery system, including the decentralisation, integration, and redistribution of functions. These services can be provided through government healthcare institutions, primary healthcare, harm reduction services, and even in prison settings, ensuring wider access and convenience for patients (WHO 2017). Routine testing for viral hepatitis B and C should become part of the healthcare and prevention system (Sputnik Radio Kyrgyzstan 2023).

The Kyrgyz Government, in collaboration with the WHO and its partners, conducts various initiatives to address viral hepatitis. These include advocating for routine hepatitis B and C testing as part of healthcare systems, promoting evidence-based prevention and treatment methods, particularly tailored for individuals who inject drugs like cocaine and amphetamines. Technical and informational support is provided to mobilize resources for implementing harm reduction measures, and efforts are made to establish a collaborative network for developing effective healthcare policies. A critical step would be the inclusion of medications for the treatment of hepatitis B and C (as well as hepatitis D) in national lists of essential and life-saving medicines for which expenses are reimbursed. This would contribute towards ensuring the availability of quality treatment at the national level (WHO 2017).

Stigmatisation

Stigmatisation occurs when people look down on others or treat others unfairly because of certain conditions or illnesses. In the case of viral hepatitis, especially chronic hepatitis B and C, stigmatisation is a big problem. It can stop people who have these conditions from seeking diagnosis and medical help. To help these people, it is important to overcome stigmatisation, get access to treatment individuals in need of help, and provide testing. Additionally, we need to raise awareness among both the general public and healthcare professionals. It is also crucial to develop ways to track what people know about hepatitis B and C and how they access healthcare services. Many people do not know much about hepatitis C, and this creates challenges for dealing with the growing epidemic.

Repressive drug control policies and careless attitudes and discrimination on the part of medical workers (Martínez-Pérez et al. 2021) push drug users away from support programmes. For many drug users, hepatitis C remains an inevitable evil.

In Kyrgyzstan, the pervasive fear of encountering law enforcement hampers both harm reduction and HIV prevention initiatives, particularly among PWID. Stigma and discrimination contribute to their hesitation in engaging with syringe service programmes (SSPs) (Deryabina/El-Sadr 2017) and undergoing HIV testing for fear of potential disclosure of their positive HIV status. Discriminatory treatment from healthcare providers and the fear of revealing their drug use status, especially near drug treatment centres, pose substantial obstacles to accessing drug treatment. These challenges underscore the necessity for a more compassionate and health-oriented approach to addressing the complex issues at the intersection of drug use, stigma, and HIV prevention (Smith et al. 2022).

Many People Who Use Drugs Are Put in Jail

Imprisonment creates additional risks for people who use drugs. At the same time, the lack of programmes to prevent diseases in places of detention can lead to outbreaks of viral infections among this vulnerable group of people. This contributes significantly the spread of hepatitis C among drug users. Also, since hepatitis C is more common and easier to spread than other types of hepatitis. This shows that the 'war on drugs' does not work and has negative consequences, making people at risk feel like they are bad and alone. Hepatitis C among drug users can be stopped and treated, but we need to change drug policies.

The Hepatitis C Epidemic is Not Getting Sufficient Attention

The hepatitis C epidemic in Kyrgyzstan does not receive the attention, resources, or support that it needs. Access to hepatitis C treatment for drug users is insufficient. As a result, this situation is causing significant damage among this vulnerable population group. Because the government's efforts to control and monitor hepatitis C are slow, the activities to improve prevention and treatment do not always work. To effectively respond to hepatitis C, Kyrgyzstan needs to strengthen harm reduction approaches.

Fear and Stigma Make Risks Worse

Focusing on law enforcement makes people scared of getting arrested or hurt by the police, but it does not stop drug use. Instead, it makes the risk of getting diseases like hepatitis C even worse and causes other problems that could have been avoided. The main result of this kind of policy is that people who use drugs are afraid to get help from important healthcare programmes. For example, police officers often go to service programmes that help drug users to find easy ways to catch possible criminals. This is a big deal, especially in countries where owning needles and syringes is against the law or where they can be used as evidence of being involved in a crime.

Despite an increase in public awareness, most governments still underestimate the importance of this area of public health and do not pay enough attention to the connection between it and harsh drug policies. The system for monitoring the hepatitis C epidemic is not well-developed, and efforts in effective prevention and treatment access are not achieving the success that has been seen in the fight against HIV. To overcome the hepatitis C epidemic, it is necessary to optimise and expand existing harm reduction methods. However, even among leading donors who support harm reduction approaches, hepatitis C remains a less noticeable public health issue.

A policy that focuses on enforcement does more harm than good. People who manage large drug markets and profit from them rarely come under the scrutiny of law enforcement. Instead, regular drug users or small-scale drug dealers become victims of the 'war on drugs'. These groups often become targets for law enforcement personnel, who often evaluate their effectiveness based solely on the number of arrests and sometimes engage in corruption and extortion for personal gain.

An emphasis on enforcement methods does not reduce drug consumption and increases the risk of spreading hepatitis C and having other harmful consequences. It discourages people who use drugs from seeking help from healthcare programmes. Places of incarceration become high-risk areas for the spread of HIV and hepatitis C, and they often deny access to necessary prevention and treatment methods, such as opioid substitution therapy and the provision of sterile injection equipment. These problems escalate in compulsory drug detention centres, where human rights violations continue despite clear signs of issues.

People who use drugs and live with hepatitis C often face a double stigma that hinders them from accessing testing, treatment, and support. This stigma can also prevent them from disclosing their hepatitis C and drug use status to healthcare workers. It is essential to combat this stigma and consider drug addiction as a chronic relapsing condition rather than a social evil. Such approaches should also include actions to prevent the criminalisation and unlawful detention of people who use drugs as this complicates their access to healthcare and support. These issues should be addressed within the framework of effective efforts to combat the HCV epidemic among drug users (Global Commission on Drug Policy 2013).

Even when support services for people who use drugs are available, these services are constantly under threat of arrests and legal prosecution by the police, which negatively affects the situation as many people are afraid to seek help. Even with the availability of hepatitis treatment for the general population, drug users often face stigmatisation and discrimination, which hinders their access to necessary medical care. Healthcare programmes are rarely adapted to meet the unique needs of drug users, despite it being well known that these individuals can successfully utilise integrated communicative services.

Strengthening efforts to create more user-friendly services leads to greater engagement and contributes to effective hepatitis prevention and liver disease prevention. Some programmes targeting drug users are limited and rely on external donor sources. Governments should reallocate resources from repressive policies to public health-oriented ones.

The level of hepatitis C transmission through medical procedures has decreased, but the infection is now associated with injection drug use, which reduces sympathy for these people. The harm reduction approach aims to reduce the negative consequences of drug use. Key goals include preventing the spread of infections, reducing the risk of overdose, and mitigating social consequences such as poverty and criminality.

Needle exchange programmes, opioid substitution therapy, informational education, medical assistance, and safe injection rooms are part of comprehensive measures. It is also essential to reduce or eliminate criminal punishment for drug-related offenses. Co-dependent individuals, such as family members and friends, also play a crucial role in providing support.

Governments should focus on public health-oriented policies, including the decriminalisation of drug use. Harm reduction programmes should be expanded to make them more accessible. Hepatitis C prevention includes safe injections, needle and syringe exchange, blood donor testing, improving the competence of healthcare staff, and using barrier methods for sexual contact. Given the absence of a vaccine, special attention should be given to high-risk groups, including drug users and people with HIV infection.

The comprehensive set of measures also includes promoting a healthy lifestyle, preventing the initiation of drug use, supporting social programmes, and distributing sterile injection equipment, including low dead space syringes. It also ensures the availability of addiction treatment, including opioid substitution therapy, risk assessment for new injection methods, and integrated services for people who use injection drugs, including testing for viral hepatitis and HIV.

Projects and NGOs

In the fight against hepatitis, the Kyrgyz Ministry of Health approved a target programme in 2016 and began vaccinating new-borns in 2021. Currently, there are no cases of hepatitis B and C among children and young people up to 23 years of age, thanks to this vaccination programme. However, some cases are possible due to vaccine refusals.

In an interview, the Director of AIDS Centre Umutkan Chokmorova said, 'The treatment of hepatitis B and C includes taking tablets, and the cost varies depending on the patient's condition. 270 million Kyrgyz Soms were allocated to combat hepatitis C, and by the end of the year, the number of affected individuals can be accurately determined' (Sputnik Radio Kyrgyzstan 2023).

HIV transmission reduction has been significant in Kyrgyzstan: vertical transmission decreased from 39% in 2016 to 2.7% in 2023. It is expected that this situation will be sustained, if people responsibly manage their health and take medication (Sputnik Radio Kyrgyzstan 2023).

The Soros-Kyrgyzstan Foundation also actively supports projects aimed at reforming the public healthcare system and expanding access to medical services for vulnerable groups. This is achieved by involving representatives of civil society in the decision-making process. The foundation also focuses its efforts on developing the potential of civil society and advancing legal aspects related to HIV (Government of the Kyrgyz Republic 2012).

Since the beginning of 2010, the foundation has been actively working to support palliative care and the treatment of viral hepatitis C.

Various UN agencies have also contributed to the fight against HIV infection. UNAIDS coordinates the efforts of UN agencies in this area. UNFPA works with youth on HIV and reproductive health issues and provides condoms. UNICEF supports HIV prevention and treatment for children. UNODC conducts HIV prevention programmes among drug users. UNESCO has developed a regulatory legal framework and strengthens the human resources of HIV prevention programmes within the education system. WHO has contributed to health policy and standards in healthcare, prevention, treatment, and care, as well as medical aspects of HIV and blood safety (Government of the Kyrgyz Republic 2012).

UNDP implements the 'Support to the Government in Responding to the HIV/AIDS Epidemic' programme. This programme is aimed at creating a favourable political environment and building the capacity of national partners. It also provides legal services, fights stigma and discrimination, improves legislation, and trains medical and non-medical workers in HIV-related areas. UNDP's role is crucial as the main recipient of the Global Fund to Fight AIDS, Tuberculosis, and Malaria (GFATM). It intends to utilize funds to enhance the capabilities of key GFATM sub-recipients and vulnerable community groups during the execution of the 10th round of the GFATM grant spanning from 2012 to 2016.

In 2010, the Healthcare Improvement Project (HIP/USAID) and PEPFAR for Central Asian Republics were launched. The project also implemented an external quality assessment programme for the laboratory diagnosis of infectious diseases, including HIV and HIV-associated infections, viral hepatitis B and C, syphilis, and others. However, these assessments face financial difficulties due to a lack of funding.

Three quarantine plasma chambers were purchased and installed in the Republican Osh and Jalal-Abad Blood Centres. Unfortunately, the chamber in the city of Osh remained non-functional for three years due to the lack of power cables (Ministry of Health of the Kyrgyz Republic 2012).

Despite the existence of a donor database and the conditions for plasma quarantine, as well as improvements in quality control programmes for HIV and viral hepatitis testing, the threat of transmission of transmissible infections such as HIV, HBV, HCV, syphilis, and others still remains. In this regard, special attention should be given to the selection of donors with low behavioural risk and limiting the clinical use of blood and its components.

The proportion of individuals who inject drugs and are HIV-positive remains relatively stable at 14.6%, similar to the rate in 2009 at 14.3%. Notably, there is a high prevalence of viral hepatitis C, affecting 50.4%

of people living with HIV, indicating risky drug use practices. Syphilis is also prevalent, affecting 6.6% of HIV-positive individuals, while among prisoners, the rates are 37.5% for HCV and 3.5% for syphilis. These findings suggest slow changes in the behaviour of this demographic group as reported by UNAIDS in 2012 (UNAIDS 2012).

Furthermore, the minimum service package is often unavailable due to limited resources. Often, only one service is provided, and there are interruptions in service delivery, which contributes to the resumption of risky practices. The integration of services for harm reduction, the provision of ART, care, and patient support remains inadequate. Harm reduction approaches in small towns and rural areas leave much to be desired, and gender aspects are not adequately considered within harm reduction programmes. Additionally, there are insufficient adequate assessments of the number of people living with HIV covered by prevention programmes.

Nevertheless, Kyrgyzstani NGOs devote less focus to HCV compared to HIV, while the Ministry of Health and medical Organisations actively engage with HCV in Kyrgyzstan.

Prevention

To ensure effective treatment, a uniform approach is applied in handling individuals with chronic viral hepatitis, involving disease assessment, regular monitoring of the patient's health status, and evaluating medication side effects. Specific focus is given to patients at advanced stages of liver disease. The next important step involves taking measures to control common coexisting conditions and concurrent infections that may accelerate the progression of liver disease or increase the risk of reinfection with viral hepatitis. Among such measures, controlling the use of alcohol and psychoactive substances is crucial.

A comprehensive set of measures for prevention and harm reduction among individuals who inject drugs includes needle and syringe exchange programmes (NSPs), opioid substitution therapy (OST), and other evidence-based methods for treating drug dependence, as well as targeted informational, educational, and communication-based activities for those who use injectable drugs.

Progress in the fight against viral hepatitis requires increasing vaccination coverage, especially among high-risk groups such as prisoners, men who have sex with men, and sex workers.

Early diagnosis plays a vital role in preventing complications and virus transmission. To achieve a reduction in disease incidence, it is necessary to implement comprehensive measures, including treating viral hepatitis, opioid substitution therapy, and harm reduction strategies.

A comprehensive set of harm reduction measures related to injection drug use is described in a technical guide developed by the WHO, UNAIDS, and UNODC. This set of measures covers a wide range of actions aimed at reducing the transmission of both HIV and hepatitis viruses, considering their common transmission route, namely through blood (WHO 2017).

Governments should also improve the quality and accessibility of data on hepatitis C and strengthen epidemiological surveillance and programme evaluation systems. This, in turn, contributes to increasing awareness among policymakers and the public about the scale of this epidemic.

In 2012, the WHO released the 'Prevention and Control of Viral Hepatitis Infection Among People Who Inject Drugs' guide, which operates based on six key principles: human rights compliance, healthcare access, justice accessibility, service acceptability for people who use drugs, health literacy, and integrated service delivery. This guide emphasises the importance of using a comprehensive harm reduction approach to combat hepatitis B and C, HIV, and tuberculosis. It includes needle and syringe exchange programmes, opioid substitution therapy (which is also effective in HIV prevention), and targeted education, prevention, diagnosis, and treatment of viral hepatitis (WHO 2017).

It is important to note that in the absence of a hepatitis C vaccine, providing sterile injection equipment and opioid substitution therapy become primary prevention methods capable of preventing the spread of the infection among people who use injection drugs. Over time, as the transmission of the hepatitis C virus through medical procedures has decreased, its connection with injection drug use has become more apparent. Attention should be given to providing support for people who use drugs and are living with hepatitis C so that they can access testing, treatment, and support while feeling free from stigma and discrimination.

Conclusion

In conclusion, Kyrgyzstan faces regional disparities in the prevalence of both HIV and HCV, with the highest concentration of cases in the Chui and Osh regions, particularly in the cities of Bishkek and Osh. While central areas have better access to testing services, peripheral and remote villages face challenges, contributing to regional variations in testing availability. Mamadzhanov's (2021) categorisation of high-, moderate-, and low-prevalence zones offers a nuanced understanding of the epidemic, with high-prevalence areas characterised by elevated infection rates, migration, unemployment, and risk behaviours among youth. Moderate-prevalence zones demonstrate lower infection rates and better HIV-related indicators, while low-prevalence regions experienced a later onset of the epidemic. Epidemiological studies on HIV and HCV lack granularity at the regional level, hindering targeted interventions. Even though containment efforts have been successful, new challenges such as rising migration rates and reduced funding levels pose a risk of increasing the epidemic.

Kyrgyzstan's response involves collaborative efforts with state institutions, international organisations, and NGOs. The Republican Centre for the Control of Hematogenous Viral Hepatitis and HIV oversees testing, treatment, and prevention, with the National Coordination Committee ensuring coordination. Financial assistance from international organisations sustains programmes, and legal frameworks guide protocols. The 2022–2027 government program emphasises comprehensive services. Despite strides in clinical protocols and expanded testing, challenges persist. Collaboration with international organisations enhances Kyrgyzstan's response, with initiatives supported by the German Development Bank, USAID, and UNAIDS. Despite challenges, Kyrgyzstan has made strides in revising clinical protocols, expanding testing, and integrating HIV services into primary healthcare.

NGOs play a crucial role in outreach, testing, and support for vulnerable groups affected by HIV and HCV, bridging healthcare gaps and addressing stigma. Challenges include sustaining diagnostics, reduced funding, and potential prevention gaps. Continuous legislative revision, NGO involvement, and comprehensive services are vital.

The text underscores HCV's global impact, with Kyrgyzstan experiencing a decrease in incidence. Government funds support diagnosis, vaccination, and treatment, but challenges persist, including HCV's association with injection drug use and stigma hindering access to treatment.

Comprehensive measures for HCV include harm reduction, needle exchange, and opioid substitution, shifting from enforcement-focused to public health-oriented drug policies. Various organisations, including the

Kyrgyz government and NGOs, play a crucial role in effective prevention and treatment for both HIV and HCV.

Challenges like stigma and discrimination require destigmatisation, increased awareness, and integrated harm reduction services. Inclusion of HCV treatment in essential lists, support from organisations like the Soros-Kyrgyzstan Foundation, and collaboration with UN agencies are crucial. Optimising harm reduction, improving policies, and expanding access to treatment are recommended for both HIV and HCV.

In conclusion, addressing the complexities of HIV and HCV requires a comprehensive strategy encompassing medical, social, legal, and economic dimensions. Kyrgyzstan demonstrates a firm commitment to safeguarding its citizens' health by integrating HIV/AIDS and HCV initiatives into its long-term national development plan. This approach is in harmony with the UN Sustainable Development Goals, emphasizing essential aspects like healthcare access, education, gender equality, and partnerships to achieve these goals effectively.

Kyrgyzstan has made significant strides in reducing hepatitis incidence, bridging gender gaps, and fostering collaborations with international bodies, underscoring its dedication to SDG objectives. However, continual efforts are vital to effectively reach key populations, educate the public, and uphold partnerships to sustain progress against HIV and HCV. The country's dedication and collaborative efforts among stakeholders play a pivotal role in achieving desired outcomes not only within Kyrgyzstan but also in broader global health initiatives.

Bibliography

AIDS Center (2022): Situation on HIV infection in the Kyrgyz Republic. www.aidscenter.kg/statistika/?lang=ru, 21.02.2024.

AIDS Center (2023): Situation on HIV infection in the Kyrgyz Republic as of 01.01.23. www.aidscenter.kg/wp-content/uploads/2023/03/01.01.2023.pdf, 21.02.2024.

Association Partnership network (2020): Results of a market study of diagnostic test systems for identifying and monitoring the treatment of HIV infection in Kyrgyzstan in 2018-2019. www.aph.org.ua/wp-content/uploads/2021/09/Kyrgystan_AnalysisOfHIVDiagnostics.pdf, 26.02.2024.

Botheju, Welathanthrige S.P./Zghyer, Fawzi/Mahmud, Sarwat/Terlikbayeva, Assel/El-Bassel, Nabila/Abu-Raddad, Laith J. (2019): The epidemiology of hepatitis C virus in Central Asia: Systematic review, meta-analyses, and meta-regression analyses. In: Scientific Reports 9, No. 2090. DOI: 10.1038/s41598-019-38853-8.

Deryabina, Anna/El-Sadr, Waafaa (2017): Uptake of needle and syringe program services in the Kyrgyz Republic: key barriers and facilitators. In: Drug and Alcohol Dependence 1, No. 179, pp. 180–186.

Eurasian Harm Reduction Association (EACB) (2021): Kyrgyz Republic: Assessing the sustainability of the response to HIV among key populations in the context of the transition from Global Fund support to government funding. www.eecaplatform.org/wp-content/uploads/2022/06/tmt-assessment-report-kyrgyzstan-ehra-2021-rus.pdf, 26.02.2024.

Global Commission on Drug Policy (2013): The War on Drugs and Its Negative Impact on Public Health: The Hidden Hepatitis C Epidemic. www.globalcommissionondrugs.org/wp-content/uploads/2016/03/GCDP_HepatitisC_2013_EN.pdf, 21.02.2024.

Government of the Kyrgyz Republic (2012): About the State program on stabilization of epidemic of HIV infection in the Kyrgyz Republic for 2012-2016 [No. 867, 29 December 2012]. www.cis-legislation.com/document.fwx?rgn=57985, 26.02.2024.

Harm Reduction Network Association (2022): Study Report People Living with HIV Stigma Index 2.0 Kyrgyz Republic. www.stigmaindex.org/country-reports/#/m/KG, 22.02.2024.

Kadyrkulova, Zhainagul (2018): Labour migration in Kyrgyzstan. In: International Journal of Humanities and Natural Sciences 2, pp. 186–189.

Kyrgyz Republic Ministry of Justice (2005): Rules for Medical Examination for the Detection of the Human Immunodeficiency Virus, Medical Record Keeping, and Monitoring of Individuals with Positive or Suspicious HIV Test Results in the Kyrgyz Republic [No. 296, 25 April 2006]. www.cbd.minjust.gov.kg/act/view/ru-ru/57394/10?mode=tekst, 22.02.2024.

Kyrgyz Republic Ministry of Justice (2006): List of Workers, Professions, Jobs, and Positions Subject to Mandatory Medical Examination [No. 296, 25 April 2006]. www.cbd.minjust.gov.kg/act/view/ru-ru/57396?cl=ru-ru, 22.02.2024.

Kyrgyz Republic Ministry of Justice (2011): Regulations on the Country Coordination Committee to Combat HIV/AIDS, Tuberculosis and Malaria [No. 617, 06 October 2011]. www.cbd.minjust.gov.kg/95360/edition/400147/ru, 22.02.2024.

Kyrgyz Republic Ministry of Justice (2017): Regulations on Psychosocial Counseling Related to HIV, approved by the Government's Resolution [No. 683, 20 October 2017]. www.cbd.minjust.gov.kg/act/view/ru-ru/11649, 22.02.2024.

Kyrgyz Republic Ministry of Justice (2017a): Program of the Government of the Kyrgyz Republic to overcome HIV infection in the Kyrgyz Republic for 2017-2021 [No. 852, 30 December 2017]. www.cbd.minjust.gov.kg/11589/edition/1146000/ru, 22.02.2024.

Mamadzhanov, Alisher (2020): Current trend in the spread of HIV infection in the Osh region. In: Mamaev, T./Mamaeva, T./Durusbekov, A./Abdykarova, A./Mamadzhanov, A. (eds.): Bulletin Osh State University. Osh: State University, pp. 104–111.

Mamadzhanov, Alisher (2021): Epidemiological features of HIV infection and measures for its prevention in a region with a high prevalence of the population [Dissertation] [unpublished].

Martínez-Pérez, Guillermo Z./Nikitin, Danil S./Bessonova, Alla/Fajardo, Emmanuel/Bessonov, Sergei/Shilton, Sonjelle (2021): Values and preferences for hepatitis C self-testing among people who inject drugs in Kyrgyzstan. In: BMC Infectious Diseases 21, No. 609. DOI: 10.1186/s12879-021-06332-z.

Ministry of Health Department of Disease Prevention and State Sanitary (2022): Epidemiological situation of viral hepatitis in the Kyrgyz Republic. www.dgsen.kg/deyatelnost/upravlenie-profilaktiki-infekcionnY/jepidemiologicheskaja-situacija-virusnogo-gepatita-v-kyrgyzskoj-respublike.html, 21.02.2024.

Ministry of Health of the Kyrgyz Republic (2012): Kyrgyzstan Country Report on Progress in Implementing the Global Response to HIV Infection 2012. www.ghdx.healthdata.org/record/kyrgyzstan-country-report-progress-implementing-global-response-hiv-infection-2012, 22.02.2024.

Ministry of Health of the Kyrgyz Republic (2014): Collection of standard operating procedures for laboratory diagnosis of HIV infection [No. 637, 26 November 2014]. Bishkek: Ministry of Health of the Kyrgyz Republic.

Miroshnik, Marina (2015): Patients with hepatitis C at the stage of cirrhosis will be able to be cured in Kyrgyzstan. www.kaktus.media/doc/330194_bolnye_gepatitom_s_na_stadii_cirroza_smogyt_izlechitsia_i_v_kyrgyzstane.html, 25.02.2024.

Regional Expert Group on Migrant Health (2023): Assessment of the current Situation: Kyrgyzstan. Secondary Data Analysis. www.ecuo.org/wp-content/uploads/2016/12/Otsenka-situatsii-analiz-vtorichnyh-dannyh-13-MB.pdf, 22.02.2024.

Republican AIDS Center/Centers for Disease Control and Prevention (CDC)/Pepfar (2021): Bio-behavioral HIV survey and population estimate among men who have sex with men and people who inject drugs in the Kyrgyz Republic. BBS MSM AND PWID IN KG. www.aidscenter.kg/wp-content/uploads/2022/07/BBS-MSM-2021-OnePager-2-1.pdf, 21.02.2024.

Republican Center for Control of Bloodborne Viral Hepatitis and Human Immunodeficiency Virus (2023b): HIV prevalence by regions of Kyrgyzstan, 2023. www.aidscenter.kg/?lang=ru, 25.02.2024.

Republican Center for Control of Bloodborne Viral Hepatitis and Human Immunodeficiency Virus (2022): HIV prevalence by regions of Kyrgyzstan. www.aidscenter.kg/?lang=ru, 22.02.2024.

Republican Center for Health Promotion and Mass Communication (2023): A vaccination campaign against hepatitis B is starting in the Kyrgyz Republic. www.saksalamat.kg/v-kr-startuet-kampaniya-po-vakcinacii-protiv-gepatita-v/, 25.02.2024.

Smith, Laramie R./Shumskaia, Natalia/Kurmanalieva, Ainura/Patterson, Thomas L./Werb, Dan/Blyum, Anna/Algarin, Angel B. et al. (2022): Cohort profile: the Kyrgyzstan InterSectional Stigma (KISS) injection drug use cohort study. In: Harm Reduction Journal 19, No. 53. DOI: 10.1186/s12954-022-00633-5.

Sputnik Radio Kyrgyzstan (2023): Treatment for hepatitis B will now be free of charge in Kyrgyzstan – doctor. www.ru.sputnik.kg/20230321/gepatit-b-gepatit-c-lechenie-analizy-kyrgyzstan-1073721326.html, 25.02.2024.

Stöver, Heino/Shadymanova, Jarkyn (2022): Syringe Exchange Points in the Penitentiary System of Kyrgyzstan. In: Pape, Ulla/Stöver, Heino/Michels, Ingo Ilja (eds.): Social Work and Health in Prisons. Studies from Central Asia and China. 7th ed., Baden-Baden: Nomos, pp. 235–256.

Sultanalieva, M.U./Aidarov, Z.A./Makhmanurov, A.A./Mamatov, S.M. (2018): HIV / AIDS, as a global problem in Kyrgyzstan. In: Bulletin of KSMA named after I.K. Akhunbaev, No. 5–6, pp. 19–24.

The Joint United Nations Programme on HIV/AIDS (UNAIDS) (2012): Country Progress Report on the Global HIV Response [Kyrgyz Republic]. Reporting period: January 2010 – December 2011. Date of submission: March 31, 2012. www.unaids.org/sites/default/files/country/documents/ce_KG_Narrative_Report_0.pdf, 22.02.2024.

The Joint United Nations Programme on HIV/AIDS (UNAIDS) (2020): Country Progress Report – Kyrgyzstan. Global monitoring of the AIDS epidemic. www.unaids.org/sites/default/files/country/documents/KGZ_2020_countryreport.pdf, 22.02.2024.

Tobokalova, Saparbu T./Zairova, Gulzada M./Bekenova, D.S./Nogoibaeva, Kalys A. (2016): Problems of liver cirrhosis in the origin of chronic viral hepatitis in Kyrgyzstan. In: Bulletin of the Kyrgyz-Russian Slavic University 16, No. 3, pp. 134–137.

World Health Organization (WHO) (2017): Action plan for the health sector response to viral hepatitis in the WHO European Region. www.who.int/europe/publications/i/item/9789289052870#:~:text=The%20goal%20of%20the%20Action,comprehensive%20prevention%2C%20recommended%20testing%2C%20care, 22.02.2024.

World Health Organization (WHO) (2023): Hepatitis C. www.who.int/ru/news-room/fact-sheets/detail/hepatitis-c, 22.02.2024.

Zheenalieva, Gulnara (2022): Features of clinical and laboratory characteristics of comorbid chronic hepatitis C [Dissertation]. www.vak.kg/wp-content/uploads/2022/06/Avtoreferat-Zheenalieva-G.M._russ.pdf, 26.02.2024.

5. HIV and Hepatitis C in Uzbekistan

Uladzimir Pikirenia, Azizbek Boltaev

Introduction

HIV and Hepatitis C remain significant public health challenges worldwide, affecting millions of people and requiring sustained attention from the global health community. While progress has been made in understanding and managing these diseases, specific regions, including Central Asia and, notably, Uzbekistan, face a number of challenges in addressing infectious diseases such as HIV and Hepatitis C. The country's distinct socio-economic and cultural landscape makes it a critical case study within the region, offering insights into the broader dynamics of the two epidemics in Central Asia.

Epidemiology of HIV/AIDS in Uzbekistan

The HIV/AIDS epidemic in Uzbekistan has traversed a complex trajectory over the past few decades. Initially, the epidemic was primarily driven by injecting drug use, a pattern common across the region due to its position on major drug trafficking routes from Afghanistan. This mode of transmission facilitated a rapid increase in HIV cases during the late 1990s and early 2000s, mirroring outbreaks in other Central Asian states and Eastern Europe. Notably, Uzbekistan experienced a significant surge in HIV diagnoses between 1999 and 2000, with people who inject drugs (PWID) and their sexual partners being the most affected groups. This period marked the beginning of what would become a persistent public health challenge for the country (Carr et al. 2005; Giyassova 2008).

By 2023, Uzbekistan had reported a total of 52,420 HIV cases, indicating a gradual yet persistent rise in the number of people living with HIV (PLHIV). The demographic breakdown of these cases revealed a slight male predominance, accounting for 55% of the total cases. Despite the number of new HIV cases stabilising at approximately 3,000 per year, certain populations remain at heightened risk. These include men who have sex with men

(MSM), PWID, and sex workers, largely due to stigma, discrimination, and barriers to accessing prevention and care services (Igamberdiev 2023; The Joint United Nations Programme on HIV/AIDS [UNAIDS] 2020).

A concerning trend is the shifting pattern of transmission, from predominantly injection drug use to heterosexual contacts. This shift underscores the changing dynamics of the epidemic, necessitating adjustments in prevention and treatment strategies. Additionally, the HIV prevalence among key populations has shown variable trends: stable among MSM, fluctuating among sex workers, and declining among PWID. Such patterns highlight the need for targeted interventions and the importance of understanding the specific risk factors affecting each group (Igamberdiev 2023).

The genetic diversity of the virus in Uzbekistan further complicates the epidemic's landscape. The presence of multiple HIV-1 subtypes, notably CRF02 AG and A6, suggests varied transmission networks and the impact of regional mobility and migration on the epidemic's dynamics. This genetic diversity indicates the necessity for tailored public health strategies to address the specific challenges posed by different viral strains (Lebedev et al. 2022).

Risk Factors and Transmission of HIV

The HIV epidemic in Uzbekistan is influenced by a confluence of behavioural, sociocultural, and economic factors that heighten the vulnerability of certain populations to HIV infection. Initially, the epidemic was largely driven by the use of contaminated injecting equipment among people who inject drugs, a common risk factor across the Central Asian region due to its proximity to major drug trafficking routes. However, as the epidemic has evolved, sexual transmission has become increasingly predominant, with heterosexual contacts now accounting for the majority of new infections. This shift underscores the changing nature of the epidemic and the importance of adapting prevention strategies accordingly.

Several sociocultural and economic factors play crucial roles in facilitating the spread of HIV in Uzbekistan. Stigmatisation and discrimination against PLHIV and key affected populations, such as MSM, sex workers, and PWID, deter many from seeking testing and treatment services. This is exacerbated by legal frameworks that criminalise behaviours associated with HIV transmission, such as drug use and sex work, further marginalising these populations and limiting their access to healthcare services.

Economic inequality, poverty of a large proportion of the population, and labour migration also contribute significantly to the HIV epidemic in Uzbekistan. Many Uzbek migrants, particularly those working in Russia and Kazakhstan, engage in high-risk behaviours such as unprotected sex with multiple partners and drug use, in contexts where they have limited access to HIV prevention and care services. Upon returning to Uzbekistan, these migrants can potentially introduce new HIV infections to their regular partners, fuelling the epidemic's spread within the general population.

People who inject drugs are at a heightened risk of HIV infection due to the sharing of contaminated injecting equipment. The historical and geographic context of Uzbekistan, lying on the 'northern route' of drug trafficking from Afghanistan to Russia and Europe, has contributed to a significant drug-using population. While there has been a decline in HIV prevalence among PWID, they remain a key population due to the enduring risks associated with injection drug use.

MSM in Uzbekistan face significant societal stigma and legal sanctions, which discourage them from accessing HIV testing, prevention, and treatment services. The criminalisation of same-sex relations in Uzbekistan exacerbates the vulnerability of MSM to HIV infection by pushing their behaviours underground and away from the reach of effective intervention (Cheburashka 2024).

Sex workers in Uzbekistan operate in an environment of legal and social vulnerability. The criminalisation of sex work and the absence of legal protection for sex workers contribute to their increased risk of HIV. These individuals often face barriers to accessing healthcare services, including HIV prevention and treatment, due to stigma, discrimination, and fear of legal repercussions.

Labour migrants constitute a particularly vulnerable group in the context of the HIV epidemic in Uzbekistan, influenced by a constellation of factors that increase their risk of HIV exposure and transmission. This vulnerabil ity is underpinned by the socio-economic dynamics of migration, limited access to health services, and the often marginalised legal and social status of migrants in host countries.

Women and young people are particularly vulnerable to HIV infection due to a combination of biological, socio-economic, and religious factors. Gender-based inequality, including limited decision-making power in sexual relationships and economic dependency on men, increases women's vulnerability to HIV. Young people, including adolescents, are at risk due to a lack of comprehensive sexual education and access to preventive services, which leaves them ill-equipped to navigate safe sexual practices.

Children are also vulnerable to HIV transmission. The sporadic information on children living with HIV in Uzbekistan suggests a growing concern, with reported cases rising from 2,500 in 2012 to 8,100 in 2021, indicating an urgent need for targeted interventions to support these children and their families (KUN.UZ 2022; O'zbekiston Milliy axborot agentligining [UzA] 2022; Institute for War & Peace Reporting [IWPR] 2012).

In conclusion, the HIV epidemic in Uzbekistan is shaped by a complex interplay of risk factors that include not only individual behaviours but also broader socio-cultural and economic dynamics. These factors contribute to the heightened vulnerability of specific populations to HIV infection. Addressing these risk factors requires a multifaceted approach that goes beyond health interventions to include social, legal, and economic reforms. Efforts must focus on reducing stigma and discrimination, reforming policies that criminalise key populations, enhancing economic opportunities, and providing targeted HIV prevention and care services. In addition, low levels of education, lack of sexual education, and the high prevalence of Muslims pose challenges for vulnerable groups (Sankar 2021).

Government and Public Health Response to HIV/AIDS

Uzbekistan's approach to combating HIV/AIDS is anchored in a series of national policies and strategic plans that prioritise prevention, testing, treatment, and care. Key among these efforts is the implementation of the Presidential Decree No. 14 'On measures to further strengthen systems for counteracting the disease caused by the human immunodeficiency virus', which underscores the government's commitment to addressing the epidemic through comprehensive and coordinated actions. Central to this strategy is the expansion of HIV testing and counselling services, enhancing the accessibility and quality of antiretroviral treatment (ART), and addressing the legal and social barriers that hinder effective HIV/AIDS prevention and care (Igamberdiev 2023).

A significant component of Uzbekistan's public health response to HIV/AIDS involves scaling up testing and treatment services. The country has made strides in increasing the availability of HIV testing, as evidenced by the expansion of testing coverage from 2,564,400 tests in 2013 to 4,137,000 in 2022. This increase in testing is crucial for early detection and linkage to care, enabling individuals to access treatment sooner and improve their health outcomes while reducing the risk of onward transmission (Igamberdiev 2023).

The treatment landscape in Uzbekistan has also evolved, with efforts to align with international standards and improve treatment outcomes for PLHIV. The adoption of the World Health Organization's (WHO) ART guidelines and the expansion of treatment coverage represent significant steps forward. However, challenges remain in achieving the desired treatment targets and ensuring that a high percentage of those on treatment achieve viral suppression, a critical factor in managing the epidemic and preventing HIV transmission.

Despite these efforts, public health initiatives in Uzbekistan face challenges related to the criminalisation of behaviours associated with HIV risk, such as drug use, sex work, and being MSM. These legal barriers can deter individuals from accessing testing and treatment services due to fear of legal repercussions, underscoring the need for policy reforms that support rather than hinder HIV prevention and care efforts.

International collaboration and the involvement of non-governmental organisations (NGOs) are pivotal components of Uzbekistan's response to HIV/AIDS. Partnerships with international bodies, including the Global Fund to Fight AIDS, Tuberculosis and Malaria (GFATM) and the Joint United Nations Programme on HIV/AIDS (UNAIDS), have been instrumental in providing the financial and technical support needed to enhance the country's HIV/AIDS programmes. These collaborations have facilitated improvements in the national HIV/AIDS response, from strengthening health systems to implementing evidence-based interventions targeting key populations.

There are four NGOs working with key populations and PLHIV: 'ISHONCH VA HAYOT' (since 2003), 'ISTIQBOLLI AVLOD' (since 2001), the Republican Information and Educational Center 'INTILISH' (since 2001), and the Anti-Cancer Society of Uzbekistan. However, there is no data on how many clients they serve per year or any other statistical information.

Treatment and Healthcare Challenges

HIV testing is a cornerstone of effective HIV management, enabling individuals to know their status and access timely treatment. In Uzbekistan, there is a network of 63 inter-district HIV laboratories and 15 regional AIDS centres. The requirement in the national HIV testing algorithm for confirmation through a series of tests, including a final confirmatory Western blot test, can delay diagnosis and increase costs, which may deter individuals from seeking testing (Ministry of Health of the Republic of Uzbekistan 2023). A household survey highlighted that less than half of women had been offered and undergone HIV tests during pregnancy, indicating gaps in the implementation of testing protocols (Uchaev et al. 2021).

In 2022, the ART was provided to approximately 45,000 patients in Uzbekistan. There are significant gaps in achieving the '90-90-90' targets set by UNAIDS: in 2020, the HIV care cascade in Uzbekistan was '83-67-59', demonstrating a major gap in reaching the declared targets with ART coverage at the level of 55% of PLHIV estimate. The government's efforts to increase public funds for HIV treatment have led to improvements in coverage, but challenges remain in ensuring that all PLHIV can access and adhere to ART (Normuratova 2022).

Most patients are transiting to dolutegravir-based regimens; currently there are 13 treatment regimens used. Uzbekistan's AIDS service is moving away from nevirapine and instead buying more FDC. The AIDS service has adopted the 2019 WHO ART treatment protocol. All pregnant women on ART are on B+ (GFATM data).

Hepatitis C in Uzbekistan

Hepatitis B and C infections are highly prevalent in Uzbekistan and are a priority of the Ministry of Health's agenda. In 2016, an estimated 2.5 million people were living with hepatitis B and 1.3 million with hepatitis C in the country (WHO 2022). Despite the scale of this public health issue, data on the spread of the hepatitis C virus (HCV) in Uzbekistan is difficult to obtain. Epidemiological data is usually published through the National Information and Analytical Center for Drug Control under the Cabinet of Ministers of the Republic of Uzbekistan. In addition, the Central Asia Drug Action Programme (CADAP) collected data on the spread of HCV in Uzbekistan.

The data on HCV prevalence among PWID in Uzbekistan varies widely. The last CADAP Country Report from the year 2018 mentioned that HCV infections had been decreasing continuously between 2005 and 2017: From

53,7% in 2005, to 36,5% in 2007, to 28,5% in 2009, to 20,9% in 2011, to 21,8% in 2013, to 15,7% in 2015 and to 12% in 2017 (Central Asia Drug Action Programme [CADAP] 2018, p. 10).

The article "The epidemiology of hepatitis C virus in Central Asia: Systematic review, meta-analyses, and meta-regression analyses" by Botheju et al. (2019), however, states that HCV prevalence is much higher. The authors argue that HCV prevalence in the general population ranged from 6.4% to 13.1%, and was 51.7% among PWID. It is therefore difficult to obtain a reliable picture of the spread of hepatitis C among the drug-using population in Uzbekistan.

Data on available treatment for HCV in Uzbekistan is also limited. In 2022, the WHO announced that the Uzbekistan government has scaled up viral hepatitis response to the national level, and passed a presidential decree offering free or subsidized treatment to all those infected with chronic hepatitis C (WHO 2022). In 2021, the government has introduced free testing in seven regions of the country. Between 2022 and 2025, an expected 2 million people in the country were screened for viral hepatitis B and C. Despite political efforts to control HCV, Uzbekistan remains a country with a very high HCV prevalence.

Discussion and Conclusion

The fight against HIV/AIDS and Hepatitis C in Uzbekistan, while marked by significant efforts and some progress, presents a complex landscape of successes and ongoing challenges. The analysis of current approaches, remaining obstacles, and potential strategies for improving outcomes highlights the multifaceted nature of the epidemic and the need for comprehensive, integrated strategies to address it effectively.

Despite the progress made, significant challenges remain in the fight against HIV/AIDS in Uzbekistan. Stigma and discrimination continue to hinder access to and uptake of HIV testing and treatment services, particularly among key populations. The criminalisation of behaviours associated with HIV transmission, such as drug use, sex work, and MSM, exacerbates this issue, creating barriers to effective prevention and care.

Improving outcomes in the response to HIV and Hepatitis C in Uzbekistan requires a multipronged strategy that addresses both the direct impacts of the two epidemics and the underlying factors that contribute to vulnerability and transmission. Key strategies can include:

- *Enhancing prevention efforts:* Expanding access to comprehensive sexual education and prevention tools, such as condoms and pre-exposure prophylaxis, particularly among key populations and young people. Tailoring prevention efforts to address the needs of labour migrants and leveraging digital platforms for education and outreach can also enhance impact. The promotion of harm reduction programmes is needed.
- *Improving access to testing and treatment:* Simplifying the HIV testing process and expanding the availability of rapid and self-testing options can facilitate early diagnosis.
- *Addressing legal and social barriers:* Reforming laws that criminalise behaviours associated with HIV risk and implementing policies that protect the rights and dignity of people living with HIV are critical for reducing structural discrimination. Good education, including sexual education and family-planning skills, is needed. It is crucial to work with religious leaders to combat family discrimination against women and increase their autonomy and independence. Engaging communities and building capacity among healthcare providers to offer non-discriminatory, supportive services can further enhance access to care.
- *Improving data transparency and accessibility:* Uzbekistan currently critically lacks good data and research on key aspects related to the HIV epidemic. A plan for community-led, international, and expert-led research needs to be developed and implemented. Data collected by the government of Uzbekistan should meet standards that allow for more in-depth study of the problem: openness, accountability, relevance, and disaggregability.

Bibliography

Botheju, Welathanthrige S.P./Zghyer, Fawzi/Mahmud, Sarwat/Terlikbayeva, Assel/El-Bassel, Nabila/Abu-Raddad, Laith J. (2019): The epidemiology of hepatitis C virus in Central Asia: Systematic review, meta-analyses, and meta-regression analyses. In: Scientific Reports 9, No. 2090, pp. 1–15.

Carr, Jean K./Nadai, Yuka/Eyzaguirre, Lindsay/Saad, Magdi D./Khakimov, Mumtaz M./Yakubov, Shavkat K./Birx, Deborah L. et al. (2005): Outbreak of a West African recombinant of HIV-1 in Tashkent, Uzbekistan. In: Journal of Acquired Immune Deficiency Syndromes 39, No. 5, pp. 570–575.

Central Asia Drug Action Programme (CADAP) (2018): 2018 Country Overview of drug situation Uzbekistan. www.eu-cadap.org/wp-content/uploads/2023/01/CSS-Uzbekistan-2018_online_final.pdf, 28.02.2024.

Cheburashka, Gena (2024): Politicking of Islam and LGBTQ+ discourse in Uzbekistan. In: Central Asian Survey 43, No. 1, pp. 151–157. DOI: 10.1080/02634937.2023.2280095.

Giyassova, G.M. (2008): National program for HIV prevention in Republic of Uzbekistan, 2007–2011. International Conference on the HIV Epidemic in Central Asia and Neighbouring Countries, Bishkek, Kyrgyzstan, 11–13 March 2008.

Igamberdiev, B.N. (2023): Data presented at a Round table: Cooperation within the framework of the implementation of Presidential Decree No. 14 "On measures to further strengthen systems for counteracting the disease caused by the human immunodeficiency virus". Tashkent, Uzbekistan, 09 June 2023.

Institute for War & Peace Reporting (IWPR) (2012): Uzbekistan: No Place for Children With HIV. www.iwpr.net/global-voices/uzbekistan-no-place-children-hiv, 28.02.2024.

KUN.UZ (2022): Number of HIV-infected citizens in Uzbekistan announced. www.kun.uz/en/news/2022/02/02/number-of-hiv-infected-citizens-in-uzbekistan-announced, 28.02.2024.

Lebedev, Aleksey/Kuznetsova, Anna/Kim, Kristina/Ozhmegova, Ekaterina/Antonova, Anastasiia/Kazennova, Elena/Tumanov, Aleksandr et al. (2022): Identifying HIV-1 Transmission Clusters in Uzbekistan through Analysis of Molecular Surveillance Data. In: Viruses 14, No. 8, p. 1675.

Ministry of Health of the Republic of Uzbekistan (2023): Узбекистон Республикасида ОИВ инфекциясини олдини олиш чора-тадбирлари ва тиббий ёрдамни ташкил этишни янада такомнллаштнриш тугрисида, ССВ буйруғм №111, 19.05.2023.

Normuratova, Gulifar (2022): Specialist: 74% of people receiving HIV treatment in our country have several times their viral load reduced [Telegram]. www.t.me/ssvuz/11540, 18.02.2024.

O'zbekiston Milliy axborot agentligining (UzA) (2022): The number of people infected with AIDS in Uzbekistan and some information about this disease have been revealed [Telegram]. www.t.me/uzauz/886, 28.02.2024.

Sankar, Deepa (2021): Uzbekistan Education Sector Analysis: 2021. www.uzbekistan.un.org/sites/default/files/2022-05/Edu%20Sit%20An_UNICEF%202022_0.pdf, 28.02.2024.

The Joint United Nations Programme on HIV/AIDS (UNAIDS) (2020): Country Progress Report – Uzbekistan. Global monitoring of the AIDS epidemic 2020. www.unaids.org/sites/default/files/country/documents/UZB_2020_countryreport.pdf, 18.02.2024.

Uchaev, Sergey/Abdullayeva, Oksana/Abdullaev, Shukhrat (2021): Assessment of access to medical services, care and health support for labour migrants living with HIV: Republic of Uzbekistan. www.migrationhealth.group/wp-content/uploads/2021/12/STUDY_Uzbekistan_RUS_FINAL.pdf, 18.02.2024.

World Health Organization (WHO) (2022): Scaling up hepatitis response in Uzbekistan. www.who.int/europe/news/item/28-07-2022-scaling-up-hepatitis-response-in-uzbekistan, 18.02.2024.

6. HIV and Hepatitis C in Tajikistan

Safarkhon Sattorov, Alijon Soliev, Umed Talbov, Sona Orbelyan, Mykyta Trofymenko

Introduction

In 2016, Tajikistan adopted the National Development Strategy for the period until 2030 (NDS–2030), which reiterates Tajikistan's commitment to the sustainable development goals (SDG) and sets out the priorities for the country's development in the coming years. To specify the targets set in NDS–2030 for the healthcare sector and the implementation of SDG No. 3, dedicated to good health and well-being, on 30th September 2021, the government of Tajikistan introduced a new National Health Strategy for the period until 2030. This article explores the HIV (Human immunodeficiency virus) and HCV (Hepatitis C Virus) response in Tajikistan as a part of the country's efforts towards implementing the SDGs. Based on the data from the national HIV Surveillance System, scientific publications, and reports from international organisations, the authors have analysed the current situation, progress, and challenges in Tajikistan's endeavors to control the spread of both HIV and HCV.

The Epidemiology of HIV in Tajikistan

According to the recent Joint United Nations Programme on HIV/AIDS (UNAIDS) estimates, there are around 15,000 people living with HIV (PLWH) in Tajikistan (UNAIDS 2022, p. 354). According to the data of the Republican AIDS Center in Tajikistan, 16,129 people were diagnosed with HIV and 4,433 of them died due to various causes from 1st of January 1991 to 1st January 2024. As of the beginning of 2024, there were 11,696 PLWH registered in the country, with 10,456 people receiving antiretroviral treatment (ART) (88.6% of whom achieved viral load suppression). In recent years, Tajikistan has made substantial progress in terms of ART coverage, improved viral load suppression, and reduction in AIDS mortality. In 2017, there were 4,948 people covered by ART, and 59% of PLWH had their viral load suppressed. After the peak of 1,421 new HIV cases registered in 2018, the annual number of new registered HIV cases reduced to 1,100 in 2023. In 2023, there were 64 AIDS-related deaths in the country, which is an almost twofold decrease in comparison with 2019 (National HIV Surveillance System/Republican AIDS Center 2024).

Tajikistan has a concentrated HIV epidemic, with 0.2% prevalence among adults (aged 15–49 years) and 0.1% prevalence among the general population. The burden of HIV is significantly higher among key populations – people who inject drugs (PWID), female sex workers (FSWs), men who have sex with men (MSM), and prisoners. Integrated biobehavioural surveys (IBBSs) are regularly conducted in Tajikistan to measure the size of key populations and behavioural trends within these groups, as well as the HIV, HCV, and syphilis prevalence. The latest IBBS among FSWs, PWID, and MSM was conducted in 2022. According to the survey, there are an estimated 18,200 PWID in Tajikistan, with an HIV prevalence of 8.9%. Among all IBBS sites, the highest HIV prevalence was observed in the capital city Dushanbe (19.9%) and the lowest in Khorog (4.7%), the main city in the remote region of Gorno-Badakhshan Autonomous Oblast (GBAO). The countrywide HIV prevalence among FSW was estimated at 2.9%, with the highest prevalence found in the city of Bokhtar (3.9%) and lowest in Kulyab (1.5%), both located in the Khatlon Region in south-western Tajikistan. The survey estimated the total number of FSWs in the country to be 18,500. Finally, according to the 2022 IBBS, there are around 12,000 MSM in the country, with an HIV prevalence of 4.3%. There were no major changes in HIV prevalence among FSWs and MSM in comparison to earlier IBBSs, but the percentage of PLWH among PWID had reduced significantly – from 23.5% in 2006 to 8.9% in 2022 (National HIV Surveillance System/Republican AIDS Center 2024). This data confirms the assumption that the predominant mode of HIV transmission has shifted from injecting drugs to in unsafe sexual practices over the past years.

In 2023, an IBBS was conducted among people in prison with a sample size of 800 people from the total prison population of 10,000. A 3.4% prevalence of HIV and 2.8% prevalence of syphilis was observed (Sattorov et al. 2023). Due to the high numbers of labour migrants in Tajikistan (mostly returning home from the Russian Federation), IBBS and operational research into HIV/tuberculosis (TB) among migrants has been planned for 2024 to collect more data about the HIV prevalence and behavioural patterns of this population group. The previous IBBS among migrants was conducted in 2020 and estimated the prevalence to be 0.4%, which is higher than among the general population but significantly lower than among PWID, FSWs, MSM, and prisoners.

HIV Policy in Tajikistan

On 27th February 2021, the government of Tajikistan adopted the National AIDS Program for 2021–2025 to set the framework for the country's AIDS response for the next five years and align it with the newly adopted National Health Strategy for the period up to 2030. The National AIDS Program reiterates the country's commitment to the SDG 3.3 target of ending the AIDS epidemic by 2030 and the goals of the UN General Assembly Political Declaration on HIV and AIDS: On the Fast Track to Accelerate the Fight Against HIV and to End the AIDS Epidemic by 2030.

The National AIDS Program outlines six strategic directions for the AIDS response:

1. preventing new HIV cases among key and vulnerable groups;
2. ensuring universal access to HIV treatment for both adults and children;
3. reducing mother-to-child transmission incidence and setting the conditions for the elimination of vertical transmission;
4. assuring blood safety and advancing infection control in healthcare institutions;
5. building awareness about and preventing HIV among young people, adolescents, young women, and girls;
6. overcoming existing barriers and strengthening the supportive environment for an effective national response to the HIV epidemic.

The basis for HIV testing and treatment in the country is the national HIV clinical protocol, which was recently reviewed, with the new version being approved by the Ministry of Health and Social Protection of the Population on 2nd June 2023. The protocol serves as guidelines for establishing HIV diagnosis, index testing, the selection of treatment options, the monitoring of treatment outcomes, strengthening patient adherence to HIV treatment, pre-exposure prophylaxis, and post-exposure prophylaxis, as well as prevention, screening, and follow-up of the most common coinfections and comorbidities. The 2023 revisions were intended to align the protocol with international standards, in particular the 2021 World Health Organization HIV Guidelines. Some of the key points included in the new protocol are as follows:

- recognition of the fact that PLWH with undetectable viral load cannot transmit HIV through any type of sexual contact, regardless of condom use (Undetectable Equals Untransmittable). This provision of the protocol was subsequently used to advocate for the decriminalisation of HIV risk exposure in Tajikistan, which resulted in the adoption of the Supreme Court Resolution of 26th December 2023, which stated that PLWH with undetectable viral load do not pose a threat of HIV transmission to their sexual partners,
- removal of limitations as regards prescribing *dolutegravir* for pregnant women and women who are trying to conceive, given the lack of evidence that using it increases the likelihood of neural tube defects in infants,
- screening of PLWH with a CD4 cell count lower than 100 cells/mm^3 and corresponding clinical symptoms for cryptococcus infection (Amirzoda et al. 2023).

As of 1st January 2024, there were 67 AIDS centres across the country at the republican (1), city (9), regional (4), and district (53) levels. Under the auspices of the AIDS centres, 24 trust points for PWID and eleven friendly sites for FSWs have been set up to provide confidential HIV prevention and testing services. An additional three trust points operate in the penitentiary system to deliver HIV prevention services to people in prisons. In 2019, following the implementation of a pilot scheme in Dushanbe, the decentralisation of HIV services has started with the provision of care for PLWH to the primary care level – multi-specially polyclinics that provide outpatient care through general physicians and various specialists, such as gynaecologists, paediatricians, cardiologists, neurologists, etc. (Lundgren et al. 2022, p. 30).

There is a network of 15 opioid substitution therapy (OST) sites covering all regions of the country, including two sites in the penitentiary system. Currently, the only OST medicine used in Tajikistan is methadone, available only in liquid form. In addition to providing opioid dependency treatment, OST sites in Tajikistan encompass additional services for PWID, such as overdose treatment, testing for HBV, HCV, and syphilis, psychological support, etc. Despite the fact that the OST system is well-established and has been operating in the country since 2010, it is still considered a pilot programme and coverage remains low (around 650 people). To explore the reasons for the underutilisation of OST sites operating in the country, a study on drug use and barriers to OST in Tajikistan was conducted between February and April 2023. Sixteen focus groups, consisting in total of 65 PWID who were receiving (30) and not receiving (35) OST, were held in eight cities across Tajikistan. The study found three main obstacles to OST access: insufficient appeal of the OST programme, e.g. the requirement to visit OST sites every day; insufficient staff capacity at the OST sites; and misleading information circulating among PWID regarding OST (Kaspirova/Malikov 2023). It should be noted that in 2023, the main institution coordinating OST programmes in Tajikistan, the Republican Clinical Narcology Center, adopted the OST Expansion Plan for the years 2024–2026, with an ambitious goal of increasing programme coverage to 2,000 people by the end of 2026. In order to achieve this goal, it is crucial to tackle the aforementioned issues.

NGOs Working in the Field of HIV in Tajikistan

Civil society and community-based organisations play a crucial role in the HIV response in Tajikistan through outreach work with key populations. There are several countrywide and regional organisations that cover almost all of the territory of Tajikistan, except for the remote mountainous GBAO region. NGOs provide a wide range of services focusing on key populations, in particular delivering harm reduction services to the hard-to-reach populations, carrying out and referring clients to HIV testing, linking clients to pre-exposure prophylaxis (PReP), raising awareness about HIV, documenting human rights violations, and providing legal support to PLWH and key populations, as well as providing medical and psychological support to clients. As of 1st January 2024 there were eight trust points for PWID, four friendly sites for FSWs, four friendly sites for MSM, and two 24/7 telephone hotlines in operation, providing confidential HIV prevention, counselling, and testing services to key populations under the auspices of NGOs. NGOs play an instrumental role in delivering prevention services to key populations, and in 2022 they provided services to 7,036 MSM (59% of the estimated population). In 2022 NGOs in collaboration with AIDS centres rendered HIV prevention services (United Nations Development Programme [UNDP] Tajikistan 2023) to 14,644 PWID (80% of the estimated population) and 12,087 FSWs (65% of the estimated population).

The Epidemiology of HCV in Tajikistan

There is not much data available on the prevalence of viral hepatitis among the general population of Tajikistan. However, the data on HCV prevalence among key populations is updated regularly, given that PWID, FSWs, MSM, and people in prison are tested for HCV during IBBSs. According to the 2022 IBBS carried out with prisoners, the prevalence of HCV among this group is 8.9%. The 2022 IBBS with PWID, FSWs, and MSM estimated the prevalence both in the country in general and at the main IBBS sites. According to the survey, the HCV prevalence among PWID in Tajikistan is 21%, with the highest rates found in the cities of Penjikent and Kulob (both 24.3%), followed by Dushanbe (19.4%), Khorog (11.1%), Vakhdat (10.4%), and Khujand (8.9%). This is a notable decrease in comparison with the 45% HCV prevalence reported in the 2006 IBBS and may be seen as evidence of a decrease in the role of injection drug use among the drivers of the HCV epidemic. The survey of FSWs estimated the prevalence at 0.9%, with the following rates at the IBBS sites – Bokhtar (2.1%), Dushanbe (1.9%), Khujand (0.9%), and Kulyab (0.8%). The highest prevalence of HCV among MSM was observed in Bokhtar (5.8%), followed by Khujand (2.7%) and Dushanbe (1.7%), with a countrywide rate of 4.3% (National HIV Surveillance System/Republican AIDS Center 2024).

Considering the progress achieved in the past decades in terms of HIV treatment and the increase in PLWH life expectancy, HCV is becoming a bigger threat for PLWH than in the past. According to the Republican AIDS Center data, HCV is the second largest cause of mortality among PLWH (9.6%), surpassed only by tuberculosis (22.2%). It should be noted that the cause of 23.8% of PLWH deaths remains unknown (National HIV Surveillance System/Republican AIDS Center 2024), which may indicate that the actual percentage of deaths that can be attributed to HCV is higher.

HCV Policy in Tajikistan

The system for responding to HCV in Tajikistan is less robust than is the case for HIV, given that in the low resource settings, HIV and TB are considered higher priorities by both state and international donors. While the National Health Strategy for the period up to 2030 and the National AIDS Program for the period of 2021–2025 acknowledge the need to respond to viral hepatitis, there is still no strategic national plan for HCV.

At a regional level, sanitary-epidemiological service departments are conducting epidemiological surveillance, and each case is assigned with its own epidemiological number. The Scientific and Research Institute for Gastroenterology is the main clinical institution for viral hepatitis in the country where the treatment of chronic cases is carried out. People who experience acute HCV symptoms are treated in the infectious disease hospitals located throughout the country. The testing and treatment of HCV is usually self-funded, including for key populations. The only exceptions that exist cover just a few categories of people, such as blood donors and clients of OST programmes. If their HCV antibody test is positive, the patient still needs to pay for a Polymerase chain reaction (PCR) test. The need for out-of-pocket expenses is the key factor that hinders access to the efficient testing and treatment of HCV in Tajikistan. To explore the possible ways to advance HCV response in the country, the Ministry of Health and Social Protection of the Population requested that the WHO Regional Office for Europe conducts the first hepatitis assessment in Tajikistan. The WHO mission visited Tajikistan in January 2023 and plans to publish the final report in early 2024. It is expected that the recommendations of the WHO will serve as the basis for the creation of a strategic national plan for viral hepatitis in Tajikistan.

The impact of potential HCV interventions in Tajikistan may be illustrated by the 2021 pilot programme on providing HCV testing and treatment to PLHIV. At the request of the Republican AIDS Center, the United Nations Development Program (UNDP) reprogrammed savings from the Global Fund to Fight AIDS, Tuberculosis and Malaria grant for the procurement of tests and HCV medication. All PLHIV with HCV were tested to confirm their diagnosis and subsequently 851 people started treatment with direct-acting antivirals. For various reasons, 27 people interrupted treatment and 824 PLHIV completed the full course of treatment. 779 of those 824 people (94.5%) achieved complete viral suppression. In addition, 140 PWID were tested and treated for HCV with a similarly high success rate of around 95% viral load suppression among those who completed the full course of treatment and reported their results to the Republican AIDS Center (National HIV Surveillance System/Republican AIDS Center 2024).

NGOs Working in the Field of HCV in Tajikistan

Civil society organisations in Tajikistan implement just a few HCV-specific activities as most of the donor funding is focused on the HIV and TB response. However, most of their interventions regarding HIV prevention among key populations play a significant role in HCV control too, since the two infections share the same risk factors and modes of transmission. Additionally, Tajik NGOs usually have medical experts among their staff who can refer clients for HCV testing. During the aforementioned HCV treatment pilot programme, NGOs played an important role in linking their PWID clients to HCV treatment provided by the Republican AIDS Center. Therefore, despite the lack of funding for HCV interventions, Tajikistan NGOs have a solid capacity for effective HCV work, given their vast experience in outreach work with the hard-to-reach populations.

Conclusions

Over the past 20 years, Tajikistan has made significant progress in its response to the HIV epidemic. The number of people covered by HIV prevention, testing, and treatment services has increased significantly, which led to a decrease in AIDS mortality. Viral load suppression rates reached almost 90% among people on ART treatment, which is evidence of positive treatment outcomes.

However, certain challenges persist and need to be tackled in order for the national HIV programme to achieve further success. The critical activities, such as HIV prevention, the testing of key populations, and the procurement of antiretroviral (ARV) medicines, laboratory consumables, etc. are almost fully supported by donors and development partners. Therefore, it is instrumental to adopt and implement a realistic transition plan, envisaging a gradual increase of the state share in the HIV response and the development of sustainable financing mechanisms, such as social contracting, to support the shift from external to domestic funding. This will ensure the uninterrupted provision of quality HIV services in the event that donor support is reduced.

Next, there is an untapped potential to further increase HIV prevention and testing coverage. Currently, only about 3.5% of PWID are receiving OST, around 78% of PLWH know their HIV status, and the coverage of PWID, FSWs, and MSM with HIV prevention services (80%, 65%, and

59% respectively) remains at a suboptimal level. The following interventions an be recommended to increase prevention and testing coverage:

- ensuring an enabling environment for HIV services by reducing stigma and discrimination against PLWH and key populations, raising public awareness about HIV, sensitising medical and law enforcement professionals to the needs of PLWH and key populations, and amending legislation related to the labour, social, and other rights of PLWH in order to increase the number of people seeking HIV services,
- adapting OST programme to the needs of PWID by introducing take-home options for stable patients and tableted OST medicines and developing the infrastructure of sites and other measures to improve the appeal of OST programmes,
- raising awareness among PWID and medical professionals about opioid dependency treatment to ensure they are in possession of verified and up-to-date information on OST,
- expanding social and outreach workers' knowledge on the specifics of working with key populations and index testing.

In recent years, Tajikistan has demonstrated its commitment to developing a system for responding to HCV by joining the Coalition for Global Hepatitis Elimination and requesting that the WHO conducts a hepatitis assessment in Tajikistan. The findings of this assessment should provide a blueprint for further work on the first strategic national hepatitis plan. The successful results of the 2021 pilot programme for HCV treatment among PLWH and PWID, as well as the broad experience of Tajik NGOs in working with key populations, may also be used to determine strategies in this field.

Bibliography

Amirzoda, Abdukholik A. et al. (2023): Guidelines for treatment and follow-up of HIV infection (adults and adolescents). Dushanbe: Ministry of Health and Social Protection of the Population.

HIV Surveillance System/Republican AIDS Center (2024): Data as of January 1, 2024. [unpublished document].

Kaspirova, Anna/Malikov, Naimdzhon (2023): Report on situation with the drug use, drug policies and existing programs on combating drug use in the Republic of Tajikistan [unpublished report]. Dushanbe: United Nations Development Programme (UNDP).

Lundgren, Jens D./Borges, Álvaro H./Stengaard, Annemarie R. (2022): Rapid Assessment of ART Implementation Plan in Tajikistan [unpublished report]. Dushanbe: United Nations Development Programme (UNDP).

Sattorov, Safarhon et al. (2023): Analytical report on 2023 HIV integrated biobehavioral survey among prisoners in the Republic of Tajikistan [unpublished report]. Dushanbe: Republican AIDS Center.

The Joint United Nations Programme on HIV/AIDS (UNAIDS) (2022): UNAIDS Data 2022. www.unaids.org/sites/default/files/media_asset/data-book-2022_en.pdf, 01.03.2024.

United Nations Development Programme (UNDP) Tajikistan (2023): UNDP Programmatic data [unpublished report]. Dushanbe: UNDP Tajikistan.

Additional Case Studies and Cross-Cutting Issues

7. Stigma

Hang Su, Yifan Xu, Jiang Du

HIV-related stigma encompasses prejudice, discounting, and discrediting directed at individuals perceived to have HIV/AIDS, as well as towards the individuals, groups, and communities associated with them. This stigma significantly influences people's decisions and behaviours, diminishing their willingness to participate in HIV testing, treatment, and prevention efforts. Over the past three decades, since the onset of the HIV/AIDS epidemic, stigma has consistently posed a formidable obstacle to HIV testing, diagnosis, treatment, and overall care (Yang et al. 2015, p. 1).

Despite the Chinese government's extensive efforts in HIV prevention over the past decades, stigmatisation against people living with HIV/AIDS (PLHIV) persists nationwide.

Li and colleagues (2018, p. 1ff.) utilised the validated Berger HIV Stigma Scale to evaluate HIV-related stigma in Zhenping County, located in Henan province, a region with a significant population of individuals affected by plasma donation-related HIV-infections. The Stigma Scale includes an overall mean score and four subscales: personalized stigma, disclosure concerns, negative self-image, and concern with public attitudes, with scores ranging from 40 to 160. The scores interpretation indicates 0–33% as no or mild stigma, 34–65% as moderate stigma, and values exceeding 66% as severe stigma.

After analysing 239 survey responses from PLHIV, the data revealed that the overall HIV stigma score ranged from 68 to 130 (indicating moderate to severe stigma), with a mean score of 105.92 ± 12.35 (95% CI: 104.34, 107.49; confidence interval [CI] is a statistical concept used to quantify the uncertainty or precision associated with a particular estimate). The scores for the four subscales were as follows: personalised stigma (48.66 ± 6.29), disclosure concerns (26.08 ± 3.48), negative self-image (34.10 ± 3.99), and concern with public attitude (53.47 ± 7.30). The results of the survey showed that participants perceived higher levels of stigma associated with personalised stigma (67.58, 95% CI: 66.47, 68.69) and comparatively lower levels of stigma related to disclosure concerns (65.20, 95% CI: 64.08, 66.30).

The finding that PLHIV in the rural areas of Henan province perceive moderate to high levels of HIV-related stigma is consistent with existing literature from both China and India, which suggest that individuals in rural settings tend to experience more stigma compared to their urban counterparts. Furthermore, the observed level of PLHIV in the rural areas of Henan province is comparatively lower than the stigma reported in a previous study conducted among the men who have sex with men (MSM) population in China. This suggests that rural former plasma donors are generally viewed within the general population with greater sympathy than is the case for those who acquired HIV through other means, such as MSM, people who inject drugs (PWID), and commercial sex workers (CSW) (Li et al. 2016, p. 1398).

Recent research indicates that individuals who contracted HIV through 'blameless' routes (e.g. blood transfusion, sex with stable partners) tend to face less stigma compared to those who acquired HIV through 'blameable' routes (e.g. injection drug use, homosexual behaviour). Consequently, the level of stigma observed in this rural sample is relatively lower than what is seen in other higher risk groups (Li et al. 2018, p. 1ff.).

Despite the fact that male–male sexual relationships have been legal in China since 1997, sociocultural factors still contribute to the stigma and discrimination experienced by this group, leading them to conceal their sexual activities from both partners and healthcare providers. The significant role of family in Chinese culture exerts considerable pressure on MSM, meaning that they have to keep their MSM identity hidden. Consequently, it appears that HIV prevention and testing rates among MSM have remained low, likely because of concerns related to disclosing personal information or facing discrimination (Wu et al. 2019, p. 461f.).

In a study conducted by Li and colleagues in Chongqing and Chengdu in 2019the objective was to identify barriers to the prevention and control of hepatitis B (HBV) and hepatitis C (HCV), as perceived by local hepatitis patients, residents, and healthcare providers. The study involved 26 participants who participated in in-depth face-to-face interviews. The findings indicated that the participants, on the whole, lacked substantial knowledge about HBV and HCV. Some hepatitis patients held misconceptions about HBV and HCV, with certain individuals erroneously believing HBV to be an inherited condition. Furthermore, the majority of the interviewed residents exhibited apathy towards HBV and HCV and displayed no proactive interest in undergoing screening for these infections (Li et al. 2019, p. 1ff.).

The study also highlighted that several workers from the Centres for Disease Control and Prevention (CDC) and community representatives have pointed out that a significant portion of residents and medical workers in community health service centres have limited knowledge about HBV and HCV. Furthermore, HBV and HCV continue to be associated with serious social discrimination and stigma. Many hepatitis patients reported encountering discrimination in their personal and professional lives to varying extents due to their condition. Workers from community health service centres also mentioned that they had witnessed cases of severe discrimination against HBV patients by their own family members (Li et al. 2019, p. 1ff.).

In summary, efforts to reduce the burden of stigma should strategically target key risk factors associated with this issue. Specifically, interventions need to be tailored to populations experiencing heightened stigma, including urban residents and individuals with depression. The implementation of psychosocial interventions to improve mental health holds promise in terms of mitigating the negative impacts of stigma on the well-being of these individuals. Recommendations encompass refining existing laws, establishing professional insurance mechanisms to protect the rights of medical staff, and addressing concerns related to service provision for HIV and HCV patients.

Additionally, crucial advocacy efforts involve expanding health education, reducing societal stigma, promoting supportive government policies, and securing funding. A significant objective is to provide social support and education for the families of patients, thus strengthening connections with potential support networks. Future strategies should focus on training health professionals and community leaders in empathy-building, stigma reduction, and discrimination elimination. This will contribute to creating a supportive clinical environment for individuals living with HIV and HCV (Yuan et al. 2023, p. 4058).

Bibliography

Li, Tingting/Su, Shu/Zhao, Yong/Deng, Runze/Fan, Mingyue/Wang, Ruoxi/Sharma, Manoj/Zeng, Huan (2019): Barriers to the Prevention and Control of Hepatitis B and Hepatitis C in the Community of Southwestern China: A Qualitative Research. In: International Journal of Environmental Research and Public Health 16, No. 2, pp. 1–11. DOI: 10.3390/ijerph16020231.

Li, Zhen/Hsieh, Evelyn/Morano, Jamie P./Sheng, Yu (2016): Exploring HIV-related stigma among HIV-infected Men who have Sex with Men in Beijing, China: A correlation study. In: AIDS Care 28, No. 11, pp. 1394–1401. DOI: 10.1080/09540121.2016.1179713.

Li, Zhen/Morano, Jamie P./Khoshnood, Kaveh/Hsieh, Evelyn/Sheng, Yu (2018): HIV-related stigma among people living with HIV/AIDS in rural Central China. In: BMC Health Services Research 18, No. 453, pp. 1–7. DOI: 10.1186/s12913-018-3245-0.

Wu, Zunyou/Chen, Junfang/Scott, Sarah Robbins/McGoogan, Jennifer M. (2019): History of the HIV Epidemic in China. In: Current HIV/AIDS Reports 16, No. 6, pp. 458–466. DOI: 10.1007/s11904-019-00471-4.

Yang, Ying/Wang, Jun/Lin, Feifei/Zhang, Tao/Yu, Feng/Zhao, Yanping/Zhang, Tiejun (2015): Stigma against HIV/AIDS among female sex workers and general migrant women in eastern China. In: BMC Women's Health 15, No. 2, pp. 1–9. DOI: 10.1186/s12905-014-0160-3.

Yuan, Guangzhe Frank/Tam, Cheuk Chi/Yang, Xueying/Qiao, Shan/Li, Xiaoming/Shen, Zhiyong/Zhou, Yuejiao (2023): Associations Between Internalized and Anticipated HIV Stigma and Depression Symptoms Among People Living with HIV in China: A four-wave Longitudinal Model. In: AIDS and Behavior 27, No. 12, pp. 4052–4061. DOI: 10.1007/s10461-023-04119-8.

8. Opioid Agonist Maintenance Treatment in Central Asia

Uladzimir Pikirenia, Medet Kudabekov, Zhyldyz Bakirova, Azizbek Boltaev

Introduction

Opioid agonist maintenance treatment (OAMT) – also known as opioid substitution treatment (OST) or methadone maintenance treatment (MMT) – is an evidence-based intervention for opiate-dependent persons that replaces illicit drug use with medically prescribed, orally administered opiates such as buprenorphine or methadone. The term 'substitution' is no longer used, in order to clarify that the term refers to treatment of opioid use disorders, not a substitution of one opioid with another (Wiessing et al. 2023).

This chapter provides an overview of the introduction of OAMT in Central Asia. The chapter discusses the developments in Kazakhstan, Kyrgyzstan, and Tajikistan. Uzbekistan and Turkmenistan do not allow OAMT and are therefore not included in this chapter.

Opioid Agonist Maintenance Treatment in Kazakhstan

The first OAMT pilot project was introduced in Kazakhstan in 2005. The first clients included 50 drug users living with HIV. Three years later, in 2008, the OAMT pilot project was expanded to three cities. 14 years later, in 2019, the OAMT programme still had the status of a pilot project. Kazakhstan had relied on financial support from the Global Fund for a large proportion of its harm reduction funding. When the country gained upper middle-income status, this (combined with its low overall HIV prevalence) led to the country's ineligibility for Global Fund grants in the 2014–2016 allocation period.

Although the national government provided support to needle and syringe programmes (NSPs),[1] only 4.7% of the country's total HIV budget went towards prevention activities and only 2.7% towards targeting people who inject drugs. In 2018, the government of Kazakhstan threatened to close the country's OAMT programmes, highlighting the political vulnerability of the service. The prompt civil society advocacy response appears to have paused this decision (Eurasian Harm Reduction Association [EHRA] 2019).

Table 1: Main indicators of the OAMT programme in Kazakhstan (EHRA 2019)

Population	18,611,100
PWID	120,500
OST	Available at ten operational sites in three cities. Reduced Global Fund funding and limited political support has recently seen OAMT restricted to pilot programmes at all sites, with less than 1% of people who use drugs accessing the programme.
NSP	Available at 144 operational sites. Civil society reports poor-quality syringes distributed by government-funded programmes, leading to the potential for increased unsafe injecting.
HIV	Prevalence among PWID (people who inject drugs) – 8.5%.
Hepatitis C	Prevalence among PWID – 58.8%.
Hepatitis B	Prevalence among PWID – 7.9%.
Tuberculosis	—
Overdose prevention	Naloxone is not accessible in Kazakhstan's pharmacies at all, or without prescription, but ambulances/hospitals have it; harm reduction projects also have Naloxone.

1 OAMT and NSP both belong to harm reduction programmes that are considered to have a potential to reduce HIV incidence among people who inject drugs and can be implemented in low- and middle-income countries (Saing 2023).

Harm reduction in closed settings	- Antiretroviral treatment (ART) is available in prisons - OAMT is not available in prisons - NSPs are not available in prisons
Criminalisation costs	- Money spent on a prisoner/per year – €1,554.90 - Money spent on harm reduction and social services – €1,382 - Average sentence for drug law offence – up to seven years
Drug laws	- Consumption in public places is a criminal offence, punishable with a fine of up to 100 monthly fine units (€0–600) or correctional work for the same amount, or community service of up to 120 hours, or arrest up to 45 days - Available alternatives: those who voluntarily refer themselves to healthcare institutions for treatment without a doctor's prescription are exempted from criminal liabilities

According to official statistics, in 1986, three to four regions in Kazakhstan, with a total of 10,000 officially registered drug users, were affected by drug addiction. In 2004, there were ten to twelve regions with about 50,000 drug users (Kazakhstan Institute for Strategic Studies under the President of the Republic of Kazakhstan 2004).

The first wave of HIV-infections among PWID was registered in the early 1990s in the city of Temirtau, Karaganda region, and by the beginning of the 21st century, the second wave had begun among PWID in the Almaty, Karaganda, and Pavlodar regions (Myrzagulova et al. 2020). In 2019, according to the Aman-Saulyk Public Foundation and the Kazakhstan Union of People Living with HIV, there were an estimated 94,600 PWID in Kazakhstan and the HIV prevalence among PWID was 7.9%. The estimated number of PWID living with HIV was 7,000 (Country Coordination Committee 2023).[2]

2 The Country Coordinating Mechanisms (CCM) are national committees that submit funding applications to the Global Fund and oversee the implementation of the grants on behalf of their countries. They are a key element in the partnership between the Global Fund and countries. The latest developments on strengthening Country Coordinating Mechanisms' contribution to health governance are in evolution phase. A CCM includes representatives of all sectors involved in the response to the HIV/

Thus, over the past 20 years, the number of people using narcotic drugs and psychotropic substances has increased almost ten times. However, the technologies for social work with PWID are not fully accepted at the state level. For example, as of 14th June 2019, less than 1% of the estimated 263 PWID were covered by the OAMT programme, of which 85 were people living with HIV and 78 of whom were receiving antiretroviral therapy. The coverage of PWID by the OAMT programme does not exceed 2%; this picture has not changed since 2008 and it does not have a significant impact on the HIV epidemiological situation in the country. As world experience shows, OAMT coverage should be at least 40% of the estimated number of opioid-dependent people in order for preventive harm reduction measures to be effective (United Nations Office on Drugs and Crime [UNODC] 2009).

The reasons for the low number of patients (2%) in OAMT in Kazakhstan can be summarised as follows. Firstly, the programme is still running in pilot mode. Furthermore, the programme has very strict requirements for enrolment. Unlike the OAMT programme in Kyrgyzstan, take-home methadone is not provided, which means that patients need to come to the site every day. However, the OAMT sites are situated very remotely, making it difficult for patients to reach them. Sometimes, shortages in the supply of methadone also occur.

In 2022, the socio-demographic characteristics of OAMT clients in Kazakhstan were as follows. 82% of clients were male and 18% were female. The average age was 44.15 years. 18.4% of clients were officially employed, while 51,08% were not working. 0.3% were convicted and 0.15% were remanded and arrested. 3.7% of clients were disabled.

State support for non-governmental organisations (NGOs) is growing every year, in the form of grants and bonuses for the introduction of new forms of work in various areas of the social sphere. This includes funding for the implementation of social projects (Kuzekbay 2021). In Kazakhstan, the development of the social protection system is focused on income protection, the stimulation of the individual's social activities, and the provision of integrated social services for vulnerable population groups. But PWID are not officially a socially vulnerable population group; they

AIDS, TB and Malaria: academic institutions, civil society, faith-based organisations, government, multilateral and bilateral agencies, non-governmental organisations, key populations, community organisations, the private sector, and technical agencies.

mainly receive social assistance and services at the onset of disability and at retirement age.

It should be emphasised that not all specialists providing social services are professional social workers; only 5.8% are qualified specialists, while 30.4% have no diploma in social work. In 2021, the average monthly salary for social workers was 150,000 Kazakh tenge, equivalent to USD 350 (Abisheva 2020). Social workers play a significant role in the primary prevention of drug addiction, in the adaptation and rehabilitation of drug users, and in helping drug users in general.

One of the main barriers to the development of affordable and high-quality social services for people living with HIV and who use drugs in Kazakhstan is the low status of the social work profession. One of the methods of attracting qualified professionals and young people to the field of social work is to raise its status in the public consciousness. Social work with PWID in Kazakhstan is at a formative stage, but development in this direction is slow. Social work with this population group is carried out mainly by local NGOs, which are financed by international donors.

Thus, the following issues need to be addressed to improve drug treatment in Kazakhstan. The low degree of primary computability of drug dependence needs to be addressed. The quality of inpatient care which is currently very low needs to be improved. New social work approaches need to be introduced. The experience of NGOs in drug treatment needs to be strengthened. The forms of interaction between the state and NGOs need to be defined and agreed upon.

In the vast majority of cases, addiction treatment focuses on complete cessation of drug use. In the process of treatment, the main emphasis is on detoxification, with the extensive use of various potent drugs that alter the consciousness of patients and, according to doctors, thus help them to endure severe withdrawal symptoms. Post-detoxification psychosocial care and rehabilitation almost only exist on paper, but are not implemented in practice. Compulsory treatment of drug (and alcohol) dependence, which is ordered by a court order and falls under the direct control of law enforcement agencies, is a common practice. There is no treatment for drug addiction in prisons (Latypov et al. 2010).

In Kazakhstan, drug treatment services apply a medical approach to addiction. Most staff members have a medical degree and focus on treatment services. Psychosocial support is not provided to the same degree, as most programmes lack staff members with social work training. The introduction of OAMT in Kazakhstan was expected in 2002, in accordance with the Order of the Ministry of Health of the Republic of Kazakhstan dated 21st August 2002 No. 791, 'On the introduction of substitution therapy', but was not launched due to the fact that for a long time, the Ministry of Internal Affairs of the Republic of Kazakhstan did not give permission for the import of the necessary drug. In comparison, substitution therapy was launched in Kyrgyzstan in 2002 and in Uzbekistan in 2006, financed by international donors (Aizberg 2008).

The first experience of medium-term planning to expand the availability of opioid substitution therapy in the Republic of Kazakhstan within the framework of the National Programme to Combat the HIV/AIDS Epidemic was implemented under the project 'Effective Prevention and Treatment of HIV Infection among Vulnerable Groups of the Population of Central Asia and Azerbaijan (2006–2010)'. The studies showed that the main task was to revise and improve the regulatory framework related to the implementation of OAMT programmes, as well as to finalise and approve the interdepartmental plan to expand the availability of OAMT for 2010–2014 (UNODC 2010).

Between 2006 and 2013, Kazakhstan established a system of services for PWID in all regions as part of the implementation of the national harm reduction strategy, based on the work of state agencies (AIDS centres) and NGOs. The components of harm reduction programmes in Kazakhstan are in line with the recommendations of UN agencies and include nine main components. In accordance with international recommendations and guidelines, the National Policy on HIV Prevention in Kazakhstan is aimed at providing the following services for PWID on the basis of trust points and harm reduction projects in Kazakhstan: needle and syringe exchange programmes, HIV testing and counselling, prevention and treatment of sexually transmitted infections, programmes to provide condoms to PWID and their sexual partners, targeted information, education, and communication (IEC) programmes for PWID and their sexual partners, antiretroviral therapy, vaccination, diagnosis, and treatment of viral hepatitis, prevention, diagnosis, and treatment of tuberculosis, and OAMT and other drug dependence treatments.

In some regions of the country, NGOs provide additional services in the form of social support for clients of harm reduction programmes, which entail greater commitment to the programme on the part of participants and positive results (Rozental et al. 2015). The use of OAMT in places of detention, general hospitals, or other institutions is not allowed in Kazakhstan, and all OAMT centres are located at regional and city narcological dispensaries (Latypov et al. 2010).

A large number of publications confirm that the use of methadone substitution therapy is associated with an increase in patient adherence to treatment, a decrease in their use of street opioids, a decrease in cravings for the use of psychoactive substances, and an improvement in their social functioning. There is also a well-documented reduction in the incidence of other drug use among patients receiving methadone substitution therapy (Pikirenia/Kopytov 2018).

There are fears in society that OAMT will lead to an increase in crime and drug use. OAMT does not eliminate addiction, but rather makes the use of the opioids less dangerous for drug users. It is known from clinical studies that the retention rate of patients in substitution therapy programmes is higher than in treatment programmes that focus on total abstinence. A disadvantage of substitution therapy programmes is the possible 'leakage' of methadone to the black market. This happens when patients are given large amounts of methadone to take at home and sell it to other drug users. The appearance of methadone on the black market indirectly indicates that there is a population of patients who need substitution therapy but for some reason are not receiving it.

From a clinical point of view, the biggest medical risk for a patient undergoing OAMT is the concomitant use of psychoactive substances (Ivanets/Altshuler 2014). A review of the literature on drug addiction and drug treatment showed that the main information on OAMT issues is provided by international organisations such as the United Nations Office on Drugs and Crime (UNODC), the World Health Organization (WHO), and the European Monitoring Centre for Drugs and Drug Addiction (EMCDDA)

An analysis of methadone and buprenorphine use, as well as the coverage of pharmacological maintenance treatment for opioid dependence, indicates that this treatment is either non existent or insufficiently available in all countries with large numbers of injecting drug users. This may be due to a lack of recognition of the efficacy of such treatments, resistance due to cultural prejudices or economic or structural problems, and/or inaction by political leadership (International Narcotics Control Board [INCB] 2020).

In many parts of the world, HIV prevention is weak or non-existent, treatment is inadequate, and there are no adequate mechanisms to combat stigma and facilitate reintegration into society. In addition, stigma is exacerbated by the disproportionate and often unjustified application of criminal measures against drug users, which is inconsistent with the principle of proportionality.

The WHO database contains information on the following indicators: access to HIV and hepatitis C counselling and treatment in institutions and services; standards of treatment and care in specialised public medical institutions; treatment programmes for women with drug use disorders; special housing services for people with drug use disorders; and employment services for people with drug use disorders (World Health Organization [WHO] 2020). However, when it comes to analysing the current situation, this data is insufficient, as some of the information is outdated. Nevertheless, these indicators can be used to study the current situation and compare it to that of previous years.

Opioid Agonist Maintenance Treatment in Kyrgyzstan

Since 2001, the number of new HIV infections has been increasing in Kyrgyzstan. During this time period, persons who inject drugs accounted for 67% of the total number of detected cases. In response to HIV/AIDS, Kyrgyzstan introduced the OAMT programme for opioid-dependent[3] persons. Since 2002, the programme has been implemented and is part of the comprehensive treatment methods for opioid users in the country.

There are two pharmacological approaches to the treatment of opioid dependence – those based on opioid withdrawal and those based on agonist maintenance therapy. In Kyrgyzstan, pharmacological treatment of opioid withdrawal is provided either through gradual discontinuation of opioid agonists (WHO 2009, p. 5ff.) (methadone is used in the country) or the use of alpha-2-adrenergic agonists to alleviate withdrawal symptoms (clonidine).

There have been a number of positive results and achievements during the time that methadone substitution treatment has been being implemented. One of them is the creation of a legislative basis for the implementation of the programme. Thus, the harm reduction strategy, which includes the implementation of the substitution therapy programme, has been reflected

3 The International Statistical Classification of Diseases and Related Health Problems, 10th Revision (ICD-10) is a version of the ICD classifier developed in 1989 and adopted by WHO in 1990 (Wikipedia 2023).

in the Anti-Drug Programme (Kyrgyz Republic Ministry of Justice 2022)[4] of the Kyrgyz Republic since 2001 (Kyrgyz Republic Ministry of Justice 2001).[5]

Since the Kyrgyz Republic includes methadone[6] in List 1 of narcotic substances subject to national control, it is not prohibited for use for medical purposes, and it is included in the list of the country's essential medicines, the following clinical guidelines and protocols have been developed, which define the procedure for providing therapy: the Clinical Protocol on Methadone Substitution Maintenance Therapy, approved by the joint order of the Ministry of Health (MoH) and the Ministry of Justice of the Kyrgyz Republic No. 147 of 8th April 2008 and No. 66, Clinical Guidelines for the Provision of Methadone Substitution Maintenance Therapy to Opioid-Dependent Persons, approved by the order of the MoH of the Kyrgyz Republic No. 497 of 11th October 2010; the Clinical Guidelines on Diagnosis and Treatment of Mental and Behavioural Disorders Caused by Opioid Use, approved by the order of the MoH, No. 703 dated 25th December 2012; and the Clinical Protocol 'Treatment of Opioid Dependence Based on Methadone Maintenance Therapy', approved by the order of the MoH, No. 372 dated 30th June 2015.

Recently, a new manual and protocol have been developed, which include additions in accordance with new scientifically proven recommendations and data, as well as changes to the order and procedures of providing maintenance therapy. Thus, the guidelines include algorithms for the management of patients using buprenorphine, which is planned to be introduced in the country in the near future, as well as details of ethical standards for treatment. In the Clinical Guidelines, the name of the programme 'Methadone Substitution Maintenance Treatment' (OST/MMT) has been changed to 'Maintenance Therapy with Opioid Agonist' (MTOA), as the use of prescribed methadone and buprenorphine drugs and therapy is understood as a treatment of drug dependency rather than a replacement of illegal opioids, as they are the central element of therapy integrating medical, psychological, and social aspects.

4 Resolution of the Government of the Kyrgyz Republic from 10th August 2022, No. 445.

5 Resolution of the Government of the Kyrgyz Republic from 13th December 2001, No. 785.

6 Methadone hydrochloride has been registered and included in the list of essential medicines of the Kyrgyz Republic in 2006.

In accordance with the Law of the Kyrgyz Republic 'On the rules of storage, accounting and reporting of narcotic drugs' (Kyrgyz Republic Ministry of Justice 2011),[7] all methadone points/sites in the Kyrgyz Republic are included in the Register of 'subjects of legal provision of narcotic substances', which is subject to state regulation and control. Thus, the existing legal framework provides an opportunity for the implementation of harm reduction programmes for substance use and is the basis for the functioning of treatment programmes such as detoxification, maintenance therapy, needle exchange programmes, and overdose prevention.

One of the positive achievements of the implementation of the substitution therapy programme is the process of decentralisation and geographical expansion. Thus, since 2005, 34 substitution therapy dispensing points have been opened in Family Medicine Centres (FMC) at the level of primary healthcare, in Bishkek and Osh, as well as in other regions[8] of the Republic. In addition, eleven substitution therapy sites were opened within the penitentiary system.

Another positive aspect was the application of the 'One Window' principle, meaning that, at the substitution therapy sites, located at TB and HIV/AIDS treatment facilities, the patient was provided with comprehensive services for the coordinated provision of treatment of the underlying disease of opioid dependence, care and treatment of HIV infection,[9] and TB therapy.[10]According to an evaluation of the OAMT programme by Subata et al. (2011), medical staff dispensed methadone to patients at home for two or more days, in isolated cases and on an individual basis. Currently, following the Covid-19 pandemic, the practice of providing methadone to a patient's home for five days is allowed.

It is necessary to mention separately the implementation of the OAMT programme in 2008 in the Ministry of Justice in Colony No. 47. The implementation and expansion of the programme into the penitentiary system led to a reduction in drug use in prisons, reduced the risk of HIV

---

7 Resolution of the Government of the Kyrgyz Republic of 18th February 2011, No. 54.

8 In different cities in Kyrgyzstan, so-called 'Family Medicine Centers' (FMCs) were opened.

9 In the city of Bishkek, the OAMT site is based at the Bishkek City Center for AIDS Prevention and Control. In the city of Osh, the OAMT site is based at Osh Territorial Clinical Hospital.

10 The OAMT is based at the City TB Hospital in Bishkek and at the TB facility at the Penal Colony No. 31.

transmission through injecting practices, and improved the quality of life of prisoners (Subata et al. 2011).

It is also positive that the hospitalisation of opioid-dependent persons in other medical institutions is well organised, in case of somatic health problems (surgery, urology, gynaecology, etc.). The process works as follows. An application is submitted to the Republican Center for Psychiatry and Narcology for the admission of a patient from the substitution therapy programme to a treatment facility, as the patients themselves are trained to provide information about their participation in the programme. The administration of the treatment facility then contacts the coordinator of the substitution treatment programme by telephone. The drug itself is kept in a safe by the head nurse of the department when it is delivered to the treatment facility.

In order to improve monitoring and the quality of record keeping, an electronic register[11] has been set up. Through the register, programme monitoring and evaluation procedures have been improved. Procedures for collecting and analysing data related to both direct service delivery and the impact of the substitution programme on patients have been streamlined. The online entry of primary documentation has been improved, and paperwork for programme staff has been reduced. In addition to storing and processing information on patients[12] enrolled in the programmes, information on patients' health status (such as comorbidities, including HIV, TB, HBV, and HCV) is shared on a tiered basis. According to epidemiological data, the increase in the number of new HIV infections decreased with the introduction of harm reduction programmes in Kyrgyzstan (Asanov 2005).

In Kyrgyzstan, OAMT is provided free of charge to the patients. Since 2002, the work of all existing substitution therapy sites has been fully funded by the Global Fund HIV project, without drawing on resources from national or local healthcare budgets. Thus, a positive moment in the implementation of the substitution therapy programme was the fact that from 2023, funding was switched from international donor organisations to the state, through the Mandatory Health Insurance Fund, according to

---

11 With technical support of ICAP "Assistance" project, all OAMT sites are equipped with an Electronic Registry of Substitution Maintenance Therapy (ERST).

12 Monitoring includes the effectiveness of therapy, including the monitoring of methadone prescriptions and of changing dosages, the monitoring of illegal substance use, drug omissions, monitoring of timely receipt of antiretroviral and TB treatment, screening and testing, information on changes regarding socio-demographic indicators and patient behaviour.

the order[13] 'On norms for the formation of the budget of health care organizations working in the Single Payer System for 2023' (Compulsory Health Insurance Fund at the Ministry of Health Kyrgyz Republic 2023). This order approved funds for the 'purchase of drugs for substitution therapy' to the value of USD 25,000.

Based on the above, the following conclusions can be drawn about the positive achievements in the implementation of substitution therapy in the Kyrgyz Republic:

1. The existing legislative framework provides an opportunity to implement harm reduction programmes for substance use, including substitution therapy programmes.
2. The substitution therapy programme has been decentralised and geographically expanded.
3. Application of the 'Single Window' principle at some substitution therapy sites located at TB and HIV/AIDS treatment facilities, which enables the provision of integrated services for the treatment of the main disease of opioid dependence as well as TB and HIV through antiretroviral therapy.
4. The practice of issuing the patient with five days' worth of methadone has been introduced.
5. The substitution therapy programme has been introduced and implemented in the penitentiary system.
6. The hospitalisation of opioid-dependent persons with somatic health problems in other treatment facilities is well organised.
7. An electronic register has been established for monitoring and evaluation.
8. HIV infection rates in the Kyrgyz Republic have reduced, including the share of injecting drug users.
9. Since 2023, the transition of funding from international donor organisations to the state has been implemented through the Mandatory Medical Insurance Fund.

Opioid Agonist Maintenance Treatment in Tajikistan

In Tajikistan, the OAMT programme was introduced in 2010. There is a network of 15 OAMT sites covering all regions of the country, including

13 Order of the Mandatory Health Insurance Fund 2nd February 2023. No. 16.

two sites in the penitentiary system. Currently, the only OAMT drug used in Tajikistan is methadone, available only in liquid form. In addition to providing opioid dependency treatment, OAMT sites in Tajikistan encompass additional services for PWID, such as overdose treatment, testing for HBV, HCV, and syphilis, providing psychological support, etc. Despite a well-developed system of OAMT sites in the country, the OAMT programme in Tajikistan is still considered to be a pilot project, and coverage remains low. At present, around 650 people are enrolled in OAMT.

To explore the reasons for the underutilisation of the potential of OAMT sites operating in the country, research on drug use and barriers to OAMT in Tajikistan was conducted between February and April 2023. Sixteen focus groups comprising 65 PWID who were both receiving OAMT (30 people) and not receiving OAMT (35 people) were held in eight cities across Tajikistan. Three main obstacles were outlined by the respondents: the insufficient appeal of the OST programme, e.g. the need for daily visits to OAMT sites; the lack of staff capacity at OST sites; and misinformation circulated among PWID about OAMT (Kaspirova/Malikov 2023).

It should be noted that in 2023, the main institution coordinating the OAMT programme in Tajikistan, the Republican Clinical Narcology Center, adopted the OAMT Expansion Plan for the years 2024–2026, with an ambitious goal of increasing programme coverage to 2,000 people by the end of 2026. In order to achieve this goal, the aforementioned barriers must be addressed.

Conclusions

Since the beginning of the 2000s, harm reduction programmes have been introduced in Central Asia. OAMT and NSPs are key strategies in harm reduction as they are believed to be able to significantly reduce HIV and hepatitis infections among the vulnerable group of PWID. Kyrgyzstan and Tajikistan have been pioneers in the adoption of harm reduction programmes as both countries have opened OAMT programmes and NSPs in the community and in the penitentiary system. However, both countries also face problems in the implementation of OAMT as coverage remains very low. In Kazakhstan, OAMT was started in 2005 but was never expanded beyond a pilot project, with less than 1% of PWID having access to OAMT in the country. In 2024, the introduction of OAMT is being actively discussed among policy makers in Kazakhstan. In line with international evidence, many argue that access to OAMT needs to be extended to effectively address the spread of HIV and hepatitis C among PWID.

Bibliography

Abisheva, K. (2020): The Role of Social Work in Managing Social Risks of Vulnerable Segments of the Population of the Republic of Kazakhstan. In: Topical Issues of Modern Science, pp. 17–26.

Aizberg, Oleg (2008): Opioid Substitution Therapy in Selected Countries of Eastern Europe and Central Asia. www.iasociety.org/Web/WebContent/File/19Jan-IASYalta-OST%20Overview_ENG%20final%20version-doc.pdf, 09.03.2024.

Asanov, Tynchtykbek (2005): Substitution maintenance therapy with methadone in the Kyrgyz Republic. Osh Conference, 2005.

Compulsory Health Insurance Fund at the Ministry of Health Kyrgyz Republic (2023): On norms for the formation of the budget of health care organizations working in the Single Payer System for 2023 [No. 16, 02 February 2023]. www.foms.kg/prikazy/, 30.10.2023.

Country Coordination Committee (2003): About CCM. www.ccmkz.kz/?lang=en, 09.03.2024.

Eurasian Harm Reduction Association (EHRA) (2019): Kazkakhstan. www.harmreductioneurasia.org/countries-and-territories/kazakhstan, 23.02.2024.

International Narcotics Control Board (INCB) (2020): Special Report: Celebrating 60 Years of the Single Convention on Narcotic Drugs of 1961 and 50 Years of the Convention on Psychotropic Substances of 1971. www.incb.org/documents/Publications/AnnualReports/AR2020/Supplement/20-07608_INCB_Supp_Ebook_R.pdf, 23.02.2024.

Ivanets, N.N./Altshuler, V.B. (2014): Substitution Therapy for Methadone and Other Opioid Drug Addiction: Origin, Essence and Trends. In: Narcology Issues 2, pp. 3–7.

Kaspirova, A./Malikov, Naimdzhon (2023): Report on situation with the drug use, drug policies and existing programmes on combating drug use in the Republic of Tajikistan [unpublished report]. Dushanbe: United Nations Development Programme (UNDP).

Kazakhstan Institute for Strategic Studies under the President of the Republic of Kazakhstan (2004): Narcotization of Society: State, Problems, Experience of Counteraction. www.kisi.kz/uploads/1/files/6LDDuGMY.pdf, 30.10.2023.

Kuzekbay, A. (2021): 16 thousand NGOs are actively working in Kazakhstan. www.inform.kz/ru/16-tysyach-npo-aktivno-rabotayut-v-kazahstane_a3754206, 23.02.2024.

Kyrgyz Republic Ministry of Justice (2001): On measures to prevent HIV/AIDS, sexually transmitted and injected infections in the Kyrgyz Republic [No. 785, 13 December 2011]. www.cbd.minjust.gov.kg/act/view/ru-ru/34692?cl=ru-ru, 29.10.2023.

Kyrgyz Republic Ministry of Justice (2011): On the order of accounting, storage and use of narcotic drugs, psychotropic substances and precursors in the Kyrgyz Republic [No. 54, 18 February 2011]. www.cbd.minjust.gov.kg/act/view/ru-ru/94051?cl=ru-ru, 29.10.2023.

Kyrgyz Republic Ministry of Justice (2022): On approval of the Anti-Drug Program of the Cabinet of Ministers of the Kyrgyz Republic and the Action Plan for its implementation for 2022-2026 years [No. 445, 10 August 2022]. www.cbd.minjust.gov. kg/act/view/en-ru-ru/159420, 29.10.2023.

Latypov, Alisher/Otiashvili, David/Aizberg, Oleg/Boltaev, Azizbek (2010): Opioid Substitution Therapy in Central Asia: Towards Diverse and Effective Drug Dependence Treatment. Vilnius: Eurasian Harm Reduction Network (EHRN).

Myrzagulova, A.O./Tastanova, S./Akzholova, N.A. (2020): Epidemiological analysis of the incidence of HIV infection in the population of Kazakhstan. In: Bulletin of the Kazakh National Medical University 1, pp. 385–388.

Pikirenia, Uladzimir/Kapytau, Andrei (2018): Adherence to methadone substitution therapy and its relationship to the socio-demographic characteristics of patients. In: Medical Journal 4, pp. 18–26. DOI: 10.13140/RG.2.2.20954.24000.

Rozental, Y.M./Yegeubayeva, S.A./Terlikbaeva, Asel/Primbetova, Sholpan/Gilbert, Louisa/El-Bassel, Nabila (2015): A randomized controlled trial to reduce the risk of HIV, viral hepatitis C and other STIs among heterosexual couples who inject drugs. Experience of Kazakhstan. In: Medicine 7, pp. 83–85.

Saing, Chan Hang (2023): OAT and NSP and their potential to reduce HIV incidence among people who inject drugs in low-and middle-income countries. In: The Lancet Regional Health – Western Pacific 34, p. 100744. DOI: 10.1016/j.lanwpc.2023.100744.

Subata, Emilis/Karymbaeva, Saliya/Møller, Lars (2011): Evaluation of opioid substitution therapy in prison. Pilot study in Kyrgyzstan. Copenhagen: WHO Regional Office for Europe.

United Nations Office on Drugs and Crime (UNODC) (2009): Technical guidance for countries to develop targets for universal access to HIV prevention, treatment and care among people who inject drugs. www.unodc.org/documents/centralasia/Expansion_OST_accessibility_in_Kazakhstan_2011_2014_RUS.pdf, 16.02.2024.

United Nations Office on Drugs and Crime (UNODC) (2010): Increasing the availability of opioid substitution therapy in the Republic of Kazakhstan in 2010-2014: a situation review, action plan and operational implementation plan. www.unodc.org/documents/centralasia/Expansion_OST_accessibility_in_Kazakhstan_2011_2014_RUS.pdf, 16.02.2024.

Wiessing, Lucas/Banka-Cullen, Prakashini/Barbaglia, Gabriela M./Belackova, Vendula/Belbaisi, Saed A.S./Blanken, Peter et al. (2023): Opioid Agonist Maintenance Treatment Outcomes – The OPTIMUS International Consensus towards Evidence-Based and Patient-Centred Care, an Interim Report. In: International Journal of Mental Health and Addiction. DOI: 10.1007/s11469-023-01213-9.

Wikipedia (2023): ICD-10. www.ru.wikipedia.org/wiki/%D0%9C%D0%9A%D0%91-10, 27.10.2023.

World Health Organization (WHO) (2009): Guidelines for psychosocial pharmacologic treatment of opioid dependence. www.who.int/publications/i/item/9789241547543, 29.02.2024.

World Health Organization (WHO) (2020): Global Health Observatory Data Repository (European Region). www.who.int/data/gho, 09.03.2024.

9. Labour Migrants – An Exploration of the New Driving Force of the HIV Epidemic in Uzbekistan

Azizbek Boltaev

HIV in Uzbekistan

According to the official data of the Ministry of Health, at the onset of 2023 a total of 52,420 cases of people living with HIV were registered in Uzbekistan (Igamberdiev 2023). From the first detected HIV infection in Uzbekistan in 1987 until 1st January 2022, around 71,000 cases have been registered, and the number of deaths among HIV-infected people is about 23,000 cases (Gazeta.uz 2022). An analysis carried out in 2022 of HIV-infected individuals, segregated by gender, revealed that 55% of HIV cases pertain to males, while 45% are attributed to females. 14% of all people living with HIV (PLWH) residing in Uzbekistan were 18 years old or younger (O'zbekiston Milliy Axborot Agentligi [UZA] 2022). HIV transmitted through sexual relations accounted for 79% of all registered cases, followed by parenteral transmission (12,7%) and mother-to-child transmission (0.6) (Uzbekistan's funding application to the Global Fund to Fight AIDS, Tuberculosis, and Malaria [GFATM] for 2020–2023).

A substantial majority (64.2%) of the registered people living with HIV (PLWH) in 2020 were geographically concentrated within four regions, namely the city of Tashkent (10,484), the Andijan region (6,870), the Tashkent region (6,560), and the Samarkand region (4,080) (Open Data Portal n.d.). Notably, in the preceding year, 2019, within the prison population, 300 persons living with HIV/AIDS (PLHA) were identified, predominantly comprising males (295 out of 300) (Uzbekistan's funding application to GFATM for 2020–2023).

The prevailing pattern of HIV transmission in the country manifests as a concentrated epidemic, with a distinct prominence of prevalence among designated key populations (KPs). The Integrated Biological and Behavioural Surveillance (IBBS) assessments reveal an upward trajectory in HIV prevalence among men who have sex with men (MSM), increasing from 3.3% in 2013 to 3.7% in 2017 and further increasing to 4.5% in 2021, as well as among sex workers (SW), increasing from 2.2% in 2011 to 3.2%

(2017) and decreasing to 1.27% in 2021. Concurrently, a discernible and consistent decline in prevalence is discernible among people who inject drugs (PWID), dropping from 8.5% in 2011 to 5.1% in 2017 and 2.9% in 2021.

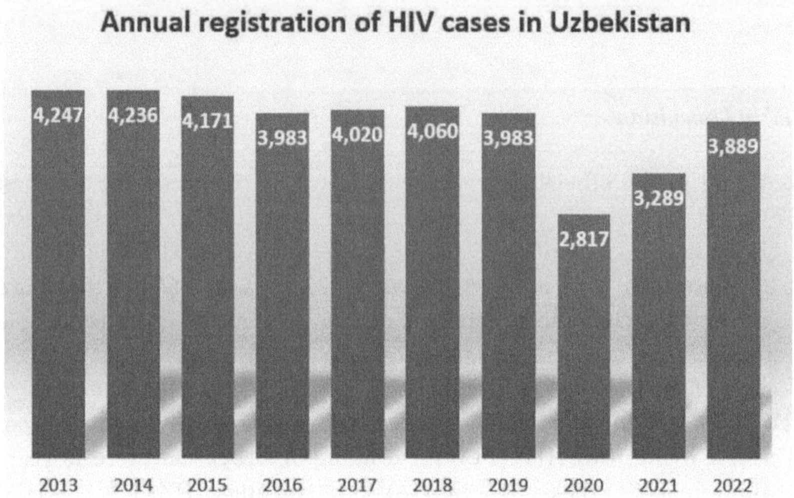

Figure 1: Annual registration of HIV cases in Uzbekistan

A noteworthy observation pertains to migrant populations, wherein 1,224 new HIV cases were identified in 2022, reflecting an almost threefold growth compared to the figures in 2013 (449 cases) (Igamberdiev 2023). Interestingly, a phylogenetic study of HIV cases in Uzbekistan carried out by Lebedev et al. (2022) suggested that the majority of HIV cases in Uzbekistan are likely to have been infected within the country through, for example, in-country migration networks. This calls for urgent attention to be paid to internal migrants as HIV prevalence appears to be growing in this group (Lebedev et al. 2022).

The IBBS assessments reveal a fluctuating trend in HIV prevalence among labour migrants (LM) over time: 0.8% in 2015, increasing to 1.3% in 2017, followed by a subsequent diminish to 1.1% in 2021. There is a particularly high HIV prevalence among LM from Samarkand (4.8%), Nukus

(1.7%), and Andijan (1.6%) (Data provided by Republican AIDS Center [RAC] to the International Organization for Migration [IOM]).

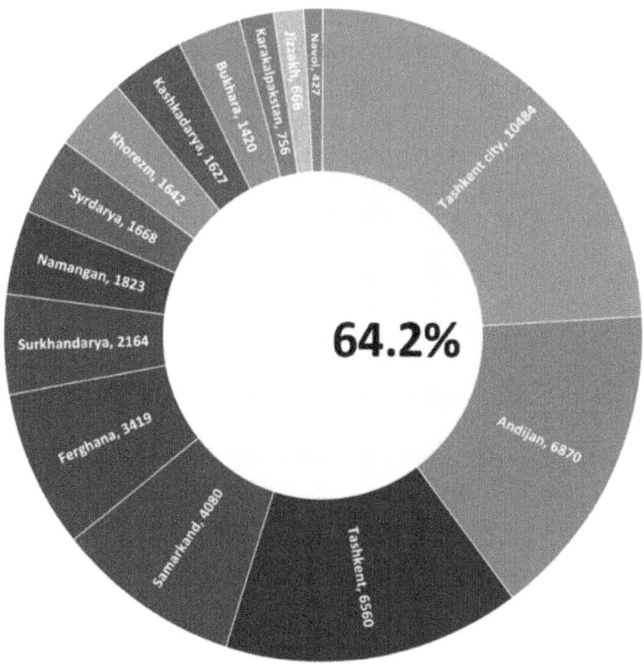

Figure 2: Distribution of HIV cases by geographical regions

Along with the prevalence of HIV among LMs, the IBBS studies revealed reductions in hepatitis C virus (HCV) and syphilis occurrences in 2021, compared to 2017. As such, HCV prevalence dropped by 20% from 2.2% to 2.0%, while the prevalence of syphilis decreased by 30% from 1.6% to 1.3%. The risk of LM contracting HIV is inflated due to the worryingly low knowledge about HIV within this group, as well the widespread engagement in risky behaviours.

Notably, the 2021 IBBS study showed that only 38.9% of LMs were able to give correct answers to all basic HIV-related questions (Data provided by RAC to IOM). Another study by Drobyshevskaya et al. (2022) that was conducted in the Moscow region, Russia in 2021 among LMs from Uzbekistan and Tajikistan revealed that about 20% of the study participants had no idea what HIV infection was. By contrast, only 4.5% of the native inhabitants of the Moscow region had similarly poor knowledge about HIV (Drobyshevskaya et al. 2022).

When it comes to LMs, injecting drugs is a practice of particular interest as it dramatically increases the likelihood of HIV infection. Therefore, it is very important to monitor the safety of injection behaviour in this group. It should be noted that drug use among LMs significantly decreased in 2021 compared to 2017: 3.5% of LM had used drugs before they migrated (2017 – 5.9%), of which 0.2% injected drugs (2017 – 1.8%) compared to 0.3% of LM who have injected drugs since migrating (2017 – 0.9%). Among those surveyed, 0.3% of LM (0.4% in 2017) indicated that they had a sexual partner who injected drugs before they migrated (Data provided by RAC to IOM).

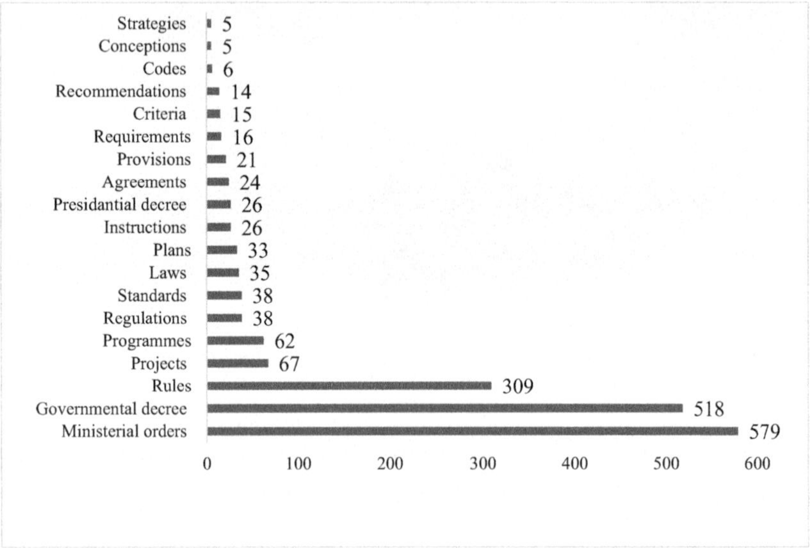

Figure 3: Annual registered cases of HIV among migrants

Of those LMs, 6.3% had at least one STI symptom when they returned home. According to a 2021 study, 28.8% of LMs with symptoms of STIs turn to a familiar health worker for medical help, 19.2% to a private doctor, and 13.1% to the STI dispensaries. 17.7% of LMs self-medicate, while 8.1% do nothing. A high proportion of LMs with at least one symptom of an STI were identified in Andijan (18.4%), Termez (14.3%), and Urgench (17%). Among such LMs, up to 35.7% (in Nukus) did nothing in relation to their

STI, while the large groups from Gulistan (40%), Urgench (38.2%), and Tashkent (33%) opted to self-medicate (ibid).

The coverage of key populations with HIV interventions increased from 2014 to 2020: PWID (estimated 39,000) from 24,552 to 32,000; SW (estimated 29,000) from 11,842 to 15,750; MSM (estimated 30,000) remained suboptimal, despite increasing from 1,491 to 2,186. The service coverage data needs to be interpreted with caution as it conflicts with other information related to the situation among the indicated key populations. As such, the increase in the coverage of PWID reported above does not correlate with the National Drug Control Committee's data that indicates a 20-fold reduction in the number of registered people who inject drugs over the last decade, falling from 7,988 in 2012 to 359 in 2021 (National Information-Analytical Center on Drug Control under the Cabinet of Ministers of Uzbekistan [NCDC] 2022).

HIV Services for Labour Migrants in Uzbekistan

In June 2021, the General Assembly of the United Nations High-Level Meeting on AIDS adopted a set of new and ambitious targets. Known as the '95–95–95' strategy, it aims to end the HIV epidemic by 2030. Within its framework, 95% of people infected with HIV should know their status, 95% of HIV-infected people should receive antiretroviral treatment (ART), and 95% of those receiving treatment should have a non-detectable viral load in their blood.

In order to implement measures in accordance with this strategy, the Government of Uzbekistan has adopted the state's 'Comprehensive programme of measures for 2023–2027 to increase the effectiveness of combating the spread of HIV infection endorsed by the President's Executive Order No. PK-14, dated 20th January 2023'. The programme envisages consolidating the funds of the state budget, the funds of the Global Fund to fight against AIDS, tuberculosis, and malaria, and the loan funds of the Asian Development Bank and the Asian Infrastructure Investment Bank and investing them strategically into reducing HIV among the population of Uzbekistan. In the next five years, a total of 120 billion Uzbek soums and 54 million US dollars will be channelled into increasing the quality of the services for the early detection, diagnosis, and treatment of HIV infection, into purchasing test systems and antiretroviral medicines, into developing the material and technical base of AIDS centres and their inter-district diagnostic laboratories, into increasing the knowledge and skills of specialists, and into carrying out extensive prevention activities, as well as implementing other organisational measures (LexUZ 2023).

HIV Prevention

Just like the general population, Uzbek LMs are eligible for preventative HIV treatment and any other HIV and healthcare services they need. However, considering the fact that LMs have become the largest subpopulation in the country, with one of the highest prevalence of HIV, the Uzbek government has implemented additional measures to ensure their safety as regards HIV both during and after their time living abroad. In particular, the state's comprehensive programme (No. PK-14, dated 20th January 2023) envisages conveyance campaigns aimed at raising awareness among migrants and their families about the risk of HIV infection, protective measures, and treatment options. Within these campaigns, importance is placed on educating LMs and preparing them for an organised departure to work abroad. These activities are being implemented under the leadership of the RAC in partnership with the Agency for Foreign Labor Migration and other interested ministries and departments (Uchaev et al. 2022).

Primary prevention programmes on HIV infection are conducted for organised youth and are integrated into the education system. Every year, in line with the joint activities planned by different sectors (the Ministry of Defense and the Ministry of Health; the Ministry of Internal Affairs and the Ministry of Health; the Security Council and the Ministry of Health, etc.), educational seminars are held in departments, educational institutions, and military units, with the involvement of specialists from the narcological service, the Ministry of Internal Affairs, representatives of the Mahalla communities, and religious figures. Information and educational materials approved by the Republican Commission for the Review and Approval of Information and Educational Materials (hereafter referred to as 'the Republican Commission') are produced for various population groups, which, in turn, are distributed by governmental and non-governmental organisations (NGOs) (ibid).

The strict requirement that all information and educational communication (IEC) materials related to HIV are approved by the Republican Commission seems to negatively affect the variety and contents of such communication. As such, the content analysis of IEC materials that are available on the internet and were developed by the Uzbek RAC and NGOs, and that target high-risk populations such as LMs, showed that while these supplies provide sufficient information about the nature of the virus and the ways it can be transmitted, too often they lack clear information on how to prevent HIV.

Prevention messages are often limited to the importance of fidelity among spouses and avoiding sexual contact outside of marriage. The author of the report failed to find any IEC materials funded by GFATM or the state budget that clearly stipulate the importance of using condoms, nor was there any material in the Uzbek language explaining the rules of correct usage of condoms. However, some training materials for NGO staff and peer educators contain safer sex-related information in Russian (Korotkova et al. 2021) and are delivered to end beneficiaries through verbal communication by social workers, peer supporters, and medical workers as part of routine counselling before and after HIV testing (Ministry of Health of the Republic of Uzbekistan 2023).

HIV Testing and Linkage to Care

HIV diagnostics are carried out by a network of 63 inter-district (*Uzb.: tumanlararo*) HIV laboratories while another 15 laboratories are located within the premises of regional AIDS centres. The Uzbek government, in its efforts to reach the '90–90–90' goal, has increased HIV testing in the last decade to 38% – from 2,564,400 tests in 2013 to 4,137,000 in 2022 (Igamberdiev et al. 2023). The current HIV testing algorithm in Uzbekistan requires HIV diagnosis to be made based on positive results from three different tests. The final confirmatory Western blotting test is also required by the national HIV testing algorithm (Ministry of Health of the Republic of Uzbekistan 2023), but its use is not recommended by the World Health Organization (WHO 2021), as it may sufficiently increase the cost of testing and delay the final diagnosis (Association of Public Health Laboratories 2015).

Upon their return to Uzbekistan after staying abroad for three months or longer, all residents of Uzbekistan (citizens and non-citizens) must undergo testing for sexually transmitted infections, including HIV. The aim of this measure is the early detection of HIV among LMs, and it is carried out jointly by the Ministry of Health, the Ministry of Internal Affairs, the Ministry of Employment and Labor Relations, the State Border Protection

Committee of the State Security Service, the Women's Committee, the Republican Council on Coordination of Activities of Self-governing Bodies, the Committee on Religious Affairs, and the Youth Union of Uzbekistan (Anonymous 2018).

Although HIV testing is conducted on a large scale, its quality and outcomes raise concerns. As such, the 2021 IBBS study showed that only half (49.5%) of the migrant cohort responded affirmatively to the question, 'Have you ever undergone an HIV test?' Conversely, a subset of 6.8% encountered difficulties in articulating their response to this question. Among those migrants who underwent testing, 44.1% indicated that they had been tested in their home country, 35.9% sought testing within the confines of Russia, and 13.9% pursued testing across both domestic and Russian locales. Notably, a noteworthy proportion of 17% of those who had taken tests remain unaware of the outcomes of testing (Data provided by RAC to IOM).

Similarly, a household survey conducted in 2020–2021 by the United Nations Children's Fund (UNICEF) and the State Committee for Statistics identified that less than half (48.3%) of women were offered and underwent HIV testing during their pregnancy. This is despite the fact that the current clinical protocol requires 100% coverage of pregnant women with HIV testing. The level of awareness of outcomes of the testing was even lower – 21.4%.

Rapid HIV tests are available through AIDS centres and HIV-service NGOs, and such testing can be performed by a trained health worker. Civil society organisations are advocating the introduction of HIV self-tests as a means of lowering the threshold to early HIV detection (Uchaev et al. 2022).

HIV Treatment and Care

The Uzbek government has taken over full responsibility for financing the procurement of antiretroviral medications from the GFATM, which had funded HIV treatment in Uzbekistan since 2004. Funds are channelled through the RAC, which coordinates HIV treatment and care through 14 regional AIDS centres and extends technical support to 137 primary healthcare facilities that dispense ART across the country (Uzbekistan's funding application to GFATM for 2020–2023).

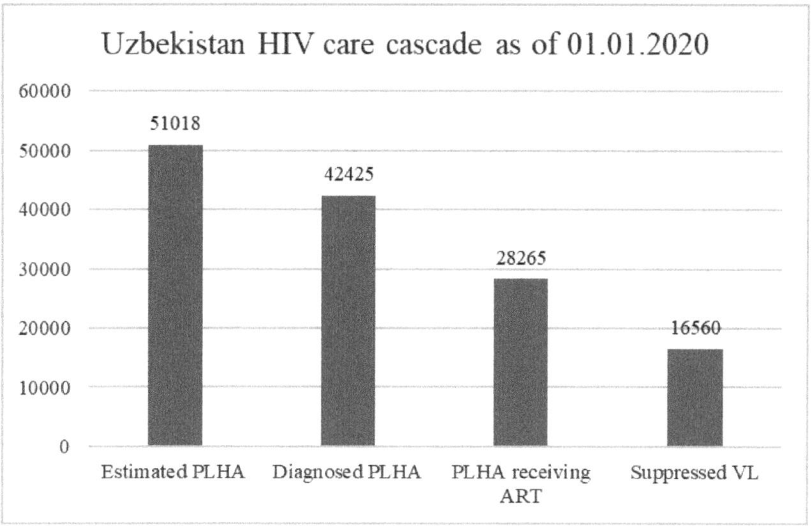

Figure 4: Uzbekistan HIV care cascade as of 01.01.2020

As the Uzbek government had indicated in its funding request to the GFATM, in 2020 the HIV care cascade in Uzbekistan was '83–67–59', demonstrating a major gap in reaching the declared targets with ART coverage at the level of 55% of PLHIV estimate (n=28,265). An increase in public funds allocated for this purpose within the framework of the adopted State Program to combat HIV infection facilitated an increase in the number of PLHIV who received treatment. The current HIV treatment protocol is based on 2019 WHO ART treatment guidelines, and according to the Ministry of Health, by 1st January 2022, ART had been provided in Uzbekistan to as many as 45,000 patients, of whom 74% were able to significantly lower their viral load levels (Ministry of Health of the Republic of Uzbekistan 2022).

All pregnant women on ART take ART during pregnancy and continue it after delivery and breastfeed their babies for at least 12 months, known as a B+ regimen.

Since 2014, PLHIV who are not able to personally visit the point of distribution of antiretroviral (ARV) drugs can receive drugs for up to three months through their authorised persons, provided they undertake the responsibility to regularly send the results of blood tests for CD-4 cells and viral load to their doctor, at their own expense. These tests are necessary to monitor the state of HIV infection and allow doctors to assess the extent of the impact of HIV infection on the body. This provision is intended to reduce the incidence of treatment interruption among individuals who travel outside the country for long periods and do not have access to ART in the destination countries (Ministry of Health of the Republic of Uzbekistan 2014). The provision of pre-exposure prophylaxis (PrEP) for discordant couples was started in mid-2019 and is now being planned for key populations (Uzbekistan's funding application to GFATM for 2020–2023).

Key Gaps in HIV Programming Targeting Migrants

1) Poor Preparation for Migration Leads to Increased HIV Vulnerability

It is typical for migrants from Central Asia to come to the Russian Federation, Kazakhstan, and Turkey without a clear understanding of the cost of living, registration requirements, employment conditions, opportunities for support, and access to healthcare. Female migrants in such circumstances are at high risk of becoming sex slaves, having unwanted pregnancies, and being denied sexual and reproductive health services (United Nations Population Fund [UNFPA] et al. 2021).

Although the Agency for Foreign Labour Migration is formally mandated to equip all Uzbek citizens with legal and healthcare-related information relevant to the country of destination, in reality only a fraction of migrants contact the Agency before their departure. For example, many LMs remain unaware of the importance and ways of obtaining a policy for Mandatory Medical Insurance when they migrate to the Russian Federation. Migrants lacking such a policy cannot benefit from the range of free healthcare services on offer, including antenatal and perinatal care (Uchaev et al. 2022).

2) Lack of HIV Prevention Programming That Is Specific to Labour Migrants' Needs

Despite the fact that LM have become the main driving force of the HIV epidemic in Uzbekistan, interventions targeting this population group are largely limited to HIV testing, with limited attention paid to HIV prevention. The lack of funding for NGO-led HIV prevention activities targeting migrants in Uzbekistan's within the largest AIDS programme funded by GFATM. LMs are not regarded as a key population with specific and multidimensional HIV-related needs, but as one that does not differ from the general population (Niginahon 2022). Although the new State Program to counteract HIV names LMs as one of the target groups, it is so far limited to HIV testing and awareness-raising as key responses to the problem, while leaving unaddressed other facets of this group's vulnerability to HIV infection such as stigma, discrimination, and access to healthcare services in the countries of migration.

3) Lack of Interventions Designed to Address the Needs of the Family Members of Migrants Who Are Left Behind

Labour migration is often associated with the separation of children from their parents. In such situations, Uzbek children are most often left with their grandparents or the families of uncles/aunts. Less frequently the children are entrusted to neighbours. In any case, children separated from their parents for extended time periods face an increased risk of emotional, physical, and sexual abuse. The Uzbek mass media regularly publishes articles and reports about such cases, which may take the form of sexual exploitation that may lead to homicides or suicides of victims of abuse (Central Asian News Service 2018; Kun.uz 2018). Irregularity of remittances sent back home may result in situations when children face several threats, ranging from reduced dietary diversity and limited access to medical services to child neglect and abuse (Murodova 2018; United Nations Children's Fund [UNICEF] 2019).

Elderly caregivers left behind by migrating family members encountered elevated levels of depression, loneliness, cognitive decline, and anxiety. Additionally, their psychological well-being, as indicated by scores, was comparatively lower compared with older parents who did not have migrant children (IOM 2020; Thapa et al. 2018).

4) Low Demand for HIV Testing among Labour Migrants

Whether in their home countries or their primary host nations such as Russia, Kazakhstan, or Turkey, LMs originating from Central Asia have access to HIV testing via ELISA (enzyme-linked immunosorbent assay) immunoassay tests and rapid diagnostic kits. Despite this availability, there is limited demand for HIV detection services among these migrants. This phenomenon suggests that LMs tend to underestimate the significance of the HIV issue and consequently do not assign high priority to undergoing testing. This perspective arises from the perception that testing does not yield immediate advantages, yet it holds the potential to engender issues linked to discrimination and deportation (UNFPA et al. 2021).

5) Limited Options for HIV Testing in Uzbekistan

While the number of HIV tests administered in Uzbekistan has demonstrated a consistent increase over time, the avenues available for individuals to ascertain their HIV status remain confined primarily to AIDS centres and other government-run healthcare establishments, as previously illustrated. Despite notable improvements in the infrastructure of private laboratories and the increasing inclination of the general populace towards seeking services from private clinics and labs, these private facilities are still not permitted to conduct HIV testing. NGOs offer rapid HIV testing but only as a joint activity conducted with medical staff members of AIDS centres, although community-led testing is recognised as a high-impact intervention and recommended to be prioritised in programmatic considerations (Wagner et al. 2023).

6) Interruptions of ART during Migration

As noted earlier, the Ministry of Health of Uzbekistan has taken an important measure to improve the adherence to ART of Uzbek PLHIV while they're working abroad by creating a mechanism to ensure they are supplied with ARV medications as needed. However, some migrants still discontinue ART for various reasons, including not being able to find a person who could receive medications from the respective AIDS centre and forward the new supplies to them abroad. Other patients discontinue ART in an attempt to hide their HIV status out of fear of being deported, as is practised in Russia (Uchaev et al. 2022; UNFPA et al. 2021).

7) Unaddressed Psychosocial Needs of Migrants with HIV

People with HIV have a significantly higher risk of depression and other mental disorders compared to persons without HIV infection (Vollmond et al. 2023), which is more evident in subpopulations of sexual minorities (White et al. 2022). Mental disturbances and a lack of specialist care to address these challenges negatively affect the quality of life of migrants and their adherence to their HIV treatment regimen. The REG report indicates that very few organisations in Uzbekistan have the capacity to offer mental health support to PLHIV who have migrated, including NGOs 'Istiqbolli Avlod', 'Ishonch va Khayot', and 'Nihol' (Uchaev et al. 2022).

8) Lack of Gender Sensitivity in HIV Interventions among Labour Migrants

Although the procedure for joint implementation of information-promoting measures for the prevention of HIV infection among groups with a high risk of HIV infection requires that all activities among migrants be carried out in accordance with national traditions and a mentality that includes differentiated approaches towards working with male and female populations, the documents that were available for this review did not provide any evidence that the gender difference of migrants is respected.

Moreover, it is questionable whether effective counselling before and after HIV testing is feasible in reality, given the fact that the majority of migrants are males whereas nearly 90% of nurses in the Uzbek health system are females (Statistical Agency under the President of the Republic of Uzbekistan 2023). The patriarchal nature of norms and traditions in Uzbekistan serves as an additional barrier for effective HIV counselling, excluding any discussions about sex with someone of the opposite sex who is not a spouse.

In cultures where it is socially acceptable for males to have multiple partners and access to sexual protection services, and where marital rape is not a crime but the norm, women are in a particularly vulnerable position (Niginahon 2022). Examples of such vulnerability are witnessed on a daily basis, when wives cannot refuse to have sex with their husbands who have returned home from abroad and are first required to undergo HIV testing.

9) Poor HIV Programming Targeting Internal Labour Migrants

Although the Uzbek government continuously scales up its efforts to control HIV among LMs, it obviously targets those who work abroad. At the same time, the labour market also involves migration within the country. Internal migrants, just like external ones, stay away from their families for extended periods of time and have an increased risk of contracting HIV by having unprotected sex with occasional partners or by using drugs. In support of this risk, a phylogenetic study conducted by Lebedev et al. (2022) challenges the assumption that the primary source of migrant-related HIV infections in Uzbekistan originates from LMs returning from abroad. Instead, the study points to the significance of in-country migration networks as a potential driver of HIV transmission (Lebedev et al. 2022).

10) Disconnect between In-Country HIV Interventions and Programmes Abroad

The review revealed the absence of funded cooperative activities between Uzbek and foreign governmental and non-governmental institutions aimed at preventing and treating HIV in the countries of migration. With the exception of sporadic social support provided by NGOs and the provision of ART medication being sent from Uzbek AIDS centres to PLHIV abroad, Uzbek LMs are largely disconnected from the HIV programming organised by the Uzbek government. In Russia, for example, migrants who test positive for HIV are deported, while those whose results are negative are left with access to no or only a minimum level of HIV prevention services. Having low access to HIV prevention services, poor HIV-related knowledge, and a lack of health and prevention-related information in their native language makes Uzbek migrants with deficient Russian language skills particularly vulnerable targets for blood-borne and sexually transmitted infections. Various sources suggest that up to a quarter of all Central Asian migrants in Russia do not speak any Russian at all, while more than half of them cannot fill in required forms in Russian (TASS Russian News Agency 2011).

Bibliography

Anonymous (2018): Procedure for joint implementation of information-promoting measures – measures for the prevention of HIV infection among groups with a high risk of HIV infection, in particular, migrants and their family members, as well as employees of beautician service institutions. Tashkent.

Association of Public Health Laboratories (2015): Limitations for use of HIV-1 Western blot in plasma/serum. www.aphl.org/aboutAPHL/publications/Documents/ID_HIV-1-1-WesternBlotBrief_62015.pdf, 06.03.2024.

Central Asian News Service (2018): In Andijan, a 60-year-old man is suspected of raping his 13-year-old niece and impregnating her. www.centralasian.org/a/29193204.html, 06.03.2024.

Drobyshevskaya, Elena V./Pronin, Alexander Y./Zhukova, Evgenia V./Sochnev, Alexey S./Vatulyan, Anush K./Terin, Dmitriy F. et al. (2022): HIV awareness among labor migrants from Central Asia States. In: Sociology and Management 8, No. 1, pp. 43–67. DOI: 10.18413/2408-9338-2022-8-1-0-5.

Gazeta.uz (2022): The annual increase in HIV-infected people in Uzbekistan has stabilized. www.gazeta.uz/ru/2022/12/01/hiv, 02.08.2023.

Igamberdiev, B.N. (2023): Data presented at a Round table: Cooperation within the framework of the implementation of Presidential Decree No. 14 "On measures to further strengthen systems for counteracting the disease caused by the human immunodeficiency virus", 09 June 2023. Tashkent.

International Organization for Migration (IOM) (2020): World Migration Report 2020. Geneva: IOM.

Korotkova, E.A./Klimashkin, A.A./Uchaev, S.S. (2021): Improvement of knowledge and skills consulting in the region reproductive health for women, living with HIV. www.plwh.uz/assets/doc/%D0%9F%D0%BE%D1%81%D0%BE%D0%B1%D0%B8%D0%B5%20%D0%92%D0%98%D0%A7%20(RU).pdf?v=c88be2e910, 02.08.2023.

Kun.uz (2018): An 11-year-old girl was raped and killed in Surkhandarya. www.kun.uz/news/2018/09/28/surhondareda-11-esli-kizca-zurlanib-uldirilgan, 06.03.2024.

Lebedev, Aleksey/Kuznetsova, Anna/Kim, Kristina/Ozhmegova, Ekaterina/Antonova, Anastasiia/Kazennova, Elena et al. (2022): Identifying HIV-1 Transmission Clusters in Uzbekistan through Analysis of Molecular Surveillance Data. In: Viruses 14, No. 8, p. 1675. DOI: 10.3390/v14081675.

LexUZ (2023): Comprehensive programme of measures for 2023–2027 to increase the effectiveness of combating the spread of HIV infection endorsed by the President's Executive Order [No. PK-14, 20 January 2023]. www.lex.uz/uz/docs/6364828#6365960, 06.03.2024.

Ministry of Health of the Republic of Uzbekistan (2014): Order of the Ministry of Health of the Republic of Uzbekistan. On standard operating procedures for managing the provision of antiretroviral drugs and diagnostics [No. 230, 05 July 2014]. Tashkent: Ministry of Health of the Republic of Uzbekistan.

Ministry of Health of the Republic of Uzbekistan (2022): Specialist: 74% of people receiving HIV treatment in our country have several times their viral load reduced [Telegram]. www.t.me/ssvuz/11540, 06.03.2024.

Ministry of Health of the Republic of Uzbekistan (2023): Узбекистон Республикасида ОИВ инфекциясини олдини олиш чора-тадбирлари ва тиббий ёрдамни ташкил этишни янада такомиллаштириш тугрисида, ССВ буйруғм №111, 19.05.2023.

Murodova, Sevilya (2018): Impact of Remittances and International Migration on Poverty in Central Asia: The cases of the Kyrgyz Republic, Tajikistan, and Uzbekistan. In: Journal of Applied Economics and Business Research 8, No. 1, pp. 38–56.

National Information-Analytical Center on Drug Control under the Cabinet of Ministers of Uzbekistan (NCDC) (2022): The Central Asian Region Information Bulletin on Drug-Related Situation for 2021. Tashkent: Baktria Press.

Niginakhon, S. (2022): Gender assessment of national responses to HIV in the Republic of Uzbekistan. National report. Geneva: The Joint United Nations Programme on HIV/AIDS (UNAIDS).

O'zbekiston Milliy Axborot Agentligi (UZA) (2022): In which regions of Uzbekistan is the incidence of AIDS increasing, or through what professions and industries can it be transmitted more? (+Video). www.uza.uz/posts/342809, 02.08.2023.

Open Data Portal (n.d.): 2-001-0265 People living with HIV. www.data.egov.uz/eng/data/610b90691a64fdd0373a8f7c, 02.08.2023.

Statistical Agency under the President of the Republic of Uzbekistan (2023): Health care. www.gender.stat.uz/uz/asosiy-ko-rsatkichlar/sog-liqni-saqlash, 06.03.2024.

TASS Russian News Agency (2011): More than 20 percent of migrants from Central Asia do not speak Russian, the Federal Migration Service reported. www.tass.ru/obschestvo/509885, 06.03.2024.

Thapa, Deependra K./Visentin, Denis/Kornhaber, Rachel/Cleary, Michelle (2018): Migration of adult children and mental health of older parents 'left behind': An integrative review. In: PLoS One 13, No. 10, p. e0205665. DOI: 10.1371/journal.pone.0205665.

Uchaev, Sergey/Abdullayeva, Oksana/Abdullaev, Shukhrat (2022): Assessment of access to medical services, care and health support for labor migrants living with HIV in the Republic of Uzbekistan. A research report. Commissioned by The Regional Expert Group (REG) on Migration and Health in Eastern Europe and Central Asia. www.migrationhealth.group/wp-content/uploads/2021/12/STUDY_Uzbekistan_RUS_FINAL.pdf, 06.03.2024.

United Nations Children's Fund (UNICEF) (2019): Study report on effects of migration on children of Uzbekistan. www.unicef.org/uzbekistan/en/reports/study-report-effects-migration-children-uzbekistan, 06.03.2024.

United Nations Population Fund (UNFPA)/International Organization for Migration (IOM)/The Joint United Nations Programme on HIV/AIDS (UNAIDS) (2021): Challenges of access to sexual and reproductive health and HIV services for internal migrants in Central Asian countries and international migrants from Central Asian countries in the Russian Federation, Kazakhstan, and Turkey during the COVID-19 pandemic. www.kazakhstan.unfpa.org/sites/default/files/pub-pdf/unfpa_eng_final.pdf, 06.03.2024.

Vollmond, Cecilie V./Tetens, Malte M./Paulsen, Fie W./Gerstoft, Jan/Kronborg, Gitte/Johansen, Isik S. et al. (2023): Risk of Depression in People With HIV: A nationwide population-based matched cohort study. In: Clinical Infectious Diseases 77, No. 11, pp. 1569–1577. DOI: 10.1093/cid/ciad415.

Wagner, Anjuli D./Njuguna, Irene N./Neary, Jillian/Lawley, Kendall A./Louden, Diana K.N./Tiwari, Ruchi et al. (2023): Demand creation for HIV testing services: A systematic review and meta-analysis. In: PLoS Med 20, No. 3, p. e1004169. DOI: 10.1371/journal.pmed.1004169.

White, Lucy C.J./Cooper, Max/Lawrence, David (2019): Mental illness and resilience among sexual and gender minority refugees and asylum seekers. In: British Journal of General Practice 69, No. 678, pp. 10–11. DOI: 10.3399/bjgp19X700349.

World Health Organization (WHO) (2021): Consolidated guidelines on HIV prevention, testing, treatment, service delivery and monitoring: recommendations for a public health approach. www.who.int/publications/i/item/9789240031593, 06.03.2024.

10. Analysis of Harm Reduction Programmes in HIV/AIDS Prevention in Kyrgyzstan: Experience, Problems, and Prospects

Tynchtyk Estebes uulu

Introduction

HIV/AIDS remains one of the most serious global threats to human health. This has a huge impact on the socio-economic development and demographic situation in different countries around the world. In recent decades, countries and international organisations have been actively working on the development and implementation of harm reduction programmes in the field of HIV prevention. Kyrgyzstan is no exception.

Kyrgyzstan emerged as one of the Central Asian countries most severely affected by the HIV epidemic. In this regard, the country is actively implementing measures and strategies aimed at preventing the spread of HIV-infection and improving public health. Harm reduction programmes are an important component of this strategy. They are a set of measures aimed at reducing the risk of HIV transmission among the most vulnerable population groups, such as people who inject drugs (PWID).

PWID are one of the most vulnerable population groups among those at risk of HIV-infection. They often face social isolation, stigmatisation, and the lack of access tohealth services. Despite the difficulties associated with this group, Kyrgyzstan is making active efforts to develop and implement harm reduction programmes for PWID. The purpose of these programmes is to prevent the spread of HIV among PWID.

Studying harm reduction programmes among PWID is not only relevant for Kyrgyzstan. It is also important for the global community in the context of the overall efforts to combat the HIV epidemic. Harm reduction programmes embody a comprehensive approach, which includes sociological, medical, and social components. An important aspect of this work is the use of sociological methods and theories. They provide a deeper understanding of the social processes associated with the spread of HIV/AIDS and the implementation of relevant programmes.

Discussion

Harm reduction is an approach or strategy aimed at reducing the negative effects of drug use, rather than eradicating drug use (Hilton et al. 2001, p. 358). In other words, harm reduction approaches focus on reducing the negative effects of certain behavioural practices, instead of banning them altogether. In terms of drug use, the main idea is the recognition that drug use cannot be completely eradicated. A more realistic and effective approach would be to reduce the harmful effects of drug use.

According to the theory of social innovation, harm reduction programmes are good examples of social innovations in the field of HIV prevention. Social innovation refers to innovative activities and services. These are often implemented by organisations or groups that are motivated to meet the identified needs of the community or population (Yang et al. 2020, p. 69). In other words, harm reduction programmes are designed to reduce the risk of transmission of HIV and other infections through intravenous drug use.

In Kyrgyzstan, examples of measures related to harm reduction theory and social innovation theory are methadone maintenance treatment (MMT) and syringe/needle exchange points (SEPs).

MMT has been implemented in Kyrgyzstan since 2002. This treatment, which uses methadone hydrochloride, is aimed at PWID. MMT is a carefully researched and scientifically based medical intervention used to treat opioid addiction (AIDS Foundation East West [AFEW] Kyrgyzstan 2019, p. 20). Based on current research (World Health Organization [WHO] 2015) in the field of treatment and prevention of opioid dependence, it can be argued that the combination of MMT and psychological support is an effective method to reduce the illegal use of psychoactive substances. Moreover, an effective harm reduction strategy also leads to a reduction in criminal behaviour and an improvement in the social adaptation of clients (AFEW Kyrgyzstan 2019, p. 20).

It is often the case that people suffering from drug use commit crimes in order to obtain ressources to purchase psychoactive substances. However, MMT combined with psychological support solves this and other problems for clients. First, it reduces the motivation to commit crimes, as clients gain access to methadone. Second, it helps clients to reintegrate into society and rebuild family and other social relations. Third, consultations with psychologists and therapists help clients to develop strategies to deal with stress, solve problems related to addiction, and improve their psychological and emotional well-being.

Sustainable financing is crucial for HIV control and ensuring public participation (Yang et al. 2020, p. 73). MMT was introduced in Kyrgyzstan in 2002 with the financial support of the Soros Foundation-Kyrgyzstan and the United Nations Development Programme (UNDP). Furthermore, since 2005, methadone sites have been funded by the Global Fund (AFEW Kyrgyzstan 2019, p. 21). On the one hand, an important aspect of the implementation of harm reduction programmes is cooperation with international organisations and foundations to maintain the level of funding and exchange best practices. On the other hand, it is also important for the country to work on strengthening national health and social care systems. Kyrgyzstan should strive to develop its own internal sources of financing for harm reduction programmes.

As mentioned above, in the context of the withdrawal of donors from the country, there is a need to convey to government officials the importance of supporting harm reduction programmes financed by the state budget. In this regard, the non-governmental organisation (NGO) 'Socium' is an active advocate for the sustainability of programmes for PWID and other vulnerable groups. It also works to mobilise and involve representatives of key communities in the development, implementation, and management of harm reduction programmes at the country level (Eurasian Harm Reduction Association [EHRA] 2017).

In Kyrgyzstan, MMT clients can undergo treatment with methadone both in the civil sector and in the prison system. They can switch from one type of treatment to another (Ivasiy et al. 2022) in case of imprisonment or release from prison.

MMT is used only in the medical institutions of the Ministry of Health of Kyrgyzstan – Republican Center of Psychiatry and Narcology (RCPN) and the State Penitentiary Service (SPS) (see Table 1).

Overall, from 2016 to 2020, the number of MMT sites decreased from 29 to 24. A significant decrease can be observed in the civil sector – RCPN (see Table 1). During the specified period, a number of MMT sites were combined, resulting in five fewer sites in total.

As of 1st October 2023, 24 MMT sites are still functioning in Kyrgyzstan (Republican Center of Psychiatry and Narcology [RCPN] 2023). 15 sites of these sites are in the civil sector and nine are located in the country's prison system.

Table 1: The number of RCPN and SPS methadone sites in Kyrgyzstan in 2016–2020 (EHRA 2021)

	2016	2017	2018	2019	2020
RCPN	20	19	15	15	15
SPS	9	10	9	9	9
Number of MMT sites – total	29	29	24	24	24

Despite the fact that MMT is carried out only by the state, it is important to note the role of NGOs in the field of HIV prevention. Over time, a powerful coalition of NGOs has been established in Kyrgyzstan. These NGOs have promoted, advocated, and implemented harm reduction programmes. MMT works effectively in the country, thanks to the strong coalition of NGOs. For example, the NGO 'Socium' was one of the first NGOs to implement and develop harm reduction programmes in Kyrgyzstan. This NGO has extensive experience in providing HIV prevention services to PWID (EHRA 2017).

The operation of SEPs is a structural component of Kyrgyzstan's harm reduction strategy. At the SEPs, prevention work is carried out among PWID. The main purpose of the SEPs is to prevent the spread of HIV infection and other infections transmitted by injection and sexually among PWID. Another goal of the SEPs is to involve key population groups in medical and social assistance programmes (AFEW Kyrgyzstan 2019, p. 19).

As in the case of MMT, the tasks of SEPs are related not only to the prevention of HIV infection but also to the provision of medical and social assistance to clients. First, SEPs deal with the exchange/distribution of used syringes/needles for sterile ones. Second, SEPs provide PWID with information on HIV infection prevention, including ways to minimise the health risks associated with substance use. Third, SEPs refer clients to medical and social services, providing specialist advice. Fourth, SEPs conduct pre-test and post-test counselling and organise access to testing for HIV and other infections (RCPN 2014).

SEPs in Kyrgyzstan operate in the RCPN, the SPS, and NGOs. However, it is worth noting that the number of SEPs has been decreasing every year (see Table 2).

Table 2: The number of SEPs in the RCPN, SPS, and NGOs in Kyrgyzstan in 2016–2020 (EHRA 2021)

	2016	**2017**	**2018**	**2019**	**2020**
RCPN	11	11	6	6	6
SPS	13	13	12	11	11
NGOs	12	12	11	8	7
Number of SEPs – total	36	36	29	25	24

According to the statistics, the total number of SEPs in Kyrgyzstan decreased from 36 in 2016 to 24 in 2020. A significant decrease in SEPs can be observed in the RCPN and NGOs. During the specified period, the number of SEPs decreased by five units in both of these sectors. In the SPS, the number of SEPs decreased by two units, or from 13 in 2016 to 11 in 2020. The reason for the decline is due to a decrease in funding from the Global Fund (EHRA 2021, p. 25).

Since the introduction of harm reduction programmes, NGOs have been engaged in the implementation of SEPs with the support of various donors (Global Fund, Soros Foundation, UNDP, etc.) (EHRA 2021, p. 18).

There is a SEP in the city of Osh, in NGO 'Roditeli protiv narkotikov' ('Parents against drugs'). In addition to issuing syringes and needles, the NGO conducts rapid HIV testing on saliva, provides social support services to clients, and distributes condoms and information materials. Clients can also get advice on HIV and safe behaviour (Osh Silk Road Provider 2024).

The Eurasian Harm Reduction Association (EHRA) notes that NGO-run SEPs reached 2.5 times more clients than government-based SEPs. Also, based on the feedback received from the clients, the range of services was wider in NGO-run SEPs compared to government service providers and clients were more satisfied. Clients reported that NGO approach was more holistic and less stigmatising (EHRA 2021, p. 25).

The EHRA additionally notes that in 2021, following the results of the country-by-country discussion of the agreement with the Global Fund for 2021–2023, the SEPs in Kyrgyzstan were implemented only in five NGOs. It is important to note a significant reduction in the number of NGOs that are involved in the implementation of programmes for PWID. Perhaps this is due to the quality of reporting required by donor organisations and the fact that NGOs are often focused mainly on the provision of services, rather than on the preparation of project documents, applications, and reports (EHRA 2021, p. 55).

Thus, harm reduction programmes provide an important foundation for combating the spread of HIV/AIDS in Kyrgyzstan and contribute to improving public health. Harm reduction programmes such as MMT and SEPs reduce the risk of HIV transmission. They provide access to testing and treatment services and help reduce stigma and discrimination. It is also important to note that the effectiveness of harm reduction programmes is closely related to sociological aspects, sociocultural factors, and interaction with society.

It is noted that adequate methadone coverage in areas where the HIV epidemic is concentrated among PWID is the most effective HIV control strategy, as well as the most cost-effective (Ivasiy et al. 2022). PWID are most vulnerable to HIV transmission due to the exchange of injecting supplies and low awareness of prevention methods.

According to the theory of social differentiation and discrimination, society differentiates and discriminates against people based on drug addiction. They may be stigmatised and alienated in society. This leads to poor health and well-being among PWID (Couto E Cruz et al. 2020). Moreover, access to healthcare and harm reduction programmes can often be limited due to discrimination by healthcare professionals.

In Kyrgyzstan, the following sociocultural factors influence the spread of HIV/AIDS among PWID. First, the low level of education about HIV/AIDS affects the ability of key groups to make informed decisions and comply with preventive measures. Second, social stigma and discrimination create barriers to access to services and information, as well as discourage those in need from seeking help. Third, low income leads to limited access to medical care and preventive measures.

Consequently, the population group most at risk of HIV transmission is PWID. Moreover, sociocultural factors have a significant impact on the spread of HIV/AIDS in Kyrgyzstan. Differentiation, stigmatisation, and discrimination can create barriers to access to harm reduction services and educational programmes.

Next, we will look at how harm reduction programmes in Kyrgyzstan affect the spread of HIV in the country. The effectiveness of MMT and SEPs will be evaluated using official statistics on the spread of HIV. When it comes to HIV prevention in Kyrgyzstan, harm reduction programmes are crucial for combating the spread of HIV infection and improving the health of vulnerable population groups. As official statistics show, over the past 15 years – from 2008 to 2022 – Kyrgyzstan has managed to significantly reduce the parenteral (when injecting drugs) pathway of HIV transmission (see Figure 1).

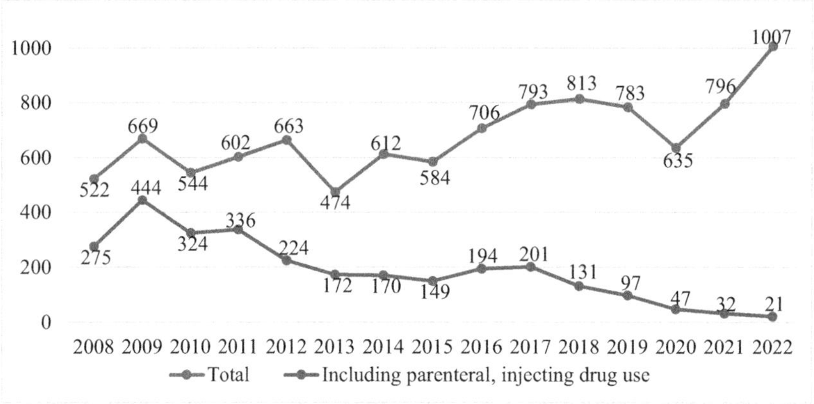

Figure 1: Ways of HIV transmission in the Kyrgyz Republic in 2008–2022 (people) – total cases and parenteral (injecting drug use) cases (AIDS Center Kyrgyzstan 2023)

In 2009, 444 cases of parenteral transmission of HIV infection were detected, which is a record high within the last 15 years. At the same time, the share of the parenteral route of transmission through injecting drug use amounted to 66.4% of all HIV transmission cases – 444 of 669 cases. By 2017, the share of the parenteral route of HIV transmission was reduced to 25.3% or 201 of 793 cases. Since 2018, a sharp decrease in the proportion of HIV transmission through injecting drug use can be seen, going from 16.1% (131 cases) in 2018 to 2.1% (21 cases) in 2022.

In general, in 2008–2022, new HIV cases among PWID and the route of HIV transmission through injecting drug use both significantly decreased in Kyrgyzstan (see Figure 2).

Due to the measures taken in the country, there has been a significant decrease in the number of cases of HIV transmission through injection routes (Kyrgyz Republic Ministry of Justice 2022). This significant reduction in HIV transmission over the past 15 years among PWID indicates that harm reduction programmes in the country are being implemented effectively. This indicates shows the positive impact these programmes have on reducing the incidence of HIV. Data analysis confirms that successful harm reduction programmes in Kyrgyzstan have a positive impact on the target audience, which indicates the important role they play in HIV prevention.

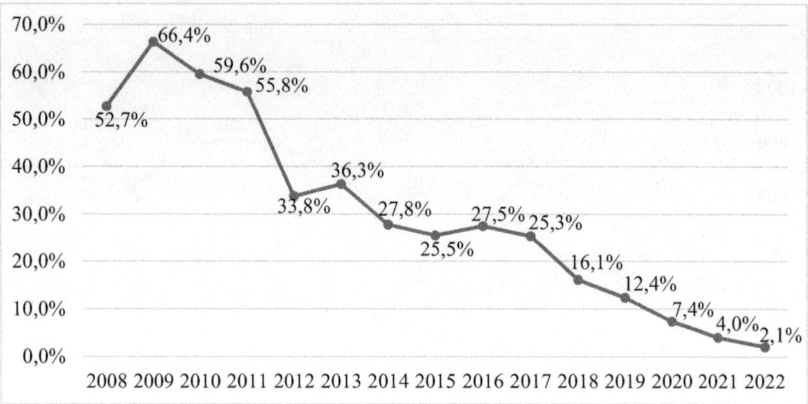

Figure 2: The share of HIV transmission through injecting drug use in the Kyrgyz Republic in 2008–2022 out of the total cases (%) (AIDS Center Kyrgyzstan 2023)

Harm reduction programmes also contribute to an increase in the number of PWID who seek out HIV testing and counselling. Statistics show that the level of rapid HIV testing among PWID has been quite high over the past five years. In 2018, 31,427 tests were conducted among PWID; in 2019, 21,618 tests; in 2020, 14,631 tests; in 2021, 18,953 tests; and in 2022, 16,507 tests (AIDS Center Kyrgyzstan 2023). Rapid HIV testing can be carried out in NGOs. In general, there are more than 30 NGOs in Kyrgyzstan where clients can take rapid HIV saliva testing (Republican Center for Control of Bloodborne Viral Hepatitis and Human Immunodeficiency Virus of the Ministry of Health of the Kyrgyz Republic 2024).

Thus, harm reduction programmes in Kyrgyzstan are effective tools in combating the spread of HIV/AIDS. An analysis of the effectiveness of harm reduction programmes shows that they have the potential to reduce the spread of HIV/AIDS and improve the health of vulnerable population groups. Despite the positive results, challenges and problems remain. In order to achieve even greater success in HIV prevention in the country, the remaining challenges and problems must be addressed and the programmes must be improved further still.

Despite the outstanding achievements in harm reduction among prisoners, there are a number of prisons that are not yet involved in harm reduction programmes. Moreover, temporary detention facilities of law enforcement agencies also do not have a system for providing important services such as MMT and antiretroviral therapy (Kyrgyz Republic Ministry of Justice 2022).

It is noted that for those who take methadone in the civil sector and end up in prison, treatment may be suspended if they are placed in prisons where there is no methadone (Ivasiy et al. 2022). When it comes to harm reduction programmes, it is important to ensure the uninterrupted receipt of MMT services. In this regard, it is necessary to ensure access to methadone for patients who are either released from prison or incarcerated in prison.

The theory of stigmatisation in the context of drug use shows that stigmatisation can come from various sources, including drug users themselves, their family members, medical professionals, and law enforcement officials (Romanyuk 2018). In other words, these different groups can contribute to the formation of negative stereotypes and bias against drug users.

It is noted that in Kyrgyzstan, people who participate in MMT face negative attitudes and stigmatisation from medical workers, prisoners and family members (Liberman et al. 2022). Other authors note that in Kyrgyzstan, PWID face a huge number of obstacles, both in prison and after release in society. The main issues are stigmatisation, poor job prospects, limited access to medical care, punitive drug policy, and harassment by law enforcement agencies (Bachireddy et al. 2022).

At the same time, it is noted that the increased activity of law enforcement agencies against participants in harm reduction programmes, including MMT and SEPs, creates barriers to access to drug treatment (Kyrgyz Republic Ministry of Justice 2022).

As noted, PWID may be concerned about the stigma associated with taking methadone or feel insecure about their ability to easily access methadone (Bachireddy et al. 2022). It is important to note that Biernacki recognised that social stigma is a serious obstacle that recovering drug users must overcome if they want to stop using drugs and change their lives (Neale et al. 2011, p. 3).

Social stigma can create physical, emotional, and psychological barriers, which makes the recovery process even more difficult. For example, encountering social stigma can cause confusion and fear among drug users. This may hinder their willingness to seek help or share their concerns.

Negative societal attitudes and social isolation can increase the levels of stress, depression, and low self-esteem among drug users. Due to fear of discrimination, drug users may refuse access to treatment, harm reduction, and psychological support services. Social stigma is a serious obstacle to the recovery and rehabilitation of drug users. This understanding is an important step in the fight against drug addiction. It helps to better develop effective strategies to support this group.

Kyrgyzstan has accomplished significant achievements in harm reduction among prisoners and people facing drug addiction. Despite this, Kyrgyzstan faces serious challenges in providing access to necessary medical and supportive services. The expansion of harm reduction programmes, the elimination of stigma, and cooperation between different sectors of society are key steps to improve the situation for drug users in the country. It is necessary to strive to ensure uninterrupted access to harm reduction and drug treatment for all, regardless of their status and location. This contributes to the health and well-being of key populations.

Resolution No. 445 of the Cabinet of Ministers of the Kyrgyz Republic dated 10th August 2022 approved the Anti-drug Program of the Cabinet of Ministers of the Kyrgyz Republic for 2022–2026 in order to reduce dependence on psychoactive substances (Kyrgyz Republic Ministry of Justice 2022).

In order to reduce harm from illegal psychoactive substances in the field of harm reduction, the state set the task of continuing to expand harm reduction programmes (Kyrgyz Republic Ministry of Justice 2022), since the harm reduction strategy has shown its effectiveness in practice.

Moreover, the task is to ensure access to services aimed at reducing harm from the use of psychoactive substances in all penitentiary institutions, including temporary detention facilities, pre-trial detention facilities, and correctional institutions. Harm reduction services include counselling, provision of sterile syringes and needles, and access to MMT (Kyrgyz Republic Ministry of Justice 2022).

In the community, educating family and community members about the use and benefits of methadone can be useful to reduce the stigma associated with methadone and those involved in MMT (Liberman et al. 2022).

Based on the analysis of harm reduction programmes in HIV prevention in Kyrgyzstan, several key perspectives and recommendations can be identified. They can contribute to improving existing programmes and planning future activities in this area.

First, harm reduction programmes should be more tailored to the specific needs and characteristics of vulnerable populations. Second, programmes should actively include elements of education and information campaigns aimed at mitigating stigma and discrimination against HIV/AIDS. Third, it is important to actively involve society and NGOs in the development and implementation of harm reduction programmes. Fourth, it is recommended to integrate harm reduction programmes into the overall health and social care system. This will help ensure more efficient use of resources and reduce barriers to access to services. Fifth, it is important to actively share experiences with other countries and regions where successful harm reduction programmes exist. A comparative analysis will identify best practices and be helpful in adapting these best practices to local conditions.

Conclusion

The analysis of harm reduction programmes in the field of HIV prevention among PWID in Kyrgyzstan underlines the importance of a sociological approach for studying and improving the effectiveness of these programmes. The study highlighted a number of key aspects that are crucial for improving the response to HIV/AIDS in Kyrgyzstan.

Harm reduction programmes – MMT and SEPs, which provide information on safe drug use – contribute to reducing the spread of HIV among PWID. Because of this, the programmes have a positive impact on public health. Furthermore, harm reduction programmes promote the social integration of PWID. They provide access to medical care and risk reduction advice, and also support community participation. This helps to reduce HIV-related stigma and discrimination.

In general, harm reduction programmes in the field of HIV prevention among PWID play an important role in maintaining health and reducing the risk of infection in Kyrgyzstan. The prospects for the development and improvement of such programmes should remain the focus of national and international efforts to combat HIV/AIDS in this vulnerable population.

Bibliography

AIDS Center Kyrgyzstan (2023): The situation of HIV infection in the Kyrgyz Republic as of 01.01.23. www.aidscenter.kg/wp-content/uploads/2023/03/01.01.2023.pdf, 03.10.2023.

AIDS Foundation East West (AFEW) Kyrgyzstan (2019): Assessment of the implementation of the Instruction "On the prevention of HIV infection by authorized state bodies of internal affairs, drug control and penal enforcement of the Kyrgyz Republic, interacting with key groups". The UNDP/Global Fund project "Effective control of tuberculosis and HIV infection in the Kyrgyz Republic". www.afew.kg/wp-content/uploads/2023/06/analitichesky-otchet-2019.pdf, 11.03.2024.

Bachireddy, Chethan/Shrestha, Roman/Bromberg, Daniel J./Azbel, Lyu/Kurmanalieva, Ainura/Wegman, Martin et al. (2022): Methadone within prison and linkage to and retention in treatment upon community release for people with opioid use disorder in Kyrgyzstan: Evaluation of a national program. In: International Journal of Drug Policy 101, p. 103558.

Couto E Cruz, Camila/Salom, Caroline/Parsell, Cameron/Dietze, Paul/Burns, Lucinda/Alati, Rosa (2020): Social domains of discrimination against people who inject drugs: Links with health and wellbeing. In: International Journal of Drug Policy 77, p. 102620.

Eurasian Harm Reduction Association (EHRA) (2017): Interview: civil society participation in decision-making processes to respond to the HIV epidemic in Kyrgyzstan. www.eecaplatform.org/intervyu-uchastie-go-v-protsessah-prinyatiya-resheniy-po-otvetu-na-epidemiyu-vich-v-kyirgyizstane/, 12.01.2024.

Eurasian Harm Reduction Association (EHRA) (2021): Changes in the Harm Reduction Packages and Unit Costs during Transition from International to Domestic Funding among Selected Countries of EECA Region. Based on the Experience of North Macedonia, Georgia, Ukraine, and the Kyrgyz Republic. Vilnius: EHRA.

Hilton, Ann B./Thompson, Ray/Moore-Dempsey, Laura/Janzen, Randy G. (2001): Harm reduction theories and strategies for control of human immunodeficiency virus: a review of the literature. In: Journal of Advanced Nursing 33, No. 3, pp. 357–370.

Ivasiy, Roman/Madden, Lynn M./Farnum, Scott O./Shumskaya, Natalia/Galvez de Leon, Samy J./Bromberg, Daniel J. et al. (2022): Implementation opportunities for scaling up methadone maintenance treatment in Kyrgyzstan: Methadone dosage and retention on treatment over two years. In: Drug and Alcohol Dependence Reports 4, p. 100075.

Kyrgyz Republic Ministry of Justice (2022): Anti-drug Program of the Cabinet of Ministers of the Kyrgyz Republic [No. 445, 10 August 2022]. www.cbd.minjust.gov.kg/act/view/ru-ru/159421?cl=ru-ru, 05.10.2023.

Liberman, Amanda R./Bromberg, Daniel J./Litz, Taylor/Kurmanalieva, Ainura/Galvez, Samy/Rozanova, Julia et al. (2022): Interest without uptake: A mixed-methods analysis of methadone utilization in Kyrgyz prisons. In: Plos one 17, No. 10, p. e0276723.

Neale, Joanne/Nettleton, Sarah/Pickering, Lucy (2011): Recovery from problem drug use: What can we learn from the sociologist Erving Goffman? In: Drugs: Education, Prevention and Policy 18, No. 1, pp. 3–9.

Osh Silk Road Provider (2024): Non-governmental organizations providing services for people living with HIV. www.med-osh.org.kg/npo/#, 12.01.2024.

Republican Center for Control of Bloodborne Viral Hepatitis and Human Immunodeficiency Virus of the Ministry of Health of the Kyrgyz Republic (2024): Non-governmental organizations (NGOs) that conduct rapid HIV testing. www.aidscenter.kg/gde-mozhno-projti-testirovanie/?lang=ru, 12.01.2024.

Republican Center of Psychiatry and Narcology (RCPN) (2014): Standards for the implementation of harm reduction programs and the provision of services to injecting drug users. Bishkek: RCPN.

Republican Center of Psychiatry and Narcology (RCPN) (2023): Healthcare organizations of the Kyrgyz Republic, on the basis of which MMT is provided. www.rcn.kg/contact, 01.10.2023.

Romanyuk, Y.V. (2018): The Problem of Social Stigma toward Persons with Drug and Psychotropic Substances Addiction and their Analogues. In: Bulletin of the Brest University, No. 1, pp. 164–169.

World Health Organization (WHO) (2015): Evaluation of opioid substitution therapy in the Kyrgyz Republic. www.rcpn.kg/2022/12/18/оценка-опиоидной-заместительной-тер/, 11.03.2024.

Yang, Fang/Janamnuaysook, Rena/Boyd, Mark A./Phanuphak, Nittaya/Tucker, Joseph D. (2020): Key populations and power: people-centred social innovation in Asian HIV services. In: The Lancet HIV 7, No. 1, pp. e69–e74.

11. Media Portrayal and Stigma: Analysing HIV/AIDS Coverage in Uzbekistan's Press

Uladzimir Pikirenia

Introduction

The media plays a powerful role in shaping public perceptions of HIV/AIDS (Aghaei et al. 2023). However, media representations of HIV/AIDS are often inaccurate and stigmatising. These representations can have a negative impact on the lives of people living with HIV, making it more difficult for them to access the services they need and leading to social isolation and discrimination (Jaspal/Nerlich 2022; Vaughan/Power 2023). Stigma has been driven by societal beliefs about the severity and contagiousness of HIV, perceptions that people who acquire HIV are blameworthy, and associations between HIV and behaviours that violate some individuals' behaviour variations, such as sex between men, having multiple partners, drug use, and sex work (Stutterheim et al. 2022). These stereotypes can have a devastating impact on the lives of people living with HIV. They can lead to social isolation, discrimination, and even violence. There are different national and international guidelines (mostly in developed countries) for media who report on HIV ('Guidelines for Reporting HIV. Advice for editors and journalists writing about HIV in the UK', National AIDS Trust [NAT] 2010; 'Media Reporting Guidelines – HIV', HIV Ireland n.d.; 'New guidelines for media reporting on HIV in India', The Joint United Nations Programme on HIV/AIDS [UNAIDS] 2008). These policies are designed to promote accurate and respectful reporting and to avoid stigmatising people living with HIV. However, media in developing countries still frequently use hate speech and stigma and have a lack of competency in reporting on HIV. This can result in a number of negative consequences, discouraging people from seeking testing and treatment, increasing perpetuating stigma and discrimination, and undermining public health efforts.

Uzbekistan Context

According to the national data, approximately 48,000 registered people were living with HIV in Uzbekistan in 2023 (KUN.UZ 2023) and according to UNAIDS estimated data, the number of people living with HIV (PLHIV) was 54,000 (UNAIDS 2020). The HIV epidemic in Uzbekistan seems to be stabilising at approximately 3,000 new cases per year, but key populations, including men who have sex with men (MSM), people who inject drugs, and sex workers, remain at risk (Gazeta.uz 2022). These populations are at increased risk of HIV infection due to many factors, including stigma, discrimination, and lack of access to prevention and care services.

HIV/AIDS is criminalised in Uzbekistan. Article 113 of the Criminal Code penalises the intentional transmission of HIV/AIDS with up to eight years in prison. This law has been used to target and prosecute PLHIV, even when there is no evidence of intentional transmission. Sexual work is subject to administrative sanctions, although clients face no penalties (UzTAG Uzbek Telegraph Agency 2019), and MSM are still considered criminal in Uzbekistan, according to Article 120 of the current criminal code (Human Rights Watch 2021): 'satisfying the sexual needs of a man with a man without violence is punishable by restriction of freedom from one year to three years or imprisonment for up to three years' (Criminal Code of the Republic of Uzbekistan, LexUZ n.d.). These laws create a climate of stigma and discrimination, making it difficult for key populations to access the prevention and care services they need.

This study will examine how HIV/AIDS is represented in the Uzbek media and analyse Uzbek media coverage of HIV/AIDS in order to explore the frequency and nature of the coverage, as well as the style used to represent HIV/AIDS.

Short Results

The research highlights the media's role in shaping public perceptions of HIV/AIDS, which are often stigmatised and inaccurate. The findings reveal that approximately 45% of the media coverage contained stigmatising language, particularly towards women and sex workers, while only 5.1% presented anti-stigmatising views. Neutral reporting, consisting mainly of statistical information, accounted for 52.6% of the articles. The study also notes a significant lack of information on HIV prophylaxis and prevention methods, with no coverage of blood transmission prevention and only a minimal focus on sexual transmission prevention. Incorrect use of HIV/AIDS terms was found in 17.9% of the articles. The study calls for media reform to ensure accurate, respectful, and stigma-free coverage of HIV/AIDS, emphasising the need for guidelines for journalists in Uzbekistan and the establishment of ethical reporting standards. It also advocates for policy changes, particularly the decriminalisation of HIV transmission and the cessation of gender-biased legal practices, to improve the lives of people living with HIV and enhance the efficacy of HIV prevention and care services in Uzbekistan.

Methods

We analysed all the publications of the 14 most popular media outlets in Uzbekistan from 1st November 2022 to 31st October 2023. There is a list of the 15 most popular media outlets according to The Nationwide Movement Yuksalish (2023). However, one media outlet from the list (www.azon.uz) was closed in the summer and is no longer available, so we excluded it from the analysis. The web pages of most media do not have user-friendly interfaces to search for old publications, so we used official Telegram channels because they are easier to search through. We used the Russian version of official channels if they had one, or the Uzbek version if they didn't.

We searched for articles with the keywords "ВИЧ" (HIV) and "СПИД" (AIDS) in Russian, and "ОИВ" (HIV) and "ОИТС" (AIDS) in Uzbek. Then we manually checked the content and excluded non-relevant articles. We found 78 relevant articles.[1]

Based on the content of the articles, we constructed a table that presents a summary of the number of articles that we defined as follows: a) articles that are stigmatising; b) articles that are anti-stigmatising; c) articles that provide only statistical (neutral) information; d) articles that provide information about effective prevention measures that should be taken to avoid HIV transmission (including but not limited to condom use, harm reduction, and other activities for key populations); and e) articles that contain incorrect usage of HIV/AIDS terms.

1 A full list of the articles we analysed, including their headlines and a summary, can be found here: www.osf.io/ahf78/files/osfstorage/6548e3bc253a740383a0e3ff (for ease of comprehension, content in Uzbek has been translated into Russian).

Articles were deemed stigmatising if they shamed people living with HIV or humiliated the dignity of any group of individuals. Articles were deemed anti-stigmatising if they contained accurate data, demonstrated vulnerabilities, and facilitated a better understanding of an individual's suffering. Articles were deemed neutral if they only contained statistical information. Example of a stigmatising headline: 'A girl who infected more than 20 men with AIDS was jailed for only three years'. Example of an anti-stigmatising headline: 'HIV and status disclosure: is it easy to live with a "hidden face"?' Example of incorrect use of HIV or AIDS terms: 'A 21-year-old girl in Bukhara deliberately infected three men with AIDS'.

Results

Table 1: Media resources and their articles on HIV/AIDS topics

Media (language: Russian or Uzbek)	N of articles, n	Stigmatising, n (%), group[1]	Anti-stigmatising, n (%)	Neutral (statistical info), n (%)	HIV prophylaxis (sexual trans-mission), n (%)	HIV prophylaxis (blood trans-mission), n (%)	Incorrect usage HIV/ AIDS, n (%)
Kun.uz (Rus.)	6	0	1 (16.7)	5 (83.3)	1 (16.7)	0	0
Qalampir.uz (Uz.)	5	2 (40), SW-women	0	3 (60)	1 (20)		1 (20)
gazeta.uz (Rus.)	5	2 (40), SW-women	0	3 (60)	0		0
daryo.uz (Rus.)	3	1 (33.3), SW-women	0	2 (67.7)	0		0
podrobno.uz (Rus.)	4	2 (50), SW-women	1 (25)	1 (25)	0	0	0
uznews.uz (Rus.)	2	2 (100), SW-women, women	0	0	0	0	2 (100)
repost.uz (Rus.)	11	6 (54.5), SW-women, women, men	0	4 (36.3)	1 (9.1)	0	3 (27.3)
xabar.uz (Uz.)	7	5 (71.4), SW-women	0	2 (28.6)	0	0	4 (57.1)
nova24.uz (Rus.)	11	7 (63.6), women	0	4 (36.4)	0	0	3 (27.3)

Media (language: Russian or Uzbek)	N of articles, n	Stigmatising, n (%), group[1]	Anti-stigma-tising, n (%)	Neutral (statis-tical info), n (%)	HIV prophylaxis (sexu-al trans-mission), n (%)	HIV prophylaxis (blood trans-mis-sion), n (%)	Incorrect us-age HIV/ AIDS, n (%)
nuz.uz (Rus.)	4	1 (25), women	0	3 (75)	0	0	0
aniq.uz (Uz.)	10	3 (30), women	0	7 (70)	1 (10)	0	1 (10)
darakchi.uz (Rus.)	7	4 (57.1), women	2 (28,6)	1 (14.3)	0	0	0
rost24.uz	0	-	-	-	-	-	-
uza.uz (Rus.)	3	0	0	3 (100)	0	0	0
Total	78	35 (44.9)	4 (5.1)	41 (52.6)	4 (5.1)	0	14 (17.9)

[1] SW-women = women involved in sex work

The analysis of the 78 relevant articles from the 14 most popular media outlets in Uzbekistan revealed a significant presence of stigmatising content. Approximately 45% of articles were defined as stigmatising, particularly towards women (in general) and sex workers. Only a small fraction, 5.1%, presented anti-stigmatising views. Neutral reporting, which primarily included statistical information, accounted for 52.6% of the coverage. Preventive measures against sexual transmission of HIV were mentioned in 5.1% of articles, while no coverage was given to blood transmission prevention methods. Incorrect usage of HIV/AIDS terms was found in 17.9% of the articles.

Examples of articles with stigmatising language: 'One more woman in Bukhara was convicted of deliberately infecting others with HIV. It was established that a 30-year-old woman living in the Romitan district of the Bukhara region deliberately infected others with HIV'; 'A 21-year-old woman was caught while travelling from Andijan to Bukhara and infected men with AIDS. The number of people infected with HIV due to contact with them is increasing'; 'In Bukhara, a young woman has been detained, despite being HIV-positive, she repeatedly engaged in sexual relations with various men'.

Examples of incorrect usage of HIV/AIDS terms: 'She had sex with men for a pin money and hid her illness from her partners. During investigation, it became known that more than twenty men were deliberately infected with AIDS'; 'A man was found in Bukhara who deliberately infected a woman with AIDS'; 'The list of professions prohibited for people with AIDS is being updated'.

Discussion

The media's portrayal of HIV/AIDS in Uzbekistan not only shapes public opinion but also reflects and potentially reinforces the stigma associated with the disease. A particularly troubling aspect of the media coverage is the emphasis on the criminal penalties faced by women under Article 113 of the Criminal Code, which penalises the transmission of HIV/AIDS. The media materials frequently highlight cases where women are prosecuted, even though: 1) the majority of registered HIV-positive individuals in Uzbekistan are men; 2) the overall number of people convicted in 2020 under Article 113 of the Criminal Code, disaggregated by gender, from the report of the organisation '*Ishonch va hayot*' with Eurasian Woman's network on AIDS, was 131; and 3) 100 criminal cases were initiated during nine months of 2021 (Ishonch va hayot 2021), desegregation by sex not available. This gendered narrative in the media perpetuates a blame culture that disproportionately targets women, exacerbating gender inequality and discrimination.

In the context of Uzbekistan, a significant concern in the criminalisation of HIV transmission lies in the legal ambiguity surrounding the concept of 'intentional transmission'. Courts typically determine intent based primarily on whether an individual has been formally notified of their HIV-positive status. Moreover, the legislation criminalises actions that put others at risk of infection, such as engaging in unprotected sex. This legal framework poses a dilemma for individuals who engage in high-risk behaviours like commercial sex work or the use of injectable drugs. In scenarios where access to condoms or new syringes is limited, and if HIV infection is suspected, individuals may be deterred from seeking official assistance due to the potential legal ramifications.

This approach to criminalisation, often echoed in media narratives and particularly in the portrayal of women, has several detrimental consequences. It can inhibit individuals from seeking HIV testing and treatment, driven by the fear of legal repercussions and societal stigma. Additionally, this narrative erroneously positions HIV as an issue predominantly concerning women, despite statistical evidence indicating that the majority of HIV cases in Uzbekistan involve men. Such a skewed representation fosters inaccurate public understanding of HIV's epidemiology, which can adversely affect the effectiveness of public health strategies. This misrepresentation necessitates a more informed and balanced public discourse to enhance the efficacy of health interventions and policies related to HIV in Uzbekistan.

An equally concerning issue is the dramatic lack of media coverage on effective HIV transmission prevention, both through sexual contact and blood. This omission is a significant oversight, given the importance of prophylaxis in HIV prevention strategies. The absence of such critical information in the media discourse deprives the public of knowledge on how to protect themselves and others from HIV transmission. It also fails to highlight the advancements in HIV treatment and prevention, such as antiretroviral therapy (ART), pre-exposure prophylaxis (PrEP), and post-exposure prophylaxis (PEP), which are essential components in the global response to HIV/AIDS.

The media's failure to adequately report on preventive measures contributes to the persistence of myths and fears about HIV transmission.

This gap in reporting needs to be addressed through comprehensive media training and the development of guidelines that ensure the inclusion of informative and life-saving medical information in media reports. By doing so, the media can play a pivotal role in educating the public and promoting health initiatives that can lead to a reduction in new HIV infections.

Furthermore, addressing the media's portrayal of HIV/AIDS must go hand in hand with policy changes, particularly the decriminalisation of HIV transmission and the cessation of gender-biased legal practices. By improving media practices and revising punitive laws, Uzbekistan can make significant strides towards improving the lives of people living with HIV, fostering a more equitable society, and enhancing the efficacy of HIV prevention and care services.

There is no public data on undetectable viral load. The UNAIDS 2020 Country Report was published without the information about the number of individuals who achieved an undetectable viral load (UNAIDS 2020). Government officials avoid discussing this issue directly and use the manipulative term 'significant reduction in viral load' instead. Only 74% of people in treatment achieve the 'significant reduction in viral load' (Ministry of Health Press service 2022).

Uzbekistan is experiencing rapid population growth (Eurasian Research Institute [ERI] 2020), resulting in a significant portion of the population being comprised of children and young adults. This age group is more prone to engaging in risky behaviours, making it crucial for them to have access to reliable information about HIV prevention and treatment. The absence of such access results in the underutilisation of available prevention methods. The challenge of effective prevention is exemplified by the existing data on condom usage, which shows a substantial drop from 80% in 2011 to 50% in 2015 (UNAIDS 2020). Unfortunately, more recent data is not available through publicly accessible sources. According to the national reporting on sustainable development goals by the Agency of Statistics under the President of the Republic of Uzbekistan, approximately 50% of women have resorted to modern contraceptive methods (indicator 3.7.1.1) in the last decade (Agency of statistics under the President of the Republic of Uzbekistan 2023). However, a global report with disaggregated data available on the United Nations website reveals a different scenario. In the latest comprehensive report (submitted for the year 2006), it is shown that only 2% of women use condoms, while the indicator for the provision of intrauterine devices (IUDs) stands at 49.7% (United Nations 2022). These data suggest a near-total lack of use of barrier methods of contraception by women. Additionally, according to the same UN data, only 2% of women use oral contraceptives. This information further substantiates the existence of gender discrimination and the subordinate status of women in Uzbekistan. The predominant reliance on intrauterine devices, which can only be administered by a medical professional, likely occurs with the consent of a male partner. This reliance on IUDs over other forms of contraception, such as condoms or oral contraceptives, underscores the limited autonomy women have in making decisions about their reproductive health.

Similarly, there is a lack of data on the annual number of new HIV cases among individuals under the age of 18, and the information on children living with HIV is sporadic in brief official reports. These reports do not provide a comprehensive understanding of the trend: in 2012, 2,500 children under 18 years were living with HIV, and in 2021, 8,100 children under 18 years were living with HIV (KUN.UZ 2022; O'zbekiston Milliy axborot agentligining [UzA] 2022; Institute for War & Peace Reporting [IWPR] 2012). Furthermore, the authors of the reports did not give an explanation for the statistics. The combination of limited awareness, difficulties in obtaining HIV prevention tools, and prevailing gender stereotypes could potentially lead to a significant rise in new cases among adolescents and young people.

Conclusions

The findings of this study call for a concerted effort to reform the media's representation of HIV/AIDS in Uzbekistan. Media professionals should be encouraged to follow guidelines for HIV reporting, ensuring that coverage is not only accurate but also respectful and free from stigmatising language. There is an urgent need in Uzbekistan to develop guidelines on ethical standards in journalism, which will also include topics related to news involving vulnerable people. It is necessary to include these standards in training programs for journalists, and monitor their compliance with various information campaigns in the media.

Furthermore, addressing the media's portrayal of HIV/AIDS must go hand in hand with policy changes in Uzbekistan, particularly the decriminalisation of HIV transmission and the cessation of gender-biased legal practices. By improving media practices and revising punitive laws, Uzbekistan can make significant progress towards improving the lives of people living with HIV, fostering a more equitable society, and enhancing the efficacy of HIV prevention and care services.

Limitations

Firstly, the selection of media outlets, though popular, may not represent the entire spectrum of Uzbek media, potentially overlooking regional and less mainstream publications that might offer different perspectives. Secondly, the reliance on digital media and official Telegram channels may introduce a selection bias, as it excludes print media and other forms of journalism not available online. Additionally, the manual selection and classification of articles also introduce a subjective element to the determination of stigmatising content. Furthermore, the study does not account for the readership's perception and interpretation of the media content, which could impact understanding the real-world influence of media portrayal on public stigma. Lastly, the focus on media content alone does not address the broader socio-political and legal context that both shapes and is shaped by media narratives, warranting a more multidisciplinary approach in order to fully grasp the complexities of HIV/AIDS stigma in Uzbekistan.

Bibliography

Agency of statistics under the President of the Republic of Uzbekistan (2023): 3 Good Health and Well-Being. Ensure healthy lives and promote well-being for all at all ages. Situation in Uzbekistan. www.nsdg.stat.uz/en/goal/6, 11.06.2023.

Aghaei, Atefeh/Sakhaei, Ayoub/Khalilimeybodi, Ali/Qiao, Shan/Li, Xiaoming (2023): Impact of Mass Media on HIV/AIDS Stigma Reduction: A Systematic Review and Meta-analysis. In: AIDS and Behavior 27, pp. 3414–3429. DOI: 10.1007/s10461-023-04057-5.

Eurasian Research Institute (ERI) (2020): A Brief Review of Uzbekistan's Demographic Profile. www.eurasian-research.org/publication/a-brief-review-of-uzbekistans-demographic-profile/, 11.07.2023.

Gazeta.uz (2022): The annual increase in HIV-infected people in Uzbekistan has stabilized. www.gazeta.uz/ru/2022/12/01/hiv/, 11.07.2023.

HIV Ireland (n.d.): Media Reporting Guidelines – HIV. www.hivireland.ie/policy-news-and-media/mediareportingguidelines/, 11.03.2023.

Human Rights Watch (2021): Uzbekistan: Gay Men Face Abuse, Prison. Ensure Rights to Personal Security, Privacy, Nondiscrimination. www.hrw.org/news/2021/03/23/uzbekistan-gay-men-face-abuse-prison, 11.06.2023.

Institute for War & Peace Reporting (IWPR) (2012): Uzbekistan: No Place for Children With HIV. www.iwpr.net/global-voices/uzbekistan-no-place-children-hiv, 11.06.2023.

Ishonch va hayot (2021): Analysis of legislation and practice regarding the criminalization of HIV infection in the Republic of Uzbekistan. Toshkent: Ishonch va hayot.

Jaspal, Rusi/Nerlich, Brigitte (2022): HIV stigma in UK press reporting of a case of intentional HIV transmission. In: Health 26, No. 3, pp. 319–337. DOI: 10.1177/1363459320949901.

KUN.UZ (2022): Number of HIV-infected citizens in Uzbekistan announced. www.kun.uz/en/news/2022/02/02/number-of-hiv-infected-citizens-in-uzbekistan-announced, 11.06.2023.

KUN.UZ (2023): More than 48 thousand people have been diagnosed with HIV in Uzbekistan. www.kun.uz/ru/news/2023/06/08/v-uzbekistane-u-boleye-chem-48-tysyach-chelovek-diagnostirovan-vich, 11.03.2023.

LexUZ (n.d.): Criminal Code of the Republic of Uzbekistan. www.lex.uz/docs/111457, 11.07.2023.

Ministry of Health Press service (2022): Ministry of Health Vaccine is the only solution! [Telegram]. www.t.me/ssvuz/11540, 11.06.2023.

National AIDS Trust (NAT) (2010): Guidelines for Reporting HIV. Advice for editors and journalists writing about HIV in the UK. London: NAT.

O'zbekiston Milliy axborot agentligining (UzA) (2022): The number of people infected with AIDS in Uzbekistan and some information about this disease have been revealed [Telegram]. www.t.me/uzauz/886, 11.06.2023.

Stutterheim, Sarah E./Kuijpers, Kyran J.R./Waldén, Moon I./Finkenflügel, Renee N.N./Brokx, Pieter A.R./Bos, Arjan E.R. (2022): Trends in HIV Stigma Experienced by People Living With HIV in the Netherlands: A Comparison of Cross-Sectional Surveys Over Time. In: AIDS Education and Prevention 34, No. 1. DOI: 10.1521/aeap.2022.34.1.33.

The Joint United Nations Programme on HIV/AIDS (UNAIDS) (2008): New guidelines for media reporting on HIV in India. www.unaids.org/en/resources/presscentre/featurestories/2008/november/20081119newguidlinesmediahivindia, 11.03.2023.

The Joint United Nations Programme on HIV/AIDS (UNAIDS) (2020): Country Progress Report – Uzbekistan. Global AIDS Epidemic Monitoring 2020. www.unaids.org/sites/default/files/country/documents/UZB_2020_countryreport.pdf, 27.02.2024.

The Nationwide Movement Yuksalish (2023): Top 15 Popular Media in Uzbekistan: People Read Less, Watch More Video. www.yumh.uz/en/news_detail/564, 11.04.2023.

United Nations (2022): World Contraceptive Use. www.un.org/development/desa/pd/data/world-contraceptive-use, 11.06.2023.

UzTAG Uzbek Telegraph Agency (2019): Uzbekistan has toughened penalties for prostitution and begging. www.uztag.info/ru/news-of-the-day/v-uzbekistane-uzhestochili-nakazanie-za-zanyatie-prostitutsiey-i-poproshaynichestvom, 11.06.2023.

Vaughan, Elena/Power, Martin (2023): The discursive construction of HIV stigma in Irish print media. In: Health 27, No. 3, pp. 398–416. DOI: 10.1177/13634593211038525.

12. The role of public organizations and non-governmental organizations (NGOs) in addressing and supporting people with HIV

Guzalkhon Zakhidova

Introduction

The Joint International Social Work Agreement defines social work as follows: 'Social work is a practice-based profession and an academic discipline that promotes social change and development, social cohesion, and the empowerment and liberation of people. Principles of social justice, human rights, collective responsibility and respect for diversities are central to social work. Underpinned by theories of social work, social sciences, humanities and indigenous knowledges, social work engages people and structures to address life challenges and enhance wellbeing' (International Federation of Social Workers [IFSW] 2024).

Non-governmental organisation (NGOs) and other civil society institutions play an important role in a democratic state by increasing the socio-political and socio-economic potential of the country.

Uzbekistan has long struggled with the need for an effective social protection system and qualified social workers to help those in need. Despite efforts to restructure ministries and address these gaps, the country still lacks a cohesive professional social work system. Recent plans led by President Shavkat Mirziyoyev aim to address these shortcomings by establishing the National Social Protection Agency. This agency, which will operate independently, is tasked with overhauling social services, creating a robust support network for various vulnerable groups, and implementing advanced international standards in social protection. The agency's objectives include training programmes for social workers, improving support for people with disabilities, expanding social insurance coverage and promoting social partnership initiatives with civil society organisations. By setting clear timelines and targets, Uzbekistan aims to reform its social protection landscape and create a more inclusive and supportive environment for its citizens.

Government Measures to Combat the Spread of HIV in Uzbekistan

By a resolution dated 20th January 2023, President of Uzbekistan Shavkat Mirziyoyev approved the Program of Comprehensive Measures to Increase the Efficiency of Combating the Spread of HIV Infection among the population for 2023–2027 (LexUZ 2023a).

The document was adopted in accordance with the political declaration '95–95–95', approved by UN member states in the summer of 2021 (The Joint United Nations Programme on HIV/AIDS [UNAIDS] 2021a). It calls on all states to ensure that 95% of the people living with HIV (PLHV) know their HIV status, 95% of the people who know their status receive HIV treatment, and 95% of the people on HIV treatment achieve suppressed viral load (meaning that the level of viral load in the blood is reduced to undetectable). The government is planning to allocate 120 billion soums and 54 million US dollars for the implementation of this strategy throughout 2023–2027 at the state budget's expense, the Global Fund to Fight AIDS, Tuberculosis and Malaria (GFATM), borrowed funds from the Asian Development Bank and the Asian Infrastructure Investment Bank (The President Republic of Uzbekistan 2023).

The Government of Uzbekistan is committed to strengthening support for essential HIV services and interventions. This commitment is demonstrated by increased government leadership and the fact that the government has increased the share of funding allocated for the HIV response. For example, the government is increasing its share in financing the purchase of antiretroviral therapy (ART) drugs to 75%. This increased commitment to the HIV response is essential to developing a new strategy that will bring services closer to people and ensures increased funding for the HIV response (World Health Organization [WHO] 2023).

The coordinating body for all activities to combat the spread of HIV infection is the Republican Commission for Coordination of Activities to Combat the Spread of HIV Infection in the Republic of Uzbekistan. At least once a quarter, the Republican Commission holds meetings that include the heads of key ministries and departments, local governments, and civil society. In order to raise the system of measures to counter the spread of HIV infection to a modern and high-quality level, the Resolution of the President of the Republic of Uzbekistan No. PP-3800 dated 22nd June 2018 'On additional measures to counter the spread of the disease caused by the human immunodeficiency virus and the prevention of nosocomial infections' (LexUZ 2018) was adopted. 'On measures to further strengthen the system for countering the disease caused by the human immunodeficiency virus' was adopted, which approved the Programme of Comprehensive Measures to Increase the Efficiency of Countermeasures against the spread of HIV infection among the population for 2023–2027 (LexUZ 2023a).

In order to further enhance the role of NGOs as active participants and partners in the reforms carried out in Uzbekistan, strengthen the protection of their rights and legitimate interests, expand the scale of state support, and create favourable conditions for them, the Resolution of the President of the Republic of Uzbekistan No. PP-5012 was approved in March 2021, entitled 'On additional measures for state support of non-governmental organizations, ensuring freedom of their activities, protection of rights and legitimate interests' (SoyuzPravoInform 2021).

This resolution of the President also defines the conditions for social partnership and state social order. This is also intended to improve the legislation in terms of introducing administrative liability for interference by government bodies and their officials in the legitimate activities of NGOs.

The resolution defines measures for the financial support of NGOs, including the provision of premises for hosting NGOs without charging rent and the introduction of social partnership and state social order. It also provides for the improvement of legislation in terms of introducing administrative responsibility for the intervention of government bodies and their officials in the legitimate activities of NGOs.

A state social order is a state assignment to carry out work or activities for the implementation of socially and publicly significant projects by concluding an agreement between a state body and an NGO or other civil society institution (Institution in the form of a non-governmental non-profit organization "Madad" 2019). The provision of state social orders is carried out through the Public Fund under the Oliy Majlis (Parliament), Public Funds for the support of NGOs and other civil society institutions under the Jokargy Kenes of the Republic of Karakalpakstan, the Kengashes of people's deputies of the regions and the city of Tashkent, as well as government bodies.

Within the framework of the social partnership provided for by this Law, state bodies shall determine the priority areas of their activities. If state bodies need the participation of NGOs and other civil society institutions to carry out their activities, they shall submit applications for the implementation of the state social order for the next fiscal year to the Public Fund under the Oliy Majlis or to the Public Support Fund for NGOs and other civil society institutions under the Jokargy Kenes of the Republic of

Karakalpakstan, the Kengashes of People's Deputies of the regions and the City of Tashkent. The application of the government body that submits the order indicates the priority areas of activity of this government body. This body also indicates the goals, objectives and conditions of the order to carry out work or carry out activities (ibid).

A parliamentary or public commission, having considered the documents submitted by the Public Support Fund under the Oliy Majlis, public foundations, NGOs and other institutions, associations under the Jokarg Kenes of the Republic of Karakalpakstan, and the Kengashes of People's Deputies of the regions of the Republic and the city of Tashkent, makes a decision on incentives in the prescribed manner; The procedure for the provision of social orders by the state and their volumes are published in the media, the list of officials and the types of state activities for which these funds are allocated, including specialized associations (including on the fight against HIV/AIDS), create equal legal rights for them and the opportunity to participate in the defence (Article 58 of the Constitution of the Republic of Uzbekistan) (ibid). These provisions are specified in the laws of the Republic of Uzbekistan 'On public associations', 'On NGOs', 'On public funds', 'On guarantees for the activities of NGOs', 'On the openness of the activities of public authorities and management', 'On social partnership', 'On environmental control', 'On public control', etc. Dissolution, prohibition, or restriction of the activities of public associations can only take place on the basis of court decisions (Article 62 of the Constitution of the Republic of Uzbekistan) (ibid). NGOs and other civil society institutions develop projects of state social orders and submit them for consideration to the Parliamentary Commissions and public commissions.

When providing a state social order, an agreement is concluded between the state body that sent the application for the provision of a state social order and an NGO or other civil society institutions. State bodies can co-finance projects of state social orders supported by the Parliamentary Commission and public commissions at the expense of extra-budgetary funds. In this case, the amount of co-financing should not exceed 20% of the total amount of financing (ibid).

In addition, the state protects the rights and legitimate interests of public associations (including those related to the fight against HIV/AIDS). For example, on 3rd March 2021, the President of Uzbekistan issued a Decree 'On additional measures of state support for NGOs in ensuring the freedom of their activities, protection of rights and legitimate interests' (O'zbekiston Milliy Axborot Agentligi [UzA] 2021), which introduced a number of changes aimed at improving the legal environment of NGOs. For example, the order increased the total amount of foreign funding that NGOs can receive annually; the period for re-registration of an NGO, as well as state registration of its symbols, has been reduced from one month to 15 days; ordered the development of a bill introducing administrative liability for interference by government bodies and other officials in the legitimate activities of NGOs (the draft was developed in 2021, but has not yet been adopted) and other important initiatives that would enhance the activities of NGOs (International Center for Not-For-Profit Law [ICNL] n.d.). The dissolution, prohibition or restriction of the activity of public associations shall take place only on the basis of a court decision (Article 70 of the Constitution of the Republic of Uzbekistan, LexUZ 2023b).

The state creates equal legal opportunities for women and men to participate in public and state life (Article 58 of the Constitution of the Republic of Uzbekistan, LexUZ 2023b). Discrimination is the establishment of any direct or indirect restrictions belonging to public associations, as well as other circumstances not related to the business qualities of employees and the results of their work (NORMA Information and legal portal 2022).

Prevention Services for Key Populations and Other Groups

Prevention services are provided through 137 Trust Rooms located in medical institutions, where services are provided mainly for persons who inject drugs (PWID); through one republican and a number of regional NGOs that provide services to sex workers, their clients and men who have sex with men (MSM); through 15 Friendly Rooms that conduct anonymous interviews with representatives of all key population groups and offer syndromic treatment of sexually transmitted infections (STIs) and a number of other services (testing, distribution of condoms, referral to other specialists, counselling on HIV and STIs); and through anonymous offices located in AIDS centres and other medical institutions. Trust rooms and friendly rooms are integrated into the healthcare system and are maintained at the healthcare budget's expense. Prevention work is funded by the Global Fund under its Behaviour Change and Prevention Services component for key populations. The Global Fund grant supports the salaries of 140 assistants and 300 outreach workers at 137 drop-in points. The Global Fund also supports the provision of services, including the distribution of needles, syringes, alcohol swabs, male condoms, printed tuberculosis (TB) screening questionnaires and rapid testing of oral fluid samples for HIV (WHO 2023).

Following the completion of the pilot project in 2006–2009, the opioid substitution therapy (OST) programme was not continued, despite promising results. During the discussions, it was assessed by the drug treatment service and was discontinued due to unfavourable results. Various stakeholders within the country viewed the programme positively, but the prospect of its implementation was considered highly unlikely. Arguments in favour of its termination included drug treatment specialists misunderstanding the goals of the programme, a lack of political support, including from key stakeholders, major changes in the drug addiction situation, and a reduction in the number of opioid injecting drug users (IDUs) (ibid). By May 2009, the working group decided that it was inappropriate to carry out OST in the country. A month later, the Ministry of Health circulated a letter to international organizations informing them of the working group's decision and the official completion of the project. On 25th June 2009, patients stopped taking replacement medications, having previously reduced their daily doses for a month. During the consultation meeting "Drug Control Policy and Public health", organized by the United Nations Office on Drugs and Crime (UNODC) on 18th August 2009 in Tashkent, the participants of this event asked representatives of the Ministry of Health to share the report of the working group, which made recommendations on the cessation of substitution therapy in Tashkent in order to familiarize themselves with the assessment methodology and on the conclusions that were made. This would have allowed them to compare the approaches used with those adopted in international practice standards. Unfortunately, the request was denied "due to the report being in the nature of a document for official use" (Latypov et al. 2010). In connection with the closure of the program, the Eurasian Harm Reduction Network conducted an international campaign to advocate for OST in Uzbekistan. An open letter was sent to the President and Minister of Health of Uzbekistan signed by 77 OST specialists and activists from Eastern Europe and Central Asia, the USA, Canada, France, Great Britain and other countries. But the program has not been resumed (Fedorova/Chingin 2014).

The coverage of prevention activities for two key population groups – PWID and women engaged in sex work (also known as female sex workers [FSW]) – has been assessed as relatively high (more than 50%). This seems significant, given the complexities of the environment and the way in which related services are provided. There is a trend towards expanding the coverage of prevention activities for key populations. However, coverage among MSM remains low (less than 11%), which may be due to the high degree of stigmatisation of this group, even by medical personnel (ibid).

Progress has been made in reaching MSM, but it is still insufficient to have a significant impact on the spread of HIV. However, coverage of PWID has increased significantly from 58.5% in 2018 to 77% in 2020–2021. It should be noted that anecdotal evidence suggests that coverage of women who inject drugs remains below 50%.

The NGO 'Intilish' project has been working with PWID for a long time and has successfully integrated this work into medical institutions. However, the majority of clients are regular participants in the programme; only 1.9% seeks help just once a year. Research shows that current coverage of PWID mainly depends on old programme clients, including former prisoners who were previously registered with drug treatment services.

The state programme to combat the spread of HIV infection in the Republic of Uzbekistan introduced the following approaches to expand the coverage of key population groups with preventive measures: HIV testing (through mobile testing units, including rapid testing), support for Friendly Rooms for syndromic treatment of STIs in representatives of key population groups, development of a comprehensive information and educational programme, and the creation of a special fund for the development of information and communication components of HIV prevention. NGOs were brought in to monitor these activities. Prevention services were provided to traditionally key population groups: FSW, MSM, and PWID. In addition, migrant workers are considered to be an important target group. The primary goal of the prevention programme among vulnerable populations is to ensure access to services aimed at reducing the risk of HIV transmission, as well as ensuring access to HIV testing and linkage to follow-up ART and other health services (WHO 2023).

All measures to combat HIV infection are carried out on the basis of the Law of the Republic of Uzbekistan No. ZRU-353 of 23rd September 2013 'On countering the spread of the disease caused by the human immunodeficiency virus (HIV infection)' (LexUZ 2013a). The most significant measures are outlined below.

Law of the Republic of Uzbekistan No. ZRU-353 of 23rd September 2013, 'On countering the spread of the disease caused by the human immunodeficiency virus (HIV infection)'

The purpose of this Law is to regulate relations in the field of combating a common disease caused by the human immunodeficiency virus (HIV infection). Below are excerpts from this law.

Article 5 of this law states that public administration in the field of combating the spread of HIV infection is carried out by: the Cabinet of Ministers of the Republic of Uzbekistan; Ministry of Health of the Republic of Uzbekistan; Ministry of Internal Affairs of the Republic of Uzbekistan; local authorities. Actions to counter the spread of HIV infection can be carried out by other institutions in accordance with the law.

Medical Examination for HIV

Medical examination for HIV (Chapter 3 'Measures to counter the spread of HIV infection. Providing medical care to HIV-infected people', LexUZ 2013a) is a study and assessment of the health status of the person being examined, which establishes the presence or absence of HIV. Medical examination for HIV can be carried out in all treatment and prevention institutions in accordance with the norms and rules established by the Ministry of Health of the Republic of Uzbekistan, on a voluntary or compulsory basis. During a medical examination for HIV, the person being examined receives both a preliminary and a follow-up consultation. Medical examination for HIV of minors and persons recognised as incompetent or partially capable is carried out with the consent of their legal representatives. At the request of the person being examined, the results of examinations conducted by laboratories of the state healthcare system to determine the presence or absence of HIV are issued at the treatment and prevention institution that conducted the preliminary consultation. For minors and persons recognised as incompetent or partially capable, the results are issued to their legal representatives. If HIV is detected in the person being examined, a follow-up consultation is carried out and the person is registered at a dispensary. This person is warned in writing about criminal liability for infecting other persons with HIV infection (Article 113 'Spread of sexually transmitted diseases or HIV/AIDS' of the Criminal Code of the Republic of Uzbekistan, LexUZ n.d.). That is, when HIV is detected, the person being examined signs a document stating criminal liability for infecting another person with HIV.

Mandatory Medical Examination for HIV

The following are subject to mandatory medical examination for HIV: donors of blood and biological fluids (Article 15 'On countering the spread of the disease caused by the human immunodeficiency virus [HIV infection]', LexUZ 2013a); persons marrying under the age of fifty (author's note: fertile age) (ibid); pregnant women; persons suspected of using drugs by injection; children born by HIV-positive mothers; medical workers who come into contact with human blood, biological fluids, organs and tissues in their activities; and persons whose sexual partner has been diagnosed with HIV.

Providing Medical Care to PLWH

The provision of medical care to PLWH is carried out after they are registered at the dispensary in AIDS centres and in treatment and preventive institutions in their place of residence. Providing medical care to PLWH includes specific treatment of HIV infection, as well as prevention of the development, diagnosis, and treatment of diseases associated with HIV infection. Free specific treatment for PLWH is prescribed based on the conclusion of a medical commission, depending on the stage of the disease, in AIDS centres and in departments for HIV-infected medical institutions. Providing medical care to HIV-infected people to prevent the development, diagnosis, and treatment of diseases associated with HIV infection is carried out by AIDS centres, together with other treatment and preventive institutions (Article 17 'On countering the spread of the disease caused by the human immunodeficiency virus [HIV infection]', LexUZ 2013a).

Social Protection of Medical Workers at Risk of Contracting HIV Infection While Performing Their Official Duties

The spreading of HIV infection among medical workers while performing their official duties is classified as an occupational disease. Medical workers providing specialised medical care for the diagnosis and treatment of PLWH, as well as ensuring the implementation of preventive and anti-epidemic measures, receive benefits provided for by law (Article 18 'Social protection of medical workers at risk of contracting HIV infection during the performance of their official duties' of the Law of the Republic of Uzbekistan 'On countering the spread of the disease caused by the human immunodeficiency virus [HIV infection]', LexUZ 2013a).

Rights and Responsibilities of PLWH

PLWH have the right to: receive the results of medical examinations for HIV and recommendations for preventing the spread of HIV; obtain information about their rights, the nature of the diseases they have, and the methods of medical care used; be treated humanely; and receive psychological support and assistance (Article 19 'Rights and obligations of HIV-infected people' of the Law of the Republic of Uzbekistan 'On countering the spread of the disease caused by the human immunodeficiency virus [HIV infection]', LexUZ 2013a).

Obligations of PLWH

PLWH are obliged to: carry out measures recommended by medical workers to prevent the spread of HIV infection; take precautions when in contact with healthy persons; and inform their sexual partner about their illness, as well as medical workers and service workers who use piercing and cutting devices in procedures that violate the integrity of the skin and mucous membranes. PLWH may have other rights and bear other responsibilities in accordance with the law (ibid).

Social Protection of PLWH

PLWH are provided with free, specific treatment. PLWH under eighteen years of age have the right to receive a monthly social benefit, regardless of the stage of the disease, and benefits for children with disabilities are established by law (Article 4 'Main directions of state policy in the field of combating the spread of HIV infection' and Article 20 'Social protection of HIV-infected people' of the Law of the Republic of Uzbekistan 'On countering the spread of the disease caused by the human immunodeficiency virus [HIV infection]', LexUZ 2013a) or a life-threatening and chronically developing rare (orphan) disease, and persons over 18 years of age with disabilities from childhood' of the Cabinet of Ministers of the Republic of Uzbekistan Decision (LexUZ 2011). Parents of HIV-infected children or persons in loco parentis have the right to stay together with their children in a treatment and prevention institution in a stationary setting, with temporary release from work and payment of temporary disability benefits in the manner prescribed by law (Article 20 'Social protection of HIV-infected people' of the Law of the Republic of Uzbekistan 'On countering the spread of the disease caused by the human immunodeficiency virus [HIV infection]', LexUZ 2013a). Legislation might also establish other measures of social protection for HIV-infected people and members of their families in the future.ibid). Legislation might also establish other measures of social protection for PLWH and members of their families in the future.

Financing Activities to Combat the Spread of HIV Infection

The financing of activities to combat the spread of HIV infection is carried out from the State Budget of the Republic of Uzbekistan, as well as from other sources not prohibited by law.

Compensation for Harm Caused to the Health of a Person Infected with HIV

Compensation for harm caused to the health of a person living with HIV as a result of failure to perform or the improper performance of their professional duties by medical workers and service workers is rewarded in the manner prescribed by law. Compensation for harm does not relieve the perpetrators from liability in accordance with the law (Article 23 'Rights and obligations of HIV-infected people', LexUZ 2013a).

'On countering the spread of the disease caused by the human immunodeficiency virus (HIV infection)' of the Law of Uzbekistan, Article 12 Participation of self-government bodies of citizens and NGOs in the field of combating the spread of HIV infection.

“Self-government bodies of citizens and NGOs can participate:

in carrying out activities to counter the spread of HIV infection, in the implementation and protection of the rights, freedoms and legitimate interests of PLWH;

in providing legal, methodological, informational and other assistance to PLWH or their legal representatives within the limits of their powers;

in organizing and conducting awareness-raising work among the population on issues of HIV prevention based on local customs and traditions.

Citizens’ self-government bodies and NGOs can participate in other activities to combat the spread of HIV infection” (LexUZ 2013a).

The Law of the Republic of Uzbekistan on Social Partnership

This law was adopted by the Legislative Chamber on 18th June 2014 and approved by the Senate on 28th August 2014. The purpose of this law is to regulate relations in the field of social partnership. Social partnership is the interaction of government bodies with NGOs and other civil society institutions in the development and implementation of programmes for the socio-economic development of the country, including sectoral and territorial programmes, as well as regulations and other decisions affecting the rights and legitimate interests of citizens (LexUZ 2014).

State Support for Social Partnership

The Parliamentary Commission or Public Commissions, having studied the documents submitted respectively by the Public Fund under the Oliy Majlis, public funds for the support of NGOs and other civil society institutions under the Jokargy Kenes of the Republic of Karakalpakstan, the Kengashes of people’s deputies of the regions and the city of Tashkent, decide on the advisability of providing state social orders and theirscopes, publish in the media a list of government customers and areas of activity to which these funds are planned to be allocated to public organisations and NGOs (including on issues of combating HIV/AIDS), and create equal legal opportunities for public organisations and NGOs to participate in public life (Article 58 of the Constitution of the Republic of Uzbekistan, LexUZ 2023b). These provisions are specified in the laws of the Republic of Uzbekistan ‘On public associations’, ‘On NGOs’, ‘On public funds’, ‘On guarantees for the activities of NGOs', 'On the openness of the activities of public authorities and management', 'On social partnership', 'On environmental control', 'On public control', etc. The dissolution, prohibition, or restriction of the activities of public associations can only take place on the basis of a court decision (Article 62 of the Constitution of the Republic of Uzbekistan, LexUZ 2023b).

A Critical Look at the Situation of NGOs

In May 2018, a decree of President Shavkat Mirziyoyev was adopted, 'On measures to radically increase the role of civil society institutions in the process of democratic renewal of the country' (LexUZ 2018b). The decree highlighted excessive bureaucratic hurdles and barriers in registering NGOs, citing outdated legislation that doesn't align with contemporary standards as a significant issue.

The development of public organizations and NGOs is hampered by various bureaucratic obstacles, a complex registration process, low legal literacy and lack of legal support, combined with illegal 'expertise' rules.

There is a reluctance to weaken control over the non-governmental sector, control over the financing and distribution of funds of NGOs, the creation of additional commissions that decide how to distribute funds from public organizations, and the adoption of important decisions behind closed doors create obstacles to the development of a free society and public organizations.

Despite the laws on NGOs, which state that the introduction of new proposals and innovations in public administration can be achieved through joint decisions, this remains the prerogative of the government. Citizens, NGOs and other factors are not sufficiently involved in this process.

This presidential decree adopted in May 2018 emphasised the inadequacy of state funds to sufficiently support expansive projects by civil society institutions. Consequently, the decree aimed to create specific public funds, funded locally, to increase assistance for NGOs and other civil society bodies from 2019 onwards. Although these public funds have been established and formally recognised in all regions of the country, their effective operation faces substantial limitations. The funds haven't been allocated, and the staff required to run these funds haven't been recruited. For instance, the Fergana regional branch of the Association of Disabled People of Uzbekistan has faced challenges securing grants and subsidies from the regional public fund meant to aid NGOs due to the fund's lack of financial resources and personnel. Similar difficulties persist across various other regions nationwide.

As per the legislation encompassing 'On NGOs' and 'On public associations', NGOs are legally entitled to obtain grants and financial support from foreign donors. However, due to constrained financial resources allocated by the state, various restrictions persist concerning the utilisation of foreign funding for NGO activities. A recent press release from the Uzbekistan Ministry of Justice highlighted that the utilisation of funds and assets acquired by NGOs from foreign states and international and foreign organisations is permitted without hindrance, provided these receipts of funds and assets are reported to the registration authority prior to their reception (LexUZ 2013b).

For NGOs, the process of obtaining grants still involves navigating bureaucratic procedures, reminiscent of what was previously referred to as the 'grant commission'. Even though this commission was not officially documented, it functioned in practice. Previously, NGOs had to open a dedicated account exclusively in branches of the National Bank for Foreign Economic Affairs of the Republic of Uzbekistan or the state-owned, joint-stock commercial bank Asaka. However, according to the Ministry of Justice, there has been a shift: now, 'grant funds are deposited into specially designated accounts of NGOs in any banking institution' (ICNL n.d.b).

Resolution of the Cabinet of Ministers No. 858 of 9th October 2019 on the procedure for NGOs to receive funds and property from international donors received by NGOs, and No. 328 of 13th June 2022 on the procedure for the interaction of NGOs with government agencies when implementing international grant projects, became invalid on 5th October 2023. The initiative group of NGOs made a collective appeal to cancel Resolution No. 328 of 13th June 2022 due to the fact that it contradicts national legislation and international standards ensuring the freedom of activity of NGOs. After a meeting of the initiative group with the leadership of the Ministry of Justice, a mutual decision was made to finalize this resolution, taking into account the proposals of representatives of civil society. However, an analysis of comments from representatives of NGOs on the portal for discussing draft regulatory legal acts shows that the draft resolution requires improvement. Experts from the International Center for Non-Commercial Law (ICNL) came to a similar conclusion, which identified a number of conceptual problems that raise reasonable concerns about Uzbekistan's compliance with international standards and national legislation. We hope that the Ministry of Justice will take into account these constructive proposals and recommendations when further editing the draft resolution of the Cabinet of Ministers (Yusupov 2023).

On 4th October, the Government of Uzbekistan adopted a resolution (No. 527) regarding the social partnership of NGOs with government agencies as part of the implementation of projects financed by international grants (LexUZ 2023c).

To this resolution, Appendix No. 527 dated 4th October 2023 was approved: Regulations on the procedure for coordinating the receipt of funds and property by non-state commercial organizations from external sources and the procedure for implementing projects in the territory of the Republic of Uzbekistan financed from external sources (LexUZ 2023c).

The new procedure to some extent simplifies the procedure for receiving funds and property from external sources and cooperation between NGOs and government agencies when implementing international grant projects.

The ICNL welcomed the adoption of the resolution, noting that it was the result of a successful advocacy campaign by Uzbek NGOs and "the first success of its kind in the last 25 years in the history of Uzbekistan". The expert organization noted that the government and the Ministry of Justice held active consultations with NGOs. The draft resolution was published for public discussion, and the Ministry of Justice organized several meetings with representatives of NGOs. Based on these consultations, a number of important recommendations from civil society were reflected in the resolution (Yusupov 2023).

Stigmatization

HIV-related discrimination – and stigma when it leads to rights violations – is a human rights issue. People have the right to protection from the church and to a life of dignity where stigmatizing attitudes do not reach others' enjoyment of their rights, including the right to education, health care, employment, access to justice, privacy, family, bodily autonomy and other rights (UNAIDS 2021b).

47 countries still have travel restrictions for PLWH (ibid). According to official information, in 25 of the 36 countries, more than 50% of people aged 15 to 49 years share discriminatory attitudes towards PLWH(UNAIDS 2020). 40% of PLWH report being forced to undergo certain medical procedures. HIV treatment depended on taking birth control pills funds (ibid).

Representatives of key populations face high levels of stigma, discrimination and violence (ibid).

More and more people in the world believe that the unstable emotional state of a person is caused by both social insecurity and the turbulent situation in the world and in the country. People who seek psychological and social services experience fear and anxiety for a variety of reasons. HIV infection is seen by society as a discreditable, inappropriate, dangerous characteristic of an infected person, i.e. it becomes a shameful stigma. People perceive PLWH as a threat to their personal safety, treat them with hostility and seek to protect themselves in a variety of ways, including outright discrimination and even isolation.

Psychosocial work is needed in segments of the population exposed to stress and depression. Public NGOs support vulnerable segments of the population. Orphans and disadvantaged segments of the population, the disabled, and those suffering from infectious or other diseases that worsen the quality of life are closely monitored by society and public organisations.

Vulnerable segments of society include those PLWH and those who engage in risky behaviour, such as sex workers who use injecting drugs, as well as MSM.

The Article 113 of the Criminal Code penalises the intentional transmission of HIV/AIDS with up to eight years in prison (LexUZ n.d.). This article constitutes a serious barrier for HIV prevention if HIV/AIDS was to be criminalised in Uzbekistan. This law has been used to target and prosecute people living with HIV, even when there is no evidence of intentional transmission. Sexual work is subject to administrative sanctions, while clients have no penalty, and men having sex with men is still considered a criminal act in Uzbekistan according to Article 120 of the current criminal code (LexUZ n.d.): 'satisfying the sexual needs of a man with a man without violence is punishable by restriction of freedom from one year to three years or imprisonment for up to three years'. These laws create a climate of stigma and discrimination, making it difficult for key populations to access the prevention and care services they need.

The Joint United Nations Program on HIV/AIDS (UNAIDS) considers gay men and other MSM, sex workers, transgender people, PWID and prisoners and other incarcerated people as the five main key population groups that are particularly vulnerable to HIV and frequently lack adequate access to services (UNAIDS 2023). At the same time, other groups, such as migrants and young people, are not part of key populations but still participate in HIV programmes and awareness-raising because of their risk behavior. According to UNAIDS' latest estimation, in Uzbekistan there are 105 needles and syringes issued per person who injects drugs, HIV prevalence among sex workers is 3.2%, and HIV prevalence among MSM is 3.7% (UNAIDS 2022).

Sexual relations between men remain illegal in Uzbekistan, despite past promises by authorities to repeal the discriminatory law. This follows on from the draft of the new Criminal Code of the Republic, published by the Prosecutor General's Office for public discussion. In Uzbekistan, voluntary sex between men is currently punishable by a prison term of one to three years in accordance with Article 120 Criminal Code (LexUZ n.d.). In the new edition of this law, the punishment for men who have sex with men only changed in terms of the article number: the wording of the new Article 154 is identical to that of its predecessor, Article 120. The position of this article within the document has also changed: where in the old article, sodomy, or 'besoqolbozlik' (Eurasian Coalition on Health, Rights, Gender and Sexual Diversity [ECOM] 2021), referred to crimes against sexual freedom, in the draft of the new document it refers to crimes 'against family, youth and morality' (ibid). Over five years (2016–2020), 44 people were prosecuted on charges of sodomy in Uzbekistan, as reported by Qalampir (2021). The persecution of MSM makes it more difficult to provide care to PLHV.

The scope of the package of services for PWID is limited and includes the distribution of 25 disposable syringes per month, 1–2 alcohol wipes for each syringe, condoms, information and educational materials, HIV testing, and a questionnaire to identify TB symptoms. In addition, legal assistance and referral to a specialist may be provided as part of the package of services. The service package does not include naloxone or other materials (UNAIDS 2022).

Condoms are provided to all target groups, to both women and men. There were no specific complaints about the quality of the condoms. Lubricants were not provided. The group of MSM and FSWs emphasised the need to provide lubricants and even suggested using them to increase the motivation of new clients to participate in the programme and get tested for HIV.

All new programme clients are clinically screened using a TB questionnaire and, if symptoms are detected, it is easy to obtain follow-up TB diagnostic services. Testing of oral fluid samples for HIV has been available since May 2022 and is considered a useful addition to the range of services provided.

NGOs Working with PLHV in Uzbekistan

There are currently 11,303 registered NGOs in Uzbekistan (Ministry of Justice of the Republic of Uzbekistan n.d.). Out of those, the following NGOs work with vulnerable segments of the population such as HIV-infected people: 'ISHONCH VA HAYOT' (since 2003), 'ISTIQBOLLI AVLOD' (since 2001), the Republican Information and Educational Center 'INTILISH' (since 2001), and the Anti-Cancer Society of Uzbekistan.

Also, Uzbekistan has specific laws governing NGOs, including 'On NGOs' and 'On public associations'. These laws outline the legal framework within which NGOs operate.

Civil Society Development: efforts have been made to encourage the development of civil society in Uzbekistan. However, the effectiveness of these efforts may vary, and NGOs, especially those in all regions of Uzbekistan, may face unique challenges in terms of resources and support.

However, NGOs make a significant contribution to the prevention of HIV infection. Communities living with and affected by HIV, including key populations, support programme development and implementation, expansion of coverage, and improvement in the quality of health services. In all regions of the country, there is a system of approach and social partnership between the government and NGOs for the prevention of HIV infection. Through the joint efforts of regional AIDS centres and NGOs in all 14 administrative regions of the Republic, preventive measures are carried out among sex workers and MSM and psychological and social support for PLHV.

Republican NGO in the Form of a Public Association in Support of People Living with HIV/AIDS and Their Loved Ones 'Ishonch va Hayot' ('Faith and Life') (Ishonch Va Hayot n.d.)

The organization carries out its activities in accordance with the Constitution of the Republic of Uzbekistan, the Law of the Republic of Uzbekistan 'On NGOs' and on the basis of laws on other public organizations. The organization is a self-governed created by individuals and (or) legal entities on a voluntary basis, not pursuing as its own the main goal of generating income (profit) and not distributing the received income (profit) among its participants (members). The organization was created and operates on the basis of voluntariness, equality of its members, self-government, legality and transparency.

Mission of the organization is unifying and comprehensive support PLHV, specially affected populations (SPAs), and their loved ones, improving the quality and dignity of their lives, fighting against stigma and discrimination, and actively participating in overcoming the development and spread of the HIV/AIDS epidemic in the Republic of Uzbekistan. Over the past 20 years, since the registration of the NGO 'Ishonch va Hayot', the organisation has provided assistance and support to more than 35,000 PLHV and their loved ones in Uzbekistan, in the form of crisis counselling, social support, and support on issues related to living with HIV infection.

In collaboration with the AIDS centres, with direct participation and involvement in various projects and programmes in the context of HIV infection, the organisation helps and supports PLHV:

- when their HIV status is confirmed;
- when they are adapting to the diagnosis;
- when it comes to complying with ART regimen;
- by providing care and support at home during the terminal stages of HIV infection (the AIDS stage);
- by expanding the access of PLHV and Maternal and Child Health (MCH) to prevention, treatment, and care; by providing support through peer counselling;
- by finding healthcare specialists who can help;
- by offering referrals to specialised institutions;
- and by providing social support and support in all areas of life.

Together with the AIDS centeres and within the framework of projects funded by the Global Fund to Fight AIDS, Tuberculosis and Malaria, the NGO 'Ishonch va Hayo' organised the first multi-disciplinary teams (MDTs) in the Republic of Uzbekistan who provide medical and psychosocial support, preparation for ART, and treatment, care, and support for PLHV.

The Republican NGO 'Ishonch va Hayot' annually organizes and hosts events dedicated to International AIDS Day (1st December), World Tuberculosis Day (24th March), World AIDS Day of Remembrance (the third Sunday of May), International Day against Drug Abuse and Illicit Drugs drug trafficking (26th June).

The Republican Social Information Center 'Istiqbolli Avlod' (established in 2001)

The activities of the 'Istiqbolli Avlod' Information and Educational Center and a number of regional NGOs aim to reduce the risk of HIV infection particularly among vulnerable segments of the population by strengthening outreach work.

The aim is to strengthen activities to achieve the '95–95–95' goal and 'Stop-TB partnership' (2019) (hosted by United Nations Office for Project Services [UNOPS]) in the Republic of Uzbekistan, focusing especially on vulnerable population groups through financial support from the Office of the Global Fund to Fight AIDS, Tuberculosis and Malaria and the Republican Center for the Fight against AIDS.

Goals of the organization are strengthening and expanding outreach activities among vulnerable groups of the population to reduce the risk of HIV infection in Uzbekistan.

The Global Fund Sub-Project is designed to promote the following: innovative solutions; new services and tools for the prevention of HIV/AIDS and STIs among key populations through outreach work; and healthy lifestyles and changing risk behaviour by providing free counselling and testing for HIV/STIs and TB screening among beneficiaries in eleven regions of Uzbekistan (the regions of Tashkent, Andijan, Bukhara, Namangan, Navoi, Syrdarya, Fergana, Samarkand, Khorezm, Republic of Karakalpakstan, and Tashkent City).

Beneficiaries: Key Vulnerable Population Groups (Sex Workers, MSM)

- 16,920 representatives of a key vulnerable group (sex workers, MSM) received information through outreach workers on the prevention of HIV/AIDS and STIs, as well as on healthy lifestyles and changing risk behaviour
- 115 representatives of a key vulnerable groups (sex workers, MSM) were provided with testing, HIV diagnosis, and registration. Because test is necessary to receive ART
- 16,906 information materials were distributed to key vulnerable groups
- 79,834 mini sessions were conducted by outreach workers on four different topics: 'HIV/AIDS', 'STIs', 'About a healthy lifestyle', and 'Testing for HIV'

- 5,760 representatives of key vulnerable groups were accompanied for tuberculosis screening

The Republican Information and Educational Center 'INTILISH' (established in 2001) (Intilish n.d.)

The organisation promotes the following: the implementation of government programmes; the implementation of programmes of NGOs and associations (both foreign and international) that focus on improving the cultural and educational level of the population and certain key groups, preventing drug addiction, and preventing the spread of HIV/AIDS and tuberculosis; the social adaptation of people who have stopped using drugs; and psychosocial support for PLHV in prisons, released PLHV, and other key groups.

The Republican Information and Educational Center 'Intilish' is an NGO operating in all 14 administrative territories of the Republic of Uzbekistan in the field of public health and social protection. NGO 'Intilish' provides support with the implementation of programmes on twelve topics. The NGO has an educational programme for executive leaders, Australian workers, and volunteers, which is conducted in the form of monthly webinars in two languages (Russian and Uzbek). It also leads the work within the harm reduction programme, preparing methodological materials on topics such as ART, Voluntary Counselling and Testing (VCT), outreach to key populations (mainly PWID), overdose prevention, safe injections, STIs, hepatitis, and tuberculosis.

The NGO 'Intilish' project has been working with PWID for a long time and has successfully integrated this work into medical institutions. However, the majority of clients are regular participants in the program; only 1.9% of clients seek help once during the year. Research shows that current coverage of PWID mainly depends on old program clients, including former prisoners who were previously registered with drug treatment services (WHO 2023).

Goals: The goals of the NGO 'Intilish' project are: improving the quality of life of the population and its vulnerable groups by maintaining health, increasing cultural and educational levels, and increasing social adaptation. Vulnerable groups include, but are not limited to, people at risk of or affected by infectious, endemic, psychiatric, drug addiction, and any other diseases, people who find themselves in difficult life situations, and people who are in prison.

The tasks of the NGO are: the implementation and management of activities that help to effectively achieve the statutory goal of the Center, promoting the development and strengthening of cooperation with state and non-state, local, foreign, and international structures interested in achieving the statutory goal of the Center, and the development of the material and technical base, personnel, and administrative potential of the Center to increase the effectiveness of the implementation of the statutory goal of the Center.

The organisation's experience is represented by working with such groups as injection drug users, people (women, men, adolescents) serving sentences in prison and those released after serving their sentences, PLHV, youth (organised, un-organised, with a high behavioural risk), professionals (senior and paramedical personnel, law enforcement officers, representatives of partner public organisations), and decision makers. Moreover, the organisation prepares and evaluates the activities of trainers of educational programmes.

NGO 'Anti-Cancer Society of Uzbekistan'

In 2013, MDTs began operating in the country, the work of which was initiated jointly by the NGO 'Anti-Cancer Society of Uzbekistan' (n.d.) and the AIDS centers. Multidisciplinary teams provide social-psychological support to PLHV when entering the clinical observation programme and when initiating antiretroviral therapy, and also provide assistance in resolving social and everyday issues. MDTs are the link between AIDS service organisations and healthcare institutions. This ensures continuity in the provision of the medical and social-psychological services provided by organisations of various levels and profiles.

Project grants and partners

The Global Fund has one core grant currently operating in Uzbekistan: the HIV and TB Joint Grant, which aims to strengthening the country's HIV response, especially for key populations, improve TB treatment, and address the high drug burden-resistant tuberculosis in the country (The

Global Fund 2022). A joint HIV and TB grant of up to 44.1 million USD is being implemented in Uzbekistan throughout 2021–2024. Our investment supports the country's goal of delivering an impactful, efficient and sustainable HIV and TB response. For HIV, the grant is aligned with the national HIV strategy and mainly focuses on providing prevention services to key populations as well as quality antiretroviral therapy, care and support. For TB, the grant focuses on diagnostics and treatment of drug-resistant TB, counseling and psychosocial support for people with TB, treatment monitoring, health information systems and monitoring and evaluation, as well as strengthening Uzbekistan's laboratory systems (ibid). The national economy of Uzbekistan constitutes the major portion of funding for the HIV response, covering roughly 72% of the AIDS budget in 2018. A projected investment of 36.6 million USD was outlined for the period spanning 2019–2022, as stated in Presidential Decree PP-3800 (LexUZ 2018a). While these funds primarily support medical care, treatment, and program management initiatives (PP-3493, 2018), significant attention is devoted to holistic development efforts, notably directed towards enhancing hospital infrastructures and broadening laboratory networks.

UNAIDS is a programme of ten UN organisations created to facilitate a comprehensive, coordinated response to the global HIV/AIDS epidemic. A country office of the UNAIDS has opened in Uzbekistan. In addition, Uzbekistan adopted a programme of additional measures to combat the spread of HIV infection for 2018–2022 worth about 50 million USD (Sputnik Uzbekistan 2019).

The Russian government and UNAIDS donated a mobile clinic worth 300 thousand USD to Uzbekistan. This was reported by the Information Department of the Sanitary and Epidemiological Service.

The UN Resident Coordinator in Uzbekistan, Helena Fraser noted that the mobile diagnostic complex is designed for rapid response and preliminary examination of patients, especially in remote regions where access to care and treatment is difficult to find (Uznews.uz 2021).

The UNAIDS Secretariat supports activities for the implementation of the Program of Assistance to EECA Countries in the field of prevention, control and surveillance of HIV/AIDS and other infectious diseases (WHO 2019).

United Nations Office on Drugs and Crime (UNODC) provides support to the Government of Uzbekistan by promoting modern international approaches and standards in the field of HIV prevention and treatment, ensuring access for people who use drugs in terms of necessary medical care based on comprehensive, evidence-based programmes, while respecting the human rights, reducing stigma and discrimination. UNODC helps to build the capacity of health and social service workers who work directly with PWID. Thus, in 2012, together with World Health Organisation (WHO) and UNAIDS, UNODC released an updated version of the technical guidance for countries to develop targets within the framework of the concept of ensuring universal access to HIV prevention, treatment, and care among IDUs (UNODC 2023), and in 2017 released practical guidance for joint efforts to implement comprehensive HIV and AIDS programmes for PWID (UNODC 2017), which can be considered as international standards on the problem (UNODC 2023).

In turn, from May to August 2018, the Monitoring and Evaluation (M&E) group of the Inter-agency Expert Council (IEC) with the support of UNODC, conducted annual monitoring of the provision of services to people with HIV infection in almost all regions of Uzbekistan. During the inspection, the M&E group visited trust rooms, regional AIDS centres, tuberculosis clinics, and NGOs providing support to PLHV and vulnerable population groups. The M&E group conducts monitoring to determine the effectiveness and quality of HIV prevention services, including harm reduction programmes (exchange of injection equipment), pre- and post-test consultation, and antiretroviral therapy (ibid).

The United Nations Children's Fund (UNICEF) is working to strengthen the capacity of Uzbekistan's health system to prevent mother-to-child transmission of HIV (PMTCT) and provide paediatric and psychosocial care to HIV-positive children.

The international non-governmental organisation Doctors without Borders, in close cooperation with the Ministry of Health, is working on the basis of the Tashkent City AIDS Center, through which it provides technical assistance in carrying out specific treatment for PLWH.

A new strategy is in the process of being developed and approved by the president of the country, which recognises the importance of ensuring access to prevention measures, treatment services, and support for PLWH.

A network of HIV/AIDS centres ensures that people across the country have access to the care and resources they need to treat the disease. With centres located in major cities and rural areas, people in every part of the country can access health services. When it comes to dispensing medications, coordination between AIDS centres and primary healthcare facilities is a valuable strategy for increasing access to healthcare. This network of centres does not experience staff shortages or problems retaining staff.

The provision of services in healthcare settings remains the norm in many settings, despite high levels of stigma and discrimination, including the criminalisation of these communities. Outreach efforts are needed to promote the need for services in communities to ensure access for the most vulnerable.

Conclusion

A comprehensive examination of Uzbekistan's legal framework and social landscape of NGOs, social partnership and the fight against HIV/AIDS provides a multifaceted picture of both progress and challenges. The legal structures governing NGOs and social partnerships show a clear intention to promote cooperation between civil society and the government to address socio-economic issues, including HIV prevention. However, the practical implementation of HIV prevention programmes faces many barriers in Uzbekistan, as illustrated by bureaucratic obstacles to NGO registration and the complex process of obtaining grants, particularly from foreign donors.

The article presents a critical assessment of HIV prevention policies in Uzbekistan, based on the information provided by experts and HIV activists. The study highlights some key concerns. Issues such as bureaucratic hurdles, lack of funding and limitations in government support schemes hamper the effectiveness of NGOs and affect their ability to provide comprehensive services to vulnerable populations, including those affected by HIV/AIDS. Stigma remains a major barrier to HIV prevention, affecting marginalised groups such as MSM and sex workers and preventing them from accessing essential treatment and prevention services. The legal environment, including laws that criminalise certain behaviours, contributes to a climate of fear and discrimination that hampers efforts to respond effectively to HIV/AIDS.

Despite these challenges, NGOs remain key actors in HIV prevention efforts in Uzbekistan. They play a pivotal role in advocacy, programme development and support services to vulnerable groups. Their collaboration with government agencies demonstrates promising advances in inter-sectoral partnerships for HIV prevention and support. Overall, the article provides a nuanced understanding of the complex landscape surrounding NGOs, social partnerships and the fight against HIV/AIDS in Uzbekistan. It highlights the need for streamlined bureaucratic processes, increased financial support, legal reforms to combat stigma, and an enabling environment for NGOs to operate effectively and drive impactful change in HIV prevention and care.

Bibliography

Eurasian Coalition on Health, Rights, Gender and Sexual Diversity (ECOM) (2021): Punishment for gays remains in the draft Criminal Code of Uzbekistan. www.ecom.ngo/news-ecom/nakazanie-dlya-geev-ostalosj-v-proekte-uk-uzbekistana, 05.03.2024.

Fedorova, Olga/Chingin, Alexey (2014): Uzbekistan. Drug situation and anti-drug policy. www.rm.coe.int/-2014-/168075f32c, 05.03.2024.

Institution in the form of a non-governmental non-profit organization "Madad" (2019): State social order and the procedure for its implementation. www.advice.uz/ru/document/2744, 05.03.2024.

International Center for Not-For-Profit Law (ICNL) (n.d.): Home. www.icnl.org/, 29.11.2023.

International Center for Not-For-Profit Law (ICNL) (n.d.b): Uzbekistan. www.icnl.org/our-work/uzbekistan, 05.03.2024.

International Federation of Social Workers (IFSW) (2024): Global Definition of Social Work. www.ifsw.org/what-is-social-work/global-definition-of-social-work/, 05.03.2024.

Intilish (n.d.): Home. www.intilish.uz/, 05.03.2024.

Ishonch Va Hayot (n.d.): PLWH – Faith and Life. www.plwh.uz/, 29.11.2023.

Latypov, Alisher/Otiashvili, David/Aizberg, Oleg/Boltaev, Azizbek (2010): Opioid substitution therapy in Central Asia: on the way to diverse and effective drug addiction treatment. https://solid-exceed.org/resources/publication/opioid-substitution-therapy-central-asia-towards-diverse-and-effective-treatment-options-drug-dependence , 05.03.2024.

LexUZ (n.d.): Criminal Code of the Republic of Uzbekistan. www.lex.uz/acts/111457, 05.03.2024.

LexUZ (2011): RESOLUTION OF THE CABINET OF MINISTERS OF THE REPUBLIC OF UZBEKISTAN. About approval of the regulatory legal acts necessary for implementation of the Law of the Republic of Uzbekistan "About modification and amendments in the Law of the Republic of Uzbekistan "About the state provision of pensions of citizens" and the Labor code of the Republic of Uzbekistan". [No. 107, 07 April 2011].

https://cis-legislation.com/document.fwx?rgn=69807#B4630K7YLE, 03.05.2024.

LexUZ (2013a): Law of the Republic of Uzbekistan. On countering the spread of the disease caused by the human immunodeficiency virus (HIV infection) [No. ZRU-353, 23 September 2013]. www.lex.uz/acts/2240472, 05.03.2024.

LexUZ (2013b): Resolution of the President of the Republic of Uzbekistan. On additional measures to assist the development of civil society institutions [No. PP-2085, 12 December 2013]. www.lex.uz/docs/2294384, 05.03.2024.

LexUZ (2014): Law of the Republic of Uzbekistan. On social partnership [No. ZRU-376, 28 August 2014]. www.lex.uz/docs/2468216, 05.03.2024.

LexUZ (2018a): Resolution of the President of the Republic of Uzbekistan. On additional measures to counter the spread of the disease caused by the human immunodeficiency virus and the prevention of nosocomial infections [No. PP-3800, 22 June 2018]. www.lex.uz/docs/3791786, 29.11.2023.

LexUZ (2018b): Decree President of the Republic of Uzbekistan. On measures to radically increase the role of civil society institutions in the process of democratic renewal of the country [No. UP-5430, 04 May 2018]. www.lex.uz/docs/3721651, 05.03.2024.

LexUZ (2021): Law of the Republic of Uzbekistan. On the Rights of the Persons with Disabilities [No. LRU-641, 15 October 2020]. www.lex.uz/docs/5049549, 05.03.2024.

LexUZ (2023a): Resolution of the President of the Republic of Uzbekistan. On measures to further strengthen the system to counteract the disease caused by the human immunodeficiency virus [No. PP-14, 20 January 2023]. www.lex.uz/docs/6364832, 29.11.2023.

LexUZ (2023b): The Constitution of the Republic of Uzbekistan. www.lex.uz/docs/6451070, 29.11.2023.

LexUZ (2023c): Resolution of the Cabinet of Ministers of the Republic of Uzbekistan. On measures to further support social partnership and international cooperation in the implementation by non-governmental non-profit organizations of socially useful programs and projects [No. 527, 04 October 2023]. www.lex.uz/ru/pdfs/6627539, 05.03.2024.

Ministry of Justice of the Republic of Uzbekistan (n.d.): Portal of non-profit non-governmental organizations of the Ministry of Justice of the Republic of Uzbekistan. www.e-ngo.uz/?lang=ru, 29.11.2023.

NGO 'Anti-Cancer Society of Uzbekistan' (n.d.): Home. www.anticancer.uz/, 29.11.2023.

NORMA Information and legal portal (2022): The President signed the Law of October 28, 2022 No. ZRU-798 "On approval of the Labor Code of the Republic of Uzbekistan". www.norma.uz/novoe_v_zakonodatelstve/utverjden_novyy_trudovoy_kodeks, 05.03.2024.

O'zbekiston Milliy Axborot Agentligi (UzA) (2021): On additional measures for state support of non-governmental non-profit organizations, ensuring freedom of their activities, protection of rights and legitimate interests. www.uza.uz/ru/posts/o-dopolnitelnyx-merax-po-gosudarstvennoy-podderzhke-negosudarstvennyx-nekommercheskix-organizaciy-obespecheniyu-svobody-ix-deyatelnosti-zaschity-prav-i-zakonnyx-interesov_245988, 05.03.2024.

Qalampir (2021): Officially: it was revealed how many people were imprisoned for homosexuality in Uzbekistan. www.qalampir.uz/uz/news/rasman-uzbekistonda-besok-olbozligi-uchun-k-amalganlar-k-anchaligi-ochik-landi-37556, 07.03.2024.

SoyuzPravoInform (2021): Resolution of the President of the Republic of Uzbekistan. About additional measures for the state support of non-state non-profit organizations, ensuring freedom of their activities, protection of the rights and legitimate interests [No. PP-5012, 03 March 2021]. www.cis-legislation.com/document.fwx?rgn=130705, 05.03.2024.

Sputnik Uzbekistan (2019): Fighting HIV: UNAIDS office opened in Uzbekistan. www.uz.sputniknews.ru/20191206/Borba-s-VICh-V-Uzbekistane-otkrylos-predstavitelstvo-YuNEYDS-12954539.html, 05.03.2024.

StopTB Partnership (2019): Tuberculosis Situation in 2020. Uzbekistan. www.stoptb.org/static_pages/UZB_Dashboard.html, 05.03.2024.

The Global Fund (2022): Datasets. Uzbekistan. www.data.theglobalfund.org/location/UZB/overview, 05.03.2024.

The Joint United Nations Programme on HIV/AIDS (UNAIDS) (2020): Don't miss the moment. Eliminate inequality to end the epidemic. www.unaids.org/sites/default/files/media_asset/2020_global-aids-report_ru.pdf, 05.03.2024.

The Joint United Nations Programme on HIV/AIDS (UNAIDS) (2021a): Political Declaration on HIV and AIDS: Ending Inequalities and Getting on Track to End AIDS by 2030. www.unaids.org/ru/resources/documents/2021/2021_political-declaration-on-hiv-and-aids, 30.10.2023.

The Joint United Nations Programme on HIV/AIDS (UNAIDS) (2021b): HIV, stigma and discrimination. www.unaids.org/sites/default/files/media_asset/07-hiv-human-rights-factsheet-stigma-discrmination_ru.pdf, 05.03.2024.

The Joint United Nations Programme on HIV/AIDS (UNAIDS) (2022): A Country. Uzbekistan. www.unaids.org/ru/regionscountries/countries/uzbekistan, 05.03.2024.

The Joint United Nations Programme on HIV/AIDS (UNAIDS) (2023): Key populations. www.unaids.org/en/topic/key-populations#:~:text=UNAIDS%20considers%20gay%20men%20and,lack%20adequate%20access%20to%20services, 05.03.2024.

The President Republic of Uzbekistan (2023): On measures to further strengthen the system to counteract the disease caused by the human immunodeficiency virus. www.president.uz/ru/lists/view/5867, 30.11.2023.

United Nations Office on Drugs and Crime (UNODC) (2017): Implementation of comprehensive programs for HIV and Hepatitis C for people, injecting drug users. Practical Guide for Council Mayors. www.inpud.net/wp-content/uploads/2022/01/IDUIT_RU_new_Final.pdf, 05.03.2024.

United Nations Office on Drugs and Crime (UNODC) (2023): Interview: Combating the spread of diseases caused by the human immunodeficiency virus in Uzbekistan. A turning point. www.unodc.org/centralasia/en/news/interview_-hiv-prevention-in-uzbekistan--a-turning-point---ru.html, 05.03.2024.

Uznews.uz (2021): Russia and UNAIDS donated a mobile clinic to Uzbekistan for $300 thousand. www.uznews-uz.webpkgcache.com/doc/-/s/uznews.uz/posts/5818, 05.03.2024.

World Health Organization (WHO) (2019): Progress report on implementation of the Action Plan for the Health Sector Response to HIV in the WHO European Region [EUR/RC69/8(A)]. www.apps.who.int/iris/rest/bitstreams/1330682/retrieve, 05.03.2024.

World Health Organization (WHO) (2023): Comprehensive review of the HIV program in Uzbekistan. Mission report. Geneva: WHO.

Yusupov, Dilmurad (2023): Has the procedure for NGOs working with international grants become simpler? www.gazeta.uz/ru/2023/10/27/ngos/, 05.03.2024.

13. Innovative Approaches in Adolescent Sexual Education: Bridging the Gap Between Awareness and Action

Tatsiana Pikirenia

The importance of targeting adolescents and schoolchildren in HIV prevention efforts and sexual education programmes is globally recognised. While it is not realistic to expect that a education programmes alone can eliminate the risk of HIV and other sexually transmitted infections (STIs), unintended pregnancy, or coercive or abusive sexual activity and exploitation, properly designed and implemented education programmes can reduce some of these risks and underlying vulnerabilities (United Nations Educational, Scientific and Cultural Organization [UNESCO] 2009).

As a United Nations member state, Uzbekistan is committed to implementing the 2030 Agenda for Sustainable Development. The Resolution of the Cabinet of Ministers of the Republic of Uzbekistan approved national goals and objectives in the field of sustainable development for the period until 2030. In this document, Target 3.7 is formulated as follows: 'By 2030, ensure universal access to sexual and reproductive health-care services, including for family planning, and raising the marriageable age for girls to eighteen years of age, and the integration of reproductive health into national strategies and programmes' (LexUZ 2018).

There have been a few policy documents developed regarding sexual education and reproductive health in Uzbekistan. The Law of the Republic of Uzbekistan on Protection of the Reproductive Health of Citizens states that sex education shall be conducted based on approved special curricula, developed jointly by education authorities and government health agencies (LexUZ 2019).

Although we could not find any national guidelines on teaching reproductive health issues in open sources in order to be able to analyse the comprehensiveness of sex education programmes in Uzbekistan, a 'Report of the Implementation of the Beijing Declaration and Platform for Action' pays attention to the formal character of existing sex education that does not meet the modern standards (United Nations Economic Commission for Europe [UNECE] 2019).

We can see a gap between the declared priorities of state programmes and the actual implementation of effective practices to reduce the incidence of STIs and risky behaviour in Uzbekistan.

As another country in the post-Soviet space, Belarus has experienced similar problems. Approaches to sexual education in schools and information on transmission risks and safe behaviour are quite similar in Belarus and Uzbekistan. Both countries prioritise the importance of reproductive health issues and the prevention of risky behaviour among adolescents. At the same time, there is a gap between setting priorities and shaping the programmes according to the needs of the youth.

Some experts even assess current approaches to sexual and reproductive health and rights education in Belarus as being outdated and reiterating gender stereotypes (Belarusian Helsinki Committee 2023).

The United Nations Population Fund (UNFPA) recommends the following areas of work:

1. Increasing public awareness about safe and risky sexual behaviour, and manifestations of risky and unsafe sexual behaviour: focus on adolescents and youth, high school students in general secondary education institutions, students in specialised vocational and secondary education institutions, and university students.
2. Addressing gaps in knowledge, including misconceptions about the risk of contracting HIV infection and STIs during various forms of sexual contact. Here, the UNFPA stresses that young people under 30 are more vulnerable than other age groups, so they are the target group (UNFPA 2022).

According to the United Nations Children's Fund (UNICEF), adolescents in Belarus reported a lack of information and knowledge about mental health issues and stigma associated with mental disorders, drug use, conflicts with the law, HIV status, and non-traditional sexual orientation among peers (Ministry of Health of the Republic of Belarus/UNICEF in the Republic of Belarus 2019).

Thus, there is a need to have some tools to monitor the success of the infrastructure for the protection of reproductive health and the prevention of risky behaviour among adolescents. It is important to monitor the extent to which official training programmes actually meet the needs of adolescents.

To achieve this goal, our team (Darya Varabyeva, economist at the NGO 'Positive Movement', Katerina Parfeniuk, an activist, Aleksandra Korotkova, a social worker, and Tatsiana Pikirenia, executive director of the NGO

'Positive Movement') created a methodology of city quests for high school students (aged 15 to 16 years old) and performed it in Belarus in 2018. The pilot project made it possible to identify problems and convey them to decision makers. Based on these results, we feel that such a practice could be successfully applied in Uzbekistan and in other countries where there is a need to monitor the success of the implementation of HIV prevention programmes among adolescents.

We believe that the methodology described below is suitable for most teenagers, regardless of their social position or academic performance. It is a good tool for educational institutions and local authorities due to its affordability, ease of organization, and the engaging and entertaining nature of the activity, which makes it easy to involve schoolchildren. The exercise is also transparent due to the use of social media as a medium for sharing the experiences with others and the fact that it can be performed in an active format; and unbiased and purposeful because it is performed by the target audience of the education programmes and healthcare infrastructure. Furthermore, there are qualitative results that could be achieved when involving adolescents in monitoring activities: participants develop the skills needed to interact with service providers and advocate for the rights of adolescents.

Methodology

The purpose of the quests is to teach teenagers the skills they need to take care of their health, receive professional help, and reduce the risk of HIV transmission. The quest involves teams of schoolchildren (15 to 16 years old, several teams per school; we had four to six teams of up to 10 people each) exploring the city to try to access services related to sexual and reproductive health in various institutions, as well as find interesting spaces to spend leisure time and communicate with peers. The quest is limited to one day (24 hours); teams compete with each other to complete the tasks and share their experience on social media.

The quests were financially supported by the UNICEF Office in Belarus. To provide competitive motivation, prizes were provided for the teams that finished in first, second, and third places. The quests were developed and conducted by activists and specialists from the public organisation 'Positive Movement' in four cities in Belarus, and 135 teenagers (70 boys, 65 girls) participated. The results of the quests were presented on 19th December 2018 in Minsk, at a round table 'The practice of socio-psychological work with youth to develop constructive life skills to overcome difficulties', which included the participation of some of the teenagers who took part in the quests (Belarusian Public Association 'Positive Movement' 2018). The event was attended by social educators, school psychologists, specialists in educational and methodological schoolwork, teachers of additional education institutions, and experts in the field of psychology of adolescent behaviour. At the round table, the NGO 'Positive Movement' suggested that educational institutions use the quest methodology, as it showed effectiveness and was positively perceived by the teenagers themselves.

In our quests, tasks were divided into the following topics:

1. Testing for HIV infection.
2. Medical counselling on sexual and reproductive health issues.
3. Help in connection with violence.
4. Leisure activities.

Testing for HIV Infection

1. The team of schoolchildren needs to fill out a questionnaire about HIV infection, take a photograph and send it to the organisers for verification. We do not provide an example of a questionnaire here, since the questions we used in 2018 are somewhat outdated. However, we would like to point out that when developing a questionnaire, it is necessary to encourage adolescents to find reliable information about prevention, treatment, and living with HIV, so that in the process of answering the questions, the teams of schoolchildren correct any misconceptions they have surrounding the issue of HIV infection and sexual and reproductive health.
2. A team needs to find at least one place where they can anonymously and freely get tested for HIV, without the presence of parents. HIV testing in Belarus is voluntary, so the task does not require teenagers to actually take the test but rather just find such an opportunity and describe on social networks whether it was easy to find such places, how clear and friendly the consultation was at the healthcare institutions, whether they received answers to their questions, how much their motivation to take the test has increased/decreased, and other personal impressions.

During our quests, some HIV prevention departments based in state epidemiology centres refused to conduct HIV testing in the absence of parents. However, the schoolchildren managed to buy an HIV test at the pharmacy and used it.

Medical Counselling on Sexual and Reproductive Health Issues

1. The team needs to try to seek advice from a gynaecologist and urologist and share on their social networks about what kind of help these specialists provide and why they are relevant for teenagers. The text must be original, written by teenagers for teenagers; copying from other sources does not count.

From our quests we learned that in all four cities, adolescents were provided with medical consultation on sexual and reproductive health by either a gynaecologist or urologist.

Help in Connection with Violence

1. Teenagers need to film a video interview on their smartphone with any adult (a passer-by, parent, teacher, older brother or sister, etc.) and ask them the following questions:
   a) What kind of violence can teenagers face?
   b) Are you allowed to beat children, and if so, up to what age?
   c) Who can help a teenager if they are faced with violence?
   d) Any other questions they would like to ask.
2. The team must find a hotline that assists with issues of violence, call them, and leave feedback about this communication on their social networks.

The teams of schoolchildren managed to shoot videos on the problem of domestic violence. The majority of adults surveyed expressed a negative attitude towards violence against children, which our quest participants were very satisfied with.

At the same time, psychological support hotlines performed poorly. They either did not answer or gave advice that the adolescents rated as useless or even inadequate to their understanding of the situation. For example, one of the teams got a recommendation from a hotline specialist to obey all the demands of a family abuser, which the teenagers found weird.

Leisure Activities

1. Teams were asked to find a place where they would like to spend their leisure time. The place should be fun for them, free of charge, and accessible for the whole team. Teenagers should take photos and shoot videos at the locations, and tag them on their social networks.
2. In addition, the teams needed to share their opinion about the availability and quality of recreation options for teenagers in the city.

In our case, the quests turned out to be a very constructive way of checking the availability of services and assessing whether the conditions for receiving them met the needs of adolescents.

In large cities like Minsk, Gomel, and Vitebsk, teenagers noted that there were a lot of beautiful places, but there were no places where you could sit inside for free when it was cold outside. They also complained about the lack of places with free internet connection.

The experience of conducting quests has shown us that any initiative can be implemented with teenagers, including programmes to inform them about the risks of unsafe behaviour, if you create an environment that matches their interests and needs. In particular, free internet and heated public spaces can be easily organised in the existing urban infrastructure: in schools, cinemas, cultural centres, sports clubs, libraries, etc. Access to these places should be low-threshold (i.e. teenagers do not need to have a specific purpose to spend time there). Social issues such as domestic violence and health are of interest to teenagers, but they say the way this information is presented in schools, i.e. in a lecture format, lags behind modern trends and is irrelevant today.

To build a constructive dialogue with adolescents on sensitive topics such as HIV, sexual behaviour, and substance use, it is necessary to answer questions honestly, provide only reliable information, demonstrate a willingness to help instead of punish, maintain confidentiality, and welcome feedback and initiative.

Furthermore, direct feedback from the people who receive information and medical services is more important when there is no critical view from other stakeholders. Organising such quests can be a good alternative in countries where feedback from communities or public organisations is poorly developed.

Conclusion

Quests allow stakeholders to look at many problems through the eyes of teenagers and assess whether the surrounding infrastructure meets their needs and how efforts can be improved to prevent destructive forms of behaviour among young people.

Addressing these risks requires a multifaceted approach, including comprehensive sexual education, youth-friendly health services, empowerment programmes, and supportive legal and social environments. By targeting adolescents and schoolchildren with appropriate interventions, it is possible to significantly reduce their risk of HIV and STI transmission and support their overall health and well-being.

Bibliography

Belarusian Helsinki Committee (2023): Belarus. The right to education, advances and challenges. www.ohchr.org/sites/default/files/documents/issues/education/cfi-hrc53/submission-education-hrc53-cso-bhc-en.pdf, 22.11.2023.

Belarusian Public Association 'Positive Movement' (2018): Forms of working with teenagers – a reboot is needed. www.pmplus.by/press-room/news/snizhenie_vreda/formy_raboty_s_podrostkami_nuzhna_perezagruzka_/, 22.11.2023.

LexUZ (2018): Resolution of the Cabinet of Ministers. On measures to implement the National Goals and Objectives in the field of sustainable development for the period until 2030 [No. 841, 20 October 2018]. www.lex.uz/docs/4013358, 21.11.2023.

LexUZ (2019): Law of the Republic of Uzbekistan. On protection of the reproductive health of citizens [No. LRU-528, 11 March 2019]. www.lex.uz/en/docs/5149968, 21.11.2023.

Ministry of Health of the Republic of Belarus/United Nations Children's Fund (UNICEF) in the Republic of Belarus (2019): Study of mental health problems and suicidal behaviour of adolescents and young people in the Republic of Belarus. Brief report. www.unicef.org/belarus/media/1571/file/suicidalnoe_povedenie_podrostkov_kratki_otchet.pdf, 22.11.2023.

The United Nations Population Fund (UNFPA) (2022): Risky sexual behaviour of Belarusians and the practice of using condoms. www.belarus.unfpa.org/sites/default/files/pub-pdf/unfpa_2023_condom_use_survey_web.pdf, 22.11.2023.

United Nations Economic Commission for Europe (UNECE) (2019): Report of the Implementation of the Beijing Declaration and Platform for Action. Uzbekistan. www.unece.org/fileadmin/DAM/Gender/Beijing_20/Uzbekistan_ENG.pdf, 22.11.2023.

United Nations Educational, Scientific and Cultural Organization (UNESCO) (2009): International Technical Guidance on Sexuality Education. An evidence-informed approach for schools, teachers and health educators. www.unesdoc.unesco.org/ark:/48223/pf0000183281, 22.11.2023.

14. Social and Psychological Assistance to Women with HIV in Kyrgyzstan

Alla Bessonova, Asel Tentigenova, Nurgul Musaeva

Introduction

According to data of the Kyrgyz AIDS centre, the percentage of women among people living with HIV in Kyrgyzstan was 37.1% in June 2023 (Republican AIDS Centre 2023). Along with people who use drugs, women and girls living with HIV are vulnerable to violence and face widespread criminalisation and discrimination. A lack of reliable statistical data, misconceptions about how HIV is transmitted, as well as stigma and societal discrimination mean that HIV-positive women and girls face many challenges in Kyrgyzstan (Prosvet 2017).

This chapter focuses on the social and psychological needs of women living with HIV in Kyrgyzstan. The chapter first describes the general situation of women living on HIV and existing services, including the prevention of mother-to-child transmission and support services for mothers and children living with HIV. The chapter highlights the many forms of violence that women with HIV are facing and the need for mental health services and care in Kyrgyzstan.

The general situation of women living with HIV in Kyrgyzstan

Women living with HIV are highlighted in Kyrgyz national documents, strategies, plans, and policies related to the HIV response. The National HIV Programme (2023–2027) highlights women and girls living with HIV; it addresses research on gender-based violence and inequality and the impact these issues have for women in terms of gaining access to HIV services. Women living with HIV and sex workers contributed to the development of this programme and participated in the working group set up to develop the national funding request to the Global Fund.

The National HIV Clinical Protocols (2022) include sexual and reproductive health for people living with HIV, including cervical cancer prevention and treatment, especially for women living with HIV. Stigma, discrimination, and the human rights of women living with HIV are also discussed in national documents. HIV and gender issues are addressed by civil society organisations, with female representatives of the community of people living with HIV representing their community and advocating and actively participating in the Country Coordinating Mechanism (CCM), which coordinates the implementation of grants from the Global Fund (EWNA 2023).

Another important coordinating and governing body in the fight against HIV/AIDS is the Coordinating Council on Public Health under the Government of the Kyrgyz Republic, which has 23 members from the public and non-public sectors. 39% of the Council is made up of representatives of key communities, namely women and men living with HIV and young people (Committee to Combat HIV/AIDS, Tuberculosis and Malaria under the Committee for Health Protection under the Government of the Kyrgyz Republic 2024). The purpose of the Council is to ensure the coordination of government agencies, as well as non-profit and public organisations in addressing HIV/AIDS issues.

Due to the criminalisation of HIV, women are particularly vulnerable to stigmatisation and discrimination. In Kyrgyzstan, HIV transmission is criminalised. The laws have a strong impact on stigma and discrimination, as they create barriers to seeking care and treatment. Women who live with HIV face many difficulties when it comes to meeting their basic needs. This has a negative impact on their quality of life. The services available to women with HIV are also not gender-specific, which often limits their access to legal, social, psychological, and medical support.

There is a lack of studies on the situation of women with HIV in Kyrgyzstan. In 2017, the NGO Prosvet conducted a study on the needs of women with HIV in Kyrgyzstan. One of the biggest issues related to accessing health services is stigma, both in society in general and by medical service providers. Other issues include the lack of peer counselling services, with a person living HIV who has received special training, as a councillor. Such a person, who understands the medical, psychological, and social aspects of HIV, can share professional knowledge and help individuals when they receive an HIV diagnosis, offer assistance with adhering to ART therapy, and provide psychosocial support. Psychological support is not always available, especially outside the capital city Bishkek. The same applies to self-help groups for women living with HIV. However, psychological care (counselling, correction, rehabilitation) is one of the most important components in HIV prevention and treatment, which is why we focus on it later in this chapter.

The majority of women with HIV also need to be aware of their rights during the process of diagnosis and treatment and be protected from unlawful actions by employers, medical staff and others. One of the biggest fears of women with HIV is related to motherhood and losing custody of their child or children. It is not always understood, but childcare is an important motivating factor for many women with HIV, encouraging them to undergo regular health check-ups and adhere to ART treatment.

Prevention of Mother-to-Child Transmission in Kyrgyzstan

The global community has set the goal of eliminating mother-to-child (or vertical) transmission of HIV by 2030. This initiative seeks to eliminate the vertical transmission of not only HIV but also syphilis and viral hepatitis B. The actual elimination of mother-to-child transmission of HIV (EMTCT) means reducing the risk of vertical transmission of HIV to 1–2% among children who are not breastfed from birth and to 5% for breastfed children (World Health Organization [WHO] 2021).

Since 2007 in Kyrgyzstan, all pregnant women have been tested for HIV upon registering their pregnancy (The Joint United Nations Programme on HIV/AIDS [UNAIDS] 2020). The testing algorithm includes rapid HIV testing when pregnant women without prior HIV testing are admitted to maternity hospitals (WHO 2021).

Since 2020, Kyrgyzstan has also been implementing a state social contracting programme, which includes HIV prevention, diagnosis, care, and support for key populations (Ministry of Health of the Kyrgyz Republic 2020). From 2017 to 2021, the number of HIV-positive pregnant women in the country increased from 144 to 195, and the number of children with a vertical route of HIV infection increased from 16 to 24 (Republican AIDS Centre of the Kyrgyz Republic 2023). These negative trends may continue against the backdrop of existing stigma and discrimination against people living with HIV. At the end of 2022, the proportion of children diagnosed with HIV for the first time was 1.7% (two new cases out of 115 children with HIV).

The prevention of vertical transmission of HIV has been included in HIV clinical protocols, which does not prohibit a mother's choice to breastfeed. As part of a comprehensive approach to preventing the vertical transmission of HIV from mother to child (PMTCT), breastmilk substitutes are provided free of charge to women living with HIV (Eurasian Women's Network on AIDS [EWNA] 2023).

The Kyrgyz healthcare system follows international recommendations and ensures that pregnant women living with HIV continue to receive ART treatment after delivery. In the implementation of strategic directions in HIV programmes, issues related to compliance with international human rights standards remain unresolved, including issues of confidentiality and access to health services. Women living with HIV face discrimination in accessing family-planning services. According to the results of the Stigma Index 2020 survey, every tenth respondent openly reported that she had been advised to terminate her pregnancy and was pressurised to choose a specific method of childbirth and child feeding. At the same time, 25–27% of respondents refused to answer these questions. This may indicate that the topic is sensitive for women; perhaps they have faced discrimination, but do not want to discuss this experience.

Social protection of families with HIV-positive children

Families with children living with HIV are entitled to social support according to a jointly developed individual plan for working with families (SoyuzPravoInform 2015). A monthly social allowance is granted to children born to mothers living with HIV or AIDS (until they reach the age of 18 months).[1] The allowance is 8,000 soms (about 89 USD) (SoyuzPravoInform 2021).

In addition, since the beginning of 2023, Kyrgyzstan introduced a lump-sum payment of 6,300 soms (USD 71) for all mothers upon the birth of a child ("Balaga sүүunchү"). To put this into context, the average salary in Bishkek at the end of 2023 was 23,085 soms (USD 262) (Social Fund of the Kyrgyz Republic 2024). Women who have children with HIV are also entitled to an additional lump-sum payment of 4,900 soms (USD 55) until the child reaches the age of majority. The amount may be revised annually, taking into account changes in the subsistence level. In this case, financial support is provided to both the mother and the relatives who are caring for

1 The allowance is paid to children born to mothers living with HIV. In October 2021, the allowance was increased from 4,000 soms to 6,000 soms and in January 2022 from 4,000 soms to 8,000 soms.

the child. This form of support is guaranteed by the law because about 60% of the population of Kyrgyzstan are migrant workers. In many families, relatives take care of children while the parents are working abroad.

The Law of the Kyrgyz Republic "On HIV/AIDS in the Kyrgyz Republic" was amended on 17 August 2020: persons who were infected in medical institutions should be paid a compensation of at least 100,000 soms (SoyuzPravoInform 2020). From 2005 to February 2021, 403 HIV-positive children were registered with AIDS Centres who had been infected in medical institutions. Most of them became infected in 2005, in hospitals in the south of the country. This as a period when there was an outbreak of HIV cases among children, due to poor handling of medical instruments and non-compliance with infection control requirements.

It is worth mentioning that some private employers often require a medical examination for HIV, which contradicts the Law of the Kyrgyz Republic on HIV/AIDS. There are documented cases where women were denied employment or dismissed because of their HIV status. Some women will not take jobs that require a health book, which often results in them working below their skill level or in a grey zone. This is an example of stigma, and it results in people being pushed into poverty. Feelings of shame affect the self-esteem of women living with HIV/AIDS, as well as their ability to accept their status, and make them particularly vulnerable to violence, depression, and self-isolation.

Gender-based violence

A major problem in Kyrgyzstan is the criminalisation of HIV, which fuels stigma and discrimination, especially against women living with HIV. Article 143 of the Criminal Code of the Kyrgyz Republic (Infection with a venereal or incurable infectious disease), provides for a prison sentence, even in cases of unintended or negligent HIV transmission of HIV infection. The decriminalisation of HIV transmission is one of the main goals of the activist and human rights community in Kyrgyzstan. The existing criminalisation equates an HIV-positive person with a criminal, which fuels existing stigma, discrimination, and violence against people living with HIV, and women in particular.

While there are few convictions for HIV transmission, the criminalisation of HIV transmission maintains entrenched stigma against people living with HIV and is a source of structural discrimination that affects all areas of life. In patriarchal environments, women are even more vulnerable, both economically and socially. Women with HIV face discrimination more often than men with HIV and are often afraid to start a family, find a job, access health services, and seek help for survivors of violence.

The global community states that violence is a key risk factor for HIV infection among women (UN Commission on the Status of Women 2016). Despite the existing legislation and measures aimed at overcoming gender-based violence, the country lacks sustainable programmes and mechanisms to overcome stereotypes and violence against women. In Kyrgyzstan, women face violence in their interaction with state agencies, local communities and in their direct social environment. Women from key population, including women living with HIV, are particularly vulnerable to violence. Violence against them is systemic and is also perpetrated by law enforcement officials and representatives of other state organisations whose functions include human rights protection and service delivery, regardless of HIV status, occupation, behavioural patterns, and a number of other factors.

According to national statistics, in 2022, women accounted for the vast majority (95–96%) of victims of domestic violence (Ministry of Internal Affairs of the Kyrgyz Republic 2024). According to the data of the Alternative Report submitted to the Committee on the Elimination of Discrimination against Women (CEDAW) in 2021, women living with HIV in Kyrgyzstan are subjected to various forms of domestic violence: psychological violence in the form of insults, humiliation from family members (e.g. by insisting on using separate dishes due to an unjustified fear of infection), the isolation of children; physical and economic violence. Sometimes women with HIV are kicked out of the house by the relatives of their husband or not accepted in the house by their own relatives. Sometimes women are excluded from ART or TB treatment, which has led to cases of women dying.

In 2018, the Campaign "There is no excuse for violence" conducted a study in twelve countries of Eastern Europe and Central Asia (EECA) (EWNA 2019). The study involved 36 women living with HIV from Kyrgyzstan. Seven out of ten women reported experiencing physical violence and half of them experienced sexual violence, with two thirds of the cases of physical violence and three quarters of the cases of sexual violence being related to HIV status. Psychological and economic violence was reported by four women out of five. Forms of psychological violence included insults, humiliation, separation of dishes, and the isolation of children; economic violence included the husband's relatives being kicked out of the house or the women's own relatives not being accepted in the house. Furthermore, these women are often banned from taking ARV therapy, being treated for tuberculosis treatment, or being seen by a doctor, which has led to cases of women dying. Only one third of women sought help after facing violence during the year preceding the survey.

In interviews, Kyrgyz women reported:

> *"My mother told me not to come too often, to prevent any scandal because of me. Nobody wants my children, they [my family members] are scared that we will infect them, and they don't want their neighbours to see me come and to think that I left my husband. I have bruises everywhere, you know"* (EWNA 2019, p. 10).

> *"[He was] drunk, [he had] no job, no money. So, he lost his temper, and I was always to blame. 'Where will you go? I'll bury you and no one will find you. No one needs you; no one will look for you'"* (EWNA 2019, p. 10).

Despite the fact that Kyrgyzstan has a law on domestic violence and has developed mechanisms to enforce this law, women avoid seeking protection and resort to it only in extreme cases. Women living with HIV, being a stigmatised group, are even less likely to seek help. This situation is fuelled by widespread stereotypes that blame women for being caught up in a violent situation (victimisation). For example, one opinion leader openly accused women suffering from domestic violence of being responsible for being repeatedly battered (Kapushenko 2021). This stereotype influences the work of law enforcement officers and judges in Kyrgyzstan. In addition, women rarely receive support from relatives in cases of domestic violence; more often they face accusations from relatives. The family is often a source of stigma for women living with HIV. In such a situation, a woman is under even greater pressure and has no resources to defend herself against violence.

Kyrgyzstan lacks mechanisms for emergency interventions of specialists in cases of violence against women (e.g. to provide medical, psychological, social, or legal assistance). Protocols for HIV-related medical care do not address violence-related issues, which include screening to determine whether a woman is currently in a situation of violence, to ascertain whether there are potential threats of violence, and to provide information about organisations that can provide support in terms of counselling, legal assistance, and shelter.

Mental well-being

Mental well-being is an integral component of human health, along with physical and social well-being. The main healthcare efforts and services (including HIV prevention and treatment) are aimed at supporting physical health, while at the same time insufficiently addressing and/or ignoring problems related to mental health.

There are no available epidemiological data on depression in Kyrgyzstan, so it is impossible to see the real situation among both the general population and HIV-positive women.

In 2021, the EWNA initiated the first rapid assessment of depression screening among HIV-positive women in EECA countries, including Kyrgyzstan (EWNA n.d.). The study was designed to obtain up-to-date information on the prevalence of depression among HIV-positive women in the region and to analyse the relationship between depression and physical health problems and life circumstances. In the rapid assessment, 720 women living with HIV were screened for depression.

Factors affecting mental well-being in HIV-positive women in Kyrgyzstan

Women living with HIV often have concomitant physical health problems and find themselves in various difficult life situations, which together negatively affect both their mental health and their adherence to ARV treatment, including during and/or after pregnancy.

Depression is one of the most common mental health problems. Based on the results of a situation assessment of depression screening in women living with HIV, it was hypothesised that depression is a real problem for the mental, physical, and social well-being of HIV-positive women.

It is important to note that the problem of depression is invisible and often remains neglected for many reasons, such as due to a lack of regular screening and subsequent diagnosis of depression; women's lack of awareness of the signs and consequences of depression; and a lack of services and self-help skills.

However, the problem has not received sufficient attention. According to the first National HIV Prevention Programme in the Kyrgyz Republic of 2012, all major public health efforts and services in the area of HIV prevention and treatment were mainly focused on supporting physical health, with insufficient focus on mental health issues (Ministry of Justice of the Kyrgyz Republic 2012).

Maternal depression

According to the World Health Organisation, depressive disorders after childbirth (maternal depression) are a serious problem for many women (WHO 2022). At present, maternal depression is an under-recognised and under-researched condition, especially in countries with a low standard of living. Increased levels of stress during pregnancy, domestic violence, and stigma due to HIV status negatively affect the psychological well-being of the mother. In the postnatal period, women often find themselves in a state of social and informational isolation, as she devotes most of her time and efforts to caring for her new-born. Factors that should be considered when discussing or attempting to diagnose maternal depression include lifestyle during pregnancy, including nutrition, the presence of nicotine, alcohol, or drug addiction, and the presence of chronic diseases. The physical condition of the woman after childbirth, including the presence of postpartum stitches, difficulty using the toilet after childbirth, and discomfort in the hospital ward, also play a significant role.

More than one third of the participants of the depression screening reported signs of moderate (15.7%) and severe (12.8%) depression. More than half of the respondents reported that they were adhering to their ARV treatment (60.2%), while the rest noted that they had missed some of their regular medication, including skipping a few days (33.7%) and skipping a few weeks (3.9%).

The emergence and development of maternal depression affects not only the health of the woman herself but also has a significant impact on the child. The interaction between mother and child is very important for the child's development. Women suffering from postpartum depression may find it difficult to interact emotionally with their baby and may negatively evaluate the baby's emotional expressions. This can lead to a disruption in the emotional bond between mother and child, and affect the development of the child's emotional regulation.

Prolonged disruption of mother–child interaction can have a negative impact on the child's future physical, mental, and emotional development. Some studies show that children whose mothers suffered from postpartum depression may experience problems with social development, anger, and aggression and have an increased risk of developing mental disorders in the future.

It is therefore important to pay timely attention to maternal depression among women living with HIV and provide support and treatment to minimise the negative impact on both their own health and that of their child. Psychotherapy, pharmacotherapy, and extensive support from others can be effective options for treating maternal depression and promoting the healthy development and well-being of mother and child.

In the Action Plan of the Cabinet of Ministers of the Kyrgyz Republic's programme on overcoming HIV infection and viral hepatitis for 2023–2027, the strategic direction for the provision of treatment, care, and support services for people living with HIV (PLHIV) takes into account the expansion of access for people living with HIV to HIV education, psychological counselling, and mental health services (Cabinet of Ministers of the Kyrgyz Republic n.d.). Psychological counselling for women living with HIV is available at AIDS centres across the country. Some mental health care is provided for women at the Republican Centre for Narcology and Psychiatry (EWNA 2023).

The results of the rapid assessment of depression in the region suggest that depression is a real problem for the mental, physical, and social well-being of women living with HIV. In order not to ignore the impact of depression on the adherence to treatment as ART for mothers living with HIV, it is recommended to provide mothers with comprehensive services consisting of psychotherapy, pharmacotherapy, and extensive support in order to prevent and treat maternal depression in women living with HIV, and to study and research the mental health situation of HIV-positive women.

It should also be noted that both women living with HIV and their children require special attention due to the stigma and stereotyping they face from society, which may affect the women's adherence to ART (antiretroviral therapy). Therefore, training programmes for parents, which motivate them and advocate for children's rights, should be part of programmes for children and their parents. Working with and caring for women is also especially important during pregnancy, childbirth, and infant care. At this stage, adherence to educational activities should be encouraged, emphasising the importance of adherence to prevention of mother-to-child transmission of HIV (PMTCT) and the importance of viral load suppression for the health of the new-born. There may also be the issue of accommodating an HIV-positive woman and her infant following discharge from the maternity hospital. Providing care and support during pregnancy and breastfeeding have a significant impact on the effectiveness of PMTCT and the health of the new-born baby (Ministry of Health of the Kyrgyz Republic 2018).

Thus, in light of the aforementioned issues, socio-psychological work in the field of HIV/AIDS can be seen as especially relevant and necessary. The health of future generations and the formation of moral foundations and societal values directly depend on the well-being of families and the state of maternal health. Maternal health is an important component of national policy.

Bibliography

Cabinet of Ministers of the Kyrgyz Republic (n.d.): Action Plan of the KR Cabinet of Ministers Programme on overcoming HIV infection and haemocontact viral hepatitis for 2023–2027 (HIV component). www.gov.kg/ru, 12.03.2024.

Committee to Combat HIV/AIDS, Tuberculosis and Malaria under the Committee for Health Protection under the Government of the Kyrgyz Republic (2024): Composition of the Committee. www.hivtbcc.kg/pages/members.html, 04.03.2024.

Eurasian Women's Network on AIDS (EWNA) (n.d.): Home. www.ewna.org, 12.03.2024.

Eurasian Women's Network on AIDS (EWNA) (2019): Study on violence against women living with HIV in Eastern Europe and Central Asia. Analytical report 2019. www.ewna.org/wp-content/uploads/2019/11/EWNA_Report_EN_preview_v5.pdf, 04.03.2024.

Eurasian Women's Network on AIDS (EWNA) (2022): Community-led screening of depression among HIV-positive women in the EECA region. www.programme.aids2022.org/PAGMaterial/PPT/3074_2268/EPD244_Community-led_screening_of_depression.pdf, 12.03.2024.

Eurasian Women's Network on AIDS (EWNA) (2023): How countries are addressing barriers to HIV services for women living with HIV, sex workers and women who use drugs. www.ewna.org/wp-content/uploads/2023/08/ewna-gender-assessment-report_ru-02.08.2023-final.pdf, 04.03.2024.

Kapushenko, Anna (2021): "Fools!" Ilim Karypbekov accused victims of domestic violence of continuing to be beaten. What's wrong with that? www.kloop.kg/blog/2021/09/07/dury-ilim-karypbekov-obvinil-postradavshih-ot-domashnego-nasiliya-v-tom-chto-ih-prodolzhayut-izbivat-chto-s-etim-ne-tak/, 04.03.2024.

Ministry of Health of the Kyrgyz Republic (2018): Standards of service delivery for key population groups within the framework of the state social order of the Kyrgyz Republic approved by the order of the Ministry of Health of the Kyrgyz Republic. www.med.kg/, 12.03.2024.

Ministry of Health of the Kyrgyz Republic (2020): On approving the program for 2021–2023 according to the state social order [No. 1093, 23 December 2020]. www.aidscenter.kg/wp-content/uploads/2023/03/prikaz-1093-ot-23.12.2020-Ob-utverzhdenii-programmy-po-gosudarstvennomu-sotsialnomu-zakazu-na-2021-2023-gody.pdf, 04.03.2024.

Ministry of Internal Affairs of the Kyrgyz Republic (2024): Information on family violence for the first 6 months of 2023. www.mvd.gov.kg/rus/domesticViolence/reports/24, 04.03.2024.

Ministry of Justice of the Kyrgyz Republic (2012): About the State Programme for Stabilizing the HIV Epidemic in the Kyrgyz Republic for 2012-2016 [No. 867, 29 December 2012]. www.cbd.minjust.gov.kg/act/view/ru-ru/93826, 04.02.2024.

Prosvet (2017): Needs and Requirements of Women Living with HIV in the Kyrgyz Republic Research Report. www.ewna.org/wp-content/uploads/2022/10/prosvet_report_2017_rus.pdf, 11.03.2024.

Republican AIDS Centre of the Kyrgyz Republic (2023): The situation of HIV infection in the Kyrgyz Republic on 01.01.23. www.aidscenter.kg/wp-content/uploads/2023/03/01.01.2023.pdf, 04.03.2023.

Social Fund of the Kyrgyz Republic (2024): Data on average monthly wages in the Kyrgyz Republic for 2023. www.socfond.kg/ru/support/payer/http-socfond-kg-ru-payers-smz/, 04.03.2024.

SoyuzPravoInform (2015): About approval of the Regulations on procedure for identification of the children and families which are in difficult life situation [No. 391, 22 June 2015]. www.cis-legislation.com/document.fwx?rgn=77569, 04.02.2024.

SoyuzPravoInform (2020): On HIV/AIDS in the Kyrgyz Republic [No. 149, 17 August 2020]. www.cis-legislation.com/document.fwx?rgn=9209, 04.03.2024.

SoyuzPravoInform (2021): About increase in the sizes of monthly social benefits to separate categories of citizens [No. 373, 01 September 2021]. www.cis-legislation.com/document.fwx?rgn=134516, 04.03.2024.

The Joint United Nations Programme on HIV/AIDS (UNAIDS) (2020): Country Progress Report – Kyrgyzstan. Global Monitoring of the AIDS Epidemic 2020. www.unaids.org/sites/default/files/country/documents/KGZ_2020_countryreport.pdf, 04.03.2024.

UN Commission on the Status of Women (2016): Report of the sixtieth session. 20 March 2015 and 14–24 March 2016 [E/2016/27-E/CN.6/2016/22]. www.documents.un.org/doc/undoc/gen/n16/101/24/pdf/n1610124.pdf?token=795Qd2baNrqG4rcVeO&fe=true, 04.03.2024.

World Health Organization (WHO) (2021): Global guidance on criteria and processes for validation: elimination of mother-to-child transmission of HIV, syphilis and hepatitis B virus. www.iris.who.int/bitstream/handle/10665/349550/9789240039360-eng.pdf?isAllowed=y&sequence=1, 04.03.2024.

World Health Organization (WHO) (2022): Recommendations according to WHO prenatal care assistance for formation positive experience pregnancy. www.who.int/ru/news/item/30-03-2022-who-urges-quality-care-for-women-and-newborns-in-critical-first-weeks-after-childbirth, 04.03.2024.

15. The Role of Social Work in the Prevention and Treatment of HIV/AIDS in Germany

Larissa Steimle, Heino Stöver, Ingo Ilja Michels, Daniel Deimel

Driven by a commitment to eliminate new HIV infections, eradicate discrimination, and reduce AIDS-related deaths to zero, significant strides have been made worldwide in the fight against HIV/AIDS over the past 15 years (Henrickson et al. 2017, p. 11). Whereas two decades ago, the AIDS pandemic seemed unstoppable, claiming two million lives a year, today 29.8 million of the 39 million people living with HIV globally are receiving life-saving treatment (Joint United Nations Programme on HIV/AIDS [UNAIDS] 2023, p. 8).

Despite this incredible success in recent years, millions of people still miss out on treatment, including 43% of children living with HIV. Adolescent girls and young women in particular still have to contend with extraordinarily high risks of HIV infection in many parts of sub-Saharan Africa. Every week, 4,000 adolescent girls and young women acquire HIV. In 2022, women and girls in sub-Saharan Africa accounted for 63% of all new HIV infections. Beyond sub-Saharan Africa, numbers of new HIV infections have reduced modestly. 23% of new HIV infections were in Asia and the Pacific, where numbers of new HIV infections are rising alarmingly in some countries. Although the prevalence has decreased among injecting drug users in Central Asia and China due to implemented harm reduction measures such as needle/syringe provision and opiate substitution treatment (OST), since 2010 the numbers of new HIV infections have continued to increase steeply in Eastern Europe and Central Asia (a 49% increase) and the Middle East and North Africa (a 61% increase). The emergence of these trends can be attributed mainly to a lack of prevention services for people from marginalised and key populations and to the barriers posed by punitive laws, violence, and social stigma and discrimination (UNAIDS 2023, p. 7ff.).

Social work is a practice-based profession and academic discipline that 'engages people and structures to address life challenges and enhance wellbeing' (International Federation of Social Workers [IFSW] 2014), and therefore has a clear mandate to face the great challenges associated with

HIV/AIDS. In addition to being tasked with taking care of people affected by HIV/AIDS, social work is perhaps uniquely positioned to address the multifarious challenges presented by HIV/AIDS because of the interdisciplinary, transdisciplinary, and even intersectional nature of the work. Social work is interdisciplinary, with practitioners often collaborating with professionals from diverse fields, each contributing unique theories, perspectives, and research interests. It is transdisciplinary, as social workers routinely transcend traditional disciplinary boundaries for the well-being of clients, patients, or service users. Additionally, social work is intersectional, addressing individual and community-level experiences to advocate for individuals, families, and communities in policymaking (Henrickson et al. 2017, p. 8f.). Alongside these two points – having a clear mandate and being uniquely positioned – social workers frequently serve as the initial and, in certain cases, sole point of interaction with vulnerable populations, who are – at least in some cases – especially threatened by the potential negative consequences of HIV/AIDS. Vulnerable populations especially affected by HIV include men who have sex with men, women, commercial sex workers, injection drug users and children (Natale et al. 2010, p. 27f.). Therefore, in 2022, compared with adults in the general population, HIV prevalence was eleven times higher among gay men and other men who have sex with men, four times higher among sex workers, seven times higher among people who inject drugs, and 14 times higher among transgender people (UNAIDS 2023, p. 13). In particular, children whose parents are living with HIV but who were born free from HIV experience more health problems and deaths than children whose parents are not living with HIV (Henrickson et al. 2017, p. 5).

Therefore, it is not surprising that social work plays a prominent role in supporting people affected by HIV/AIDS. Subsequently, the history of social work and HIV/AIDS will be briefly described, followed by an overview of the current situation. Additionally, the situation as regards social work in Germany will be presented as an example of how Germany has dealt with HIV. From this, future challenges will be derived.

History of Social Work and HIV/AIDS

When HIV/AIDS first became visible within healthcare systems in the early 1980s, social workers, like everyone else, were unprepared, knew little, and had to approach these events through the lens of their own experiences working with clients. Therefore, the evidence bases for many interventions haven't been fully developed and social workers had to be adept at formulating best practices from what was available in their settings and communities (Linsk 2011, p. 219f.). Although, at that time, little could be done on a medical level, the need for social care was overwhelming (Linsk 2011, p. 220), which is why social workers – and especially self-help groups from the gay community and later from the drug user community – were at the forefront of the AIDS epidemic, providing support for those suffering in hospitals and hospices, and carrying out pioneering prevention work (Bowen 2013). Even though the persons carrying out these tasks were not always called social workers, the activities of those providing support fit squarely in the social work domain. The essential skills demonstrated by these individuals included crisis management, assisting with adjustment to illness, medical compliance, decision-making about disclosure, addressing family conflicts, legal-ethical issues, and linkage to the limited other available services (Linsk 2011, p. 220). Furthermore, social workers advocated for clients' rights, participated in policy and programme development, and ensured stakeholder engagement of people affected by HIV/AIDS (Hampton et al. 2017, p. 92). These social work skills and interventions had enormous applicability to HIV (Linsk 2011, p. 220). Even though the first decade of the HIV epidemic was characterised by overwhelm and helplessness, social workers became increasingly involved in the prevention and treatment of HIV across the globe (Natale et al. 2010, p. 28). Despite this positive role that social work played, there is also criticism of it: according to Bowen (2013), in the first decade of the epidemic, the profession fell short in preparing most social workers to address the crisis and there was a significant knowledge gap amongst social workers when it came to HIV/AIDS (Bowen 2013).

Significant medical advances during the second and third decades reshaped the role of social work in responding to HIV/AIDS. With the emergence of powerful new antiretroviral medications in 1995, changing the prognosis of HIV/AIDS from a terminal illness to a chronic health condition, social work with people living with HIV and their families was no longer centred on death and dying, although that continued to be an aspect of clinical work in some settings. Social workers began to focus on assisting HIV-positive people with complex psychosocial challenges, such as negotiating intimate relationships and partner notification, deciding whether to have children and following protocols to avoid maternal HIV transmission, and dealing with medical confidentiality in the workplace and personal settings. Prevention remained a further challenge (Bowen 2013). Therefore, social work became active on two different levels. On one hand, it supported vulnerable populations and individuals through targeted interventions. On the other hand, social work became active on a structural level by contributing to the abolition of inequalities, stigmatisation, and discrimination, for example by improving the availability and accessibility of treatment (Stöver et al. 2017, p. 102). Within the social work profession, a stronger international networking within the social work profession began. Accordingly, the International Association of Schools of Social work (IASSW) and the Joint United Nations Programme on HIV/AIDS (UNAIDS) declared in 2014 the goal of working together to achieve zero new HIV infections, zero discrimination, and zero AIDS-related deaths (Henrickson et al. 2017, p. 7).

Even though HIV/AIDS is now considered a treatable long-term chronic illness (Chandra/Shang 2021, p. 7), millions still miss out on treatment (UNAIDS 2023, p. 13). Especially amongst vulnerable populations and in specific regions, infection rates remain high (UNAIDS 2023, p. 13). Therefore, AIDS remains a life-threatening illness that requires timely, complex, costly, and at times difficult treatment (Natale et al. 2010, p. 29). Examples of social work interventions include helping people access therapy and supporting them to remain in treatment; assisting people to get access to condoms, opioid substitution therapy or sterile needles, food, housing and employment, and transport support for clinic appointments; protecting the rights of vulnerable people; and helping to prevent and treat gender- and sexual-based violence (Sidibé 2017, p. 5). Even though social workers are, in many countries and regions, a key part of this treatment (Natale et al. 2010, p. 28), social work differs tremendously around the globe. Therefore, using the example of Germany, strategies are presented that have helped to deal with HIV in support of two vulnerable groups disproportionately affected by HIV: gay men and other men who have sex with men, and people who use drugs.

Germany: A Case Study

In Germany, social work relating to HIV has mainly focused on gay men and other men who have sex with men, and people who use drugs, who have been supported on an individual and structural level (Stöver et al. 2017, p. 102). For both target groups, social work has contributed massively to the containment of the HIV epidemic (Stöver et al. 2017, p. 106).

In the early eighties, when HIV emerged, the German health system was divided between doctors and patients, with the latter excluded from planning, decision-making, and operational processes. This lack of a participatory approach hindered access to the target group of drug user, as the health system was built on patient exclusion in both operational and policy areas (Stöver et al. 2017, p. 107). Even with the release of the WHO Ottawa Charter in 1986 (World Health Organization [WHO] 1986), there was no shift within the health system. It took years until the health system began to change and a participatory approach came into force. HIV was one factor that substantially changed the system (Stöver et al. 2017, p. 108).

HIV posed a significant societal health threat, and the absence of a convincing strategy, even with aim among doctors, prompted people living with HIV, along with their friends and families, to advocate for medicines, rights, and involvement. ACT UP groups, primarily from the gay movement, called for increased research, counselling, and treatment efforts, shedding light on stigma and discrimination. The emergence of HIV, affecting mainly young men, underscored the need for swift interventions such as free access to syringes, needles, and condoms, with the aim of reducing stigma, discrimination, and criminalisation of drug possession (Rosenbrock 1987; Stöver et al. 2017, p. 108).

When it came to addressing the HIV threat, the main dispute in Germany revolved around conflicting strategies. In Bavaria, politicians advocated for mandatory testing for 'risk groups', focusing on a search and control strategy. In contrast, other states supported an educational strategy emphasising inclusion and support, which ultimately proved successful (Stroh 2012; Wicht 2012). It was evident that a resource-oriented approach, rather than inducing panic, was more successful in reaching and maintaining contact with target groups. The integration of the power and expertise of the target groups became paramount for an adequate and successful response to the HIV threat, following the principle of 'nothing about us without us'. Social workers played a crucial role in creating supportive environments for improved access to testing services and effective prevention, treatment, and care, often providing the framework for communities to voice their demands (for example, by supporting court cases or confronting politicians and media with gaps in services or adequate healthcare delivery, etc.) (Stöver et al. 2017, p. 108f.). Therefore, social work has built up a structure of harm reduction services to empower vulnerable people to protect themselves from acquiring the virus. Six central interventions will be presented below.

1. Installing needle and syringe dispensing machines

Over the last 30 years, needle and syringe programmes (NSPs) have become an essential and integral part of the pragmatic public health response to the risk of HIV and hepatitis transmission among people who inject drugs and the general public, not only in Germany but also in many other countries (WHO et al. 2007). Extensive studies on their effectiveness show that providing sterile injection equipment is a crucial preventive health measure. NSPs have been implemented in 82 countries, with varying regional and national coverage (Mathers et al. 2010; Deimel et al. 2018).

In 1987, five years after the virus was first identified in Germany, an initiative began to enhance access to prevention materials and sterile injection equipment. Many pharmacies and drug counselling agencies faced moral and legal constraints that hindered them from providing sterile injection equipment to drug users. Consequently, activists and social workers initiated the early provision of clean injection equipment and condoms to ensure easy 24/7 access to prevention materials for around USD 1. Cigarette vending machines, abundant in Germany (340,000 of them across the country at the time), were repurposed and stocked with boxes of syringes and needles in various sizes, condoms, sterile water, ascorbic acid, bandages, etc. The diverse assortments were tailored to meet the specific needs of local drug users (Schuller/Stöver 1989). These packages are predominantly filled by drug users themselves, who utilise this opportunity to pay community fines or earn money. Social workers and activists in drug or HIV counselling agencies operate and maintain the dispensing machines (Stöver et al. 2017, p. 109). A significant number of machine users obtain their needles and syringes exclusively through this method due to the anonymity it provides; they might never seek assistance from a drug counselling agency or drop-in centre (Kaplan et al. 2014). Installing these dispensing machines is challenging, often facing opposition and occasional damage from local residents. Social workers organise discussions with neighbours to garner support and acceptance for the initiative (Deimel et al. 2020).

Today, many public needle- and syringe-dispensing machines have been installed. By 2013 there were more than 170 machines providing 400,000 packages annually (Die Drogenbeauftragte der Bundesregierung 2013, p. 156).

2. Prison-Based Needle Exchange Projects

In Germany, approximately 30%–40% of inmates use drugs, and many continue injecting drugs during incarceration (Stöver 2012). While injection frequency may decrease in prison, people who live in prisons often resort to using and sharing unsterile injecting equipment (Stöver 2016; Stöver et al. 2021). Imprisonment is associated with risk factors, primarily related to injecting drug use; unsafe needle use practices including injecting, tattooing, and piercing; and unprotected sexual contact (Stöver et al. 2017, p. 110).

Despite the clear link between injecting drug use and the spread of HIV and hepatitis C in prisons, effective prevention measures, such as prison-based needle and syringe programmes (PNSPs), are rarely implemented globally. Only about 60 out of over 10,000 prisons worldwide provide needle exchange services, limiting prevention efforts to verbal advice, leaflets, and cognitive-behavioural change strategies (Arain et al. 2014).

In Germany, PNSPs have been successfully implemented in both men's and women's prisons. Various methods of syringe distribution are utilised, tailored to the specific needs and environment of each institution. These methods range from automatic dispensing machines to hand-to-hand distribution by prison physicians/healthcare staff or external community health workers, along with programmes involving prisoners trained as peer outreach workers (Lines et al. 2006; Stöver et al. 2017, p. 111; Lazarus et al. 2018). Contrary to existing fears, PNSPs have not increased drug use or injecting drug use and are not misused, and disposal of used syringes is uncomplicated. Furthermore, the sharing of syringes among drug users has decreased (Stöver/Nelles 2003).

Therefore, clear evidence exists that these programmes are feasible and affordable in a wide range of prison settings, have been effective in reducing the risk of HIV transmission, have not been associated with increased attacks on prison staff or other prisoners, and have not led to an increase in injections. They can therefore contribute to workplace safety, can lead to reduced overdose risks and a decrease in abscesses, and facilitate referral to and utilisation of drug dependence treatment programmes. They can also employ any of several different methods of needle distribution successfully in response to staff and inmate needs and can coexist with other drug prevention and treatment programmes (Lines et al. 2006). For these programmes to be successful in prisons, people living in prison need to have easy, confidential access to syringes and equipment, and both prisoners and staff should be involved in the design and implementation of the PNSP.

Successful PNSPs also feature a rigorous mechanism for the safe disposal of syringes and good monitoring, evaluation, and quality control (Stöver et al. 2017, p. 112).

Apart from political challenges in implementing and legitimising prison-based needle and syringe programmes, a significant issue is the lack of guaranteed confidentiality for prisoners, which often hinders their participation. Furthermore, because of the decrease in HIV infections in many countries, including Western Europe, over the past 20 years, HIV and opioid consumption no longer represent the central debate in prisons in Germany, with new psychoactive substances and steroids now taking centre stage. Despite this, hepatitis C (HCV), the most prevalent infectious disease, has been overlooked by policymakers, making it difficult to mobilise concerted action for disease prevention (Stöver et al. 2017, p. 112f.). However, a nationwide manual for tackling the threats of HCV in closed settings has been drawn up by social workers, together with user groups, medical doctors, and lawyers, funded by the Federal Ministry of Health (Aktionsbündnis Hepatitis und Drogengebrauch 2019).

In Germany, activists and social workers have focused on introducing needle and syringe programmes in prisons. However, due to political reasons (Stöver 2018), six out of seven programmes have been shut down. Only one out of over 180 custodial institutions in Germany provides needles and syringes via dispensing machines to female prisoners (the Women's Prison in Berlin Lichtenberg), which has been running successfully for approximately 20 years without issues (Stöver/Knorr 2014). The stark contrast between the success of PNSPs and their low acceptance and implementation spread is noteworthy.

3. Drug Consumption Rooms

Drug consumption rooms (DCRs) facilitate a supervised hygienic intake of drugs with additional assistance in health and social matters (European Monitoring Centre for Drugs and Drug Addiction [EMCDDA] 2018). Approximately 90 facilities have been set up in Europe to date (see Figure 1).

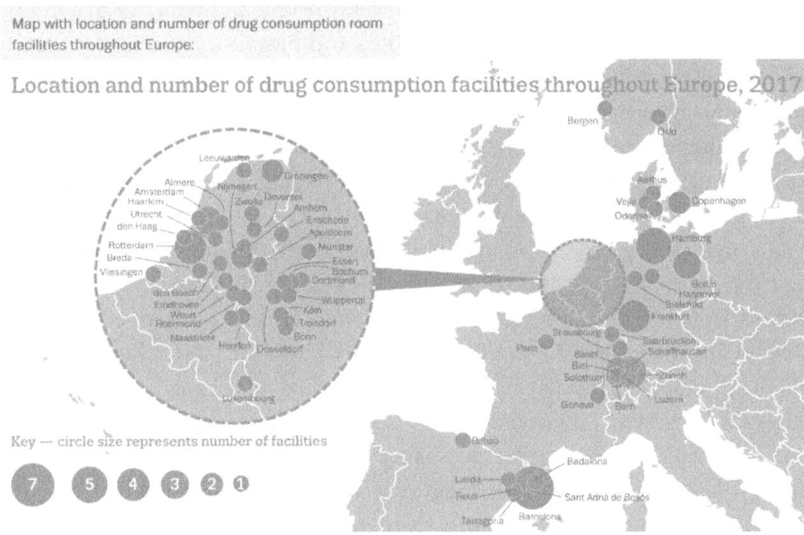

Figure 1: Location and number of DCRs throughout Europe (EMCDDA 2018)

In Germany, DCRs were initially implemented in the late 1980s in a juridical grey area, without official permission, by social workers, medical doctors, and nurses, in order to get into contact with drug users and to provide low-threshold social and health services (Stöver 1991; Michels/Stöver 2012). Yet, due to sustained advocacy efforts by social workers and activists, Germany amended its national opium law in 2000, permitting the establishment of DCRs under specific conditions (Stöver 2002). DCRs have to be legally sanctioned by each of the 16 federal states in Germany, resulting in a diverse landscape, because only eight out of 16 permitted DCRs to be implemented. Despite resistance, DCRs have significantly reduced drug-related mortality in cities where they have been implemented (Stöver et al. 2017, p. 115).

4. Psychosocial Support for People Who Use Drugs

For nearly 40 years, social workers and activists have advocated for client-based opioid substitution therapy (OST) in Germany, which was first introduced in 1987. By 2022, approximately 81,200 patients, covering 40%–50% of people who inject drugs (PWID) in Germany, benefitted from OST (Bundesinstitut für Arzneimittel und Medizinprodukte [BfArM] 2023).

Even though there is still some controversy about the benefits of OST in some parts of Germany, results of studies and practical experiences clearly show significant improvements in physical and psychological health among individuals who have received OST (Michels et al. 2007). Methadone maintenance therapy (MMT) demonstrates high retention rates and plays a vital role in accessing and maintaining ongoing medical treatment for HIV and hepatitis (Zippel-Schultz et al. 2016).

Germany's regulations mandate patient participation in psychosocial care during OST, even though empirical evidence for the universal necessity of psychosocial support remains inconclusive (Haasen et al. 2007; Deimel 2013; Deimel/Stöver 2015b/2015d). These regulations lack guidance on the frequency, mode, and scope of psychosocial care, leading to nationwide variations in organisation, structure, and quality. Psychosocial care encompasses diverse services, such as legal advice, financial management, recreational activities, crisis intervention, group sessions, housing and job assistance, and education and vocational training. There are great variations in psychosocial provision between different federal states and communities, and variations in quality and funding (Deimel 2013; Deimel/Stöver 2015c).

Nevertheless, psychosocial counselling can assist patients in reconstructing their lives with changed values, alleviating the pressure to seek drugs. However, it may also uncover significant problems, leading to crises due to painful confrontations with past injuries and negative experiences. Patients may experience depression, often resorting to alcohol and benzodiazepines as self-medication, with limited family support complicating the situation. Professional psychological support is essential for understanding and addressing the family dynamics that are crucial to successful treatment (Deimel 2013).

5. Promoting a Change in Opiate Consumption Patterns: From Injecting to Inhaling

Historically, since the early 1970s when illegal heroin use emerged in Germany, the injecting of drugs has been the predominant consumption method. Social workers and activists have actively promoted a shift in opiate consumption patterns, encouraging clients to transition from injecting to inhaling to reduce the transmission risks of HIV and other diseases and lower the risk of overdose. Despite potential strain on the respiratory system caused by smoking, inhaled use is therefore deemed less dangerous than injection.

The 'Smoke IT!' project (to support injecting drug users to change their injecting habit to smoke Heroin to avoid infectious diseases), with its accompanying evaluation study (Stöver/Schäffer 2014), aimed to influence consumption patterns by supplying smoking foils and tubes, along with informational materials. The study, conducted in five German cities, revealed that 82.5% of respondents favoured thick aluminium foils, with two thirds using them for inhaling instead of injecting. Participants cited perceived health benefits, reduced risk of hepatitis or HIV infection, and overdose prevention as reasons for the switch. Media and personal interventions, coupled with dispensing attractive drug use equipment, proved effective in motivating opiate users to change their consumption method. Smoking foils emerged as valuable additions to risk reduction strategies in drop-in centres. The survey results underscore the impact of providing new, high-quality prevention tools and a target-group-specific approach, showcasing users' interest in preserving their health (Stöver et al. 2017, p. 117).

Professionalism is crucial in addressing safer-use issues within drug consumption rooms and other services, with social workers using new mediums, such as thicker foils, to engage with users during their daily routines. The thicker foils not only allow for the reinforcement of prevention messages but also provide an opportunity to reconnect with users who were previously unreachable or with whom contact had been lost. This approach demonstrates the effectiveness of innovative harm reduction strategies in influencing drug use patterns positively (Stöver et al. 2017, p. 116f.).

6. Campaigns and Support for and with Gay Men and Other Men Who Have Sex with Men

Men who have sex with men (MSM) have faced heightened vulnerability since the onset of the HIV epidemic, constituting the group with the highest proportion of new HIV infections in Germany, with 55,100 of the estimated 90,800 people living with HIV belonging to this group (an der Heiden et al. 2022). In addition to higher HIV infection rates, MSM suffer from discrimination and exclusion, and report significantly higher psychological burdens and experiences of violence than the general population (Drewes/Kruspe 2016). In Germany, sex between men was a punishable offence between 1935 and 1994, which has contributed to the stigma against MSM both in the past and today (Steinke 2005).

At the beginning of the AIDS epidemic in Germany in 1983, HIV was synonymously called 'gay disease'. At about the same time, local AIDS self-help groups emerged, leading to the creation of the national umbrella organisation 'Deutsche AIDS Hilfe', focusing on anti-discrimination efforts and providing direct support. Unique in Europe, this organisation – which developed within self-help groups – is financed by and collaborates closely with the Federal Centre for Health Education (BZgA) and the Federal Ministry of Health (Stöver et al. 2017, p. 118f.).

Social workers in local AIDS assistance centres play a crucial role, by educating people on HIV and other sexually transmitted infections (STIs), supporting HIV testing and antiretroviral therapy, conducting crisis interventions, and supporting individuals applying for benefits and assistance. They offer face-to-face and anonymous counselling via phone and online; assist self-help groups; collaborate with MSM on HIV prevention; conduct prevention events in schools; help reduce stigma within the society; assist with 'coming out'; offer advice regarding legal issues, social assistance, and employment law; support elderly individuals and male sex workers living with HIV; and closely collaborate with other professionals on prevention and intervention concepts (Stöver et al. 2017; Deimel/Stöver 2023, p. 119).

This nationwide support structure has been established over the past 30 years, but challenges persist in reaching specific groups, such as drug-using MSM. Drug consumption in the context of sex is of increasing importance (Deimel/Stöver 2015a; Deimel et al. 2016; Schecke et al. 2019; Bohn et al. 2020; Brunt et al. 2024), which corresponds with experiences in other European countries such as the UK and Sweden (Bourne et al. 2015; Petersson et al. 2016). Because MSM often do not identify themselves as drug-dependent, they do not show up in the institutions of drug services. In response, Deutsche AIDS Hilfe initiated the QUADROS project in 2015, aiming to connect local counselling agencies in AIDS and addiction services. Besides a transfer of knowledge, counsellors have been trained in motivational interviewing and living-environment-oriented counselling (Dichtl et al. 2016) (also see Chapter 12).

Conclusions and Future Challenges

The current goal of the UNAIDS is to end AIDS as a public health threat by 2030 (UNAIDS 2023). Even though a lot of progress has been made, this does not apply to all regions and groups. Therefore, HIV is likely to still be with us for quite some time, and even if progress continues in terms of developing a vaccine and finding a cure, there will still be people who are already infected and living with HIV (Linsk 2011, p. 227).

Social work continues to play a central role in dealing with HIV/AIDS. Substantial efforts are still needed, on an individual as well as on a structural and political level. There are certain challenges for social work that we believe are particularly relevant:

(1) Reducing stigma

With the introduction of antiretroviral treatments, there was optimism that stigma and discrimination could be addressed (Chambers et al. 2015, p. 1). However, HIV-related stigma remains a common social phenomenon all over the world (Hossain et al. 2022, p. 1), even though progress has been made over the past years (Stangl et al. 2013, p. 11).

Stigma can be enacted, anticipated, or internalised and can be followed by awkward social interactions, avoidance, exclusion, rejection, isolation, social ostracism, blaming, violence, service denial, physical distance, and indifference (Hossain et al. 2022, p. 1). People living with HIV and AIDS encounter tangible stigmatisation on both personal and community fronts. Therefore, stigma and discrimination against people living with HIV/AIDS, and patients' related fears around disclosure, are the key barriers to effective care, treatment, and prevention (Chandra/Shang 2021, p. 7). According to Hossain (2022), research suggests that people living with HIV/AIDS also encounter discrimination from healthcare staff. This is reflected in care providers paying less attention to HIV/AIDS-positive people, skipping physical examinations, or making unnecessary referrals, which makes them even more vulnerable (Hossain et al. 2022, p. 2). Therefore, one of the most important tasks of social work with people living with HIV is to address stigma on different levels (also see Chapter 7).

(2) Educating social workers

According to Labra et al. (2023) who conducted a quantitative cross-sectional study with 674 university students enrolled in social work programmes in Belgium, Canada, Chile, and Switzerland, the results indicate low levels of knowledge on HIV/AIDS, which is why we argue that social work education and training programmes should more comprehensively address HIV/AIDS within their curricula. Future social workers need to be better equipped to challenge stigmatising and exclusionary practices rooted in a long-standing lack of knowledge and erroneous beliefs about the disease (Labra et al. 2023, p. 1030f.). Both current and future social workers need to be prepared and have the necessary skills to assist those infected with and affected by HIV (Natale et al. 2010, p. 27). Special training is required to be able to work with vulnerable populations (Natale et al. 2010, p. 33).

(3) Contributing to the evidence base

Evidence-informed research and monitoring are crucial for making informed political decisions (Stöver et al. 2017, p. 122). Social workers need to contribute to the evidence base through applied research projects so that we may demonstrate which psychosocial interventions are valuable and effective and can be successfully targeted at specific populations (Linsk 2011, p. 228; Deimel 2019). One example is a study by Eaton et al. (2017), surveying and interviewing people living with HIV who were over the age of 50 about their cognitive concerns and recommendations for social work intervention development. A larger evidence base would contribute to a stronger focus on the 'social aspects' of the disease within a biopsychosocial understanding of health. Furthermore, evidence-based interventions would contribute to better support for people with HIV and also strengthen the legitimacy of social work interventions.

(4) Addressing HIV/AIDS on an Institutional and Political Level

Until now, social work with people affected by HIV/AIDS has largely focused on micro interventions, such as providing medical care, prevention, and support to clients and their families and linking them with relevant service providers, such as health, social support, and educational service providers (Chandra/Shang 2021, p. 7). However, according to Chandra and Shang (2021), a macro-level perspective is also needed to not only focus on caring for and treating clients but also on employing multi-sectoral strategies to create favourable conditions and institutions to deliver innovative and sustainable solutions (Chandra/Shang 2021, p. 7).

Services for people from key populations are scarce, inaccessible, or entirely absent in many countries. Furthermore, despite some positive changes, laws that criminalise people from key groups or their behaviour are still in force in many parts of the world (UNAIDS 2023, p. 13). For example, the vast majority of countries still criminalise the use or possession of small amounts of illicit psychoactive substances. Additionally, 168 countries criminalise some aspect of sex work, 67 countries criminalise consensual same-sex intercourse, 20 countries criminalise transgender people, and 143 countries criminalise or otherwise prosecute HIV exposure, non-disclosure, or transmission (UNAIDS 2023, p. 13). Furthermore, funding for prevention programmes, especially among key populations, is badly needed (UNAIDS 2023, p. 14). Moreover, even though studies show the effectiveness of harm reduction services like needle and syringe programmes opioid substitution treatment (OST), and drug consumption rooms (DCRs), these services often face insufficient, patchy, or non-existent coverage, often due to lacking political will, ideological barriers, and inadequate funds allocation for vulnerable populations (Stöver et al. 2017, p. 122).

In some settings, harm reduction measures are hardly available, for example in custodial settings (Stöver et al. 2021). Social work is called upon to draw attention to these structural problems. The groups affected by these problems are often not in a position to advocate for change on their own, which is why social workers can engage in a participatory process with vulnerable groups, partners, and families. The future approach should embrace the motto 'Nothing about us without us' to ensure inclusive decision-making (Stöver et al. 2017, p. 122)

All in all, social workers play an important role in the prevention and treatment of HIV. However, social problems are rarely purely a national or regional phenomenon. HIV/AIDS is a social problem with obvious global scope and effect (Bowen 2013). To properly address the challenges – to reduce stigma, educate social workers, and address HIV/AIDS on an institutional and political level – social work is well advised to take an international perspective, by cooperating with and learning from different countries.

Bibliography

Aktionsbündnis Hepatitis und Drogengebrauch (eds.) (2019): Hepatitis C und Drogengebrauch. Grundlagen, Therapie, Prävention, Betreuung und Recht. 3rd ed. www.hepatitis-aktion.de/wp-content/uploads/2019/05/190508_Hepatitis_Handbuch_gesamt.pdf, 16.01.2024.

Arain, Amber/Robaeys, Geert/Stöver, Heino (2014): Hepatitis C in European prisons: a call for an evidence-informed response. In: BMC Infectious Diseases 14, No. S6, p. S17. DOI: 10.1186/1471-2334-14-S6-S17.

Bohn, Annette/Sander, Dirk/Köhler, Thorsten/Hees, Nico/Oswald, Felix/Scherbaum, Norbert/Deimel, Daniel et al. (2020): Chemsex and Mental Health of Men Who Have Sex With Men in Germany. In: Frontiers in Psychiatry 11, p. 542301. DOI: 10.3389/fpsyt.2020.542301.

Bourne, Adam/Reid, David/Hickson, Ford/Torres-Rueda, Sergio/Weatherburn, Peter (2015): Illicit drug use in sexual settings ("chemsex") and HIV/STI transmission risk behaviour among gay men in South London: findings from a qualitative study: Table 1. In: Sexually Transmitted Infections 91, No. 8, pp. 564–568. DOI: 10.1136/sextrans-2015-052052.

Bowen, Elizabeth A. (2013): AIDS at 30: Implications for Social Work Education. In: Journal of Social Work Education 49, No. 2, pp. 265–276. DOI: 10.1080/10437797.2013.768116.

Brunt, Tibor M./Graf, Niels/Deimel, Daniel/Schecke, Henrike/van Amsterdam, Jan/Knoops, Leon/van den Brink, Wim (2024): Mental Health Among Men Who Have Sex with Men Under the Influence of Psychoactive Substances: a Systematic Review. In: International Journal of Mental Health and Addiction. DOI: 10.1007/s11469-023-01230-8.

Bundesinstitut für Arzneimittel und Medizinprodukte (BfArM) (2023): Bericht zum Substitutionsregister (Januar 2023). www.bfarm.de/SharedDocs/Downloads/DE/Bundesopiumstelle/SubstitReg/Subst_Bericht2023.html, 22.02.2024.

Chambers, Lori A./Rueda, Sergio/Baker, Nico D./Wilson, Michael G./Deutsch, Rachel/Raeifar, Elmira/Rourke, Sean B. et al. (2015): Stigma, HIV and health: a qualitative synthesis. In: BMC Public Health 15, No. 1, p. 848. DOI: 10.1186/s12889-015-2197-0.

Chandra, Yanto/Shang, Liang (2021): Social entrepreneurship interventions in the HIV/AIDS sector: A social entrepreneurship-social work perspective. In: International Social Work 64, No. 1, pp. 5–23. DOI: 10.1177/0020872818807735.

Deimel, Daniel (2013): Psychosoziale Behandlung in der Substitutionstherapie. Praxis Klinischer Sozialarbeit. 1st ed., Marburg: Tectum Wissenschaftsverlag.

Deimel, Daniel/Stöver, Heino/Hößelbarth, Susann/Dichtl, Anna/Graf, Niels/Gebhardt, Viola (2016): Drug use and health behaviour among German men who have sex with men: Results of a qualitative, multi-centre study. In: Harm Reduction Journal 13, No. 36. DOI: 10.1186/s12954-016-0125-y.

Deimel, Daniel (2019): Evidenzbasierte Klinische Sozialarbeit: Gegenstand und Perspektiven. In: Das Gesundheitswesen 81, No. 7, pp. 570–574. DOI: 10.1055/s-0044-101354.

Deimel, Daniel/Oswald, Felix/Bock, Carolin/Stöver, Heino (2020): Harm reduction 24/7: Evaluation of the vending machine program for drug users in North Rhine-Westphalia, Germany. In: Heroin Addiction and Related Clinical Problems 22, No. 4, pp. 29–38.

Deimel, Daniel/Bersch, Brigitte/Stöver, Heino (2018): Infektionsrisiken bekämpfen – Spritzenautomaten realisieren. In: akzept e.V. (ed.): 5. Alternativer Drogen- und Suchtbericht. Lengerich: Pabst Science Publishers, pp. 174–193.

Deimel, Daniel/Stöver, Heino (2015a): Drogenkonsum und Gesundheitsverhalten in der homo- und bisexuellen Community. In: akzept e.V./Deutsche Aidshilfe/JES Bundesverband (eds.): 2. Alternativer Drogen- und Suchtbericht. Lengerich: Pabst Science Publishers, pp. 66–70.

Deimel, Daniel/Stöver, Heino (2015b): Psychosocially assisted pharmacological treatment of opioid dependence in Germany: problems and perspectives. In: Heroin Addiction and Related Clinical Problems 17, No. 2–3, pp. 51–58.

Deimel, Daniel/Stöver, Heino (2015c): Psychosoziale Behandlung substituierter Opiatabhängiger – Theoretische Verortung, Behandlungspraxis und Entwicklungsaufgaben. In: Praxis Klinische Verhaltensmedizin und Rehabilitation 28, No. 95, pp. 19–26.

Deimel, Daniel/Stöver, Heino (2015d): Therapeutische Ziele und Evidenz der psychosozialen Behandlung Opiatabhängiger. In: Praxis Klinische Verhaltensmedizin und Rehabilitation 28, No. 95, pp. 27–36.

Deimel, Daniel/Stöver, Heino (2023): Sexualität in der Suchthilfe. Weinheim Basel: Beltz Juventa.

Dichtl, Anna/Graf, Niels/Sander, Dirk (2016): QUADROS. Modellprojekt Qualitätsentwicklung in der Beratung und Prävention im Kontext von Drogen und Sexualität bei schwulen Männern (QUADROS). Berlin: Deutsche AIDS-Hilfe.

Die Drogenbeauftragte der Bundesregierung (2013): Drogen- und Suchtbericht. www.bundesgesundheitsministerium.de/fileadmin/Dateien/5_Publikationen/Drogen_und_Sucht/Broschueren/BMG_Drogen-_und_Suchtbericht_2013_WEB_Gesamt.pdf, 16.01.2024.

Drewes, Jochen/Kruspe, Martin (2016): Schwule Männer und HIV 2013. Schutzverhalten und Risikomanagement in den Zeiten der Behandelbarkeit von HIV. Berlin: Deutsche Aidshilfe.

Eaton, Andrew D./Craig, Shelley L./Wallace, Robert (2017): The intersecting cognitive and aging needs of HIV-positive older adults: Implications for social work practice. In: Social Work in Health Care 56, No. 8, pp. 733–747. DOI: 10.1080/00981389.2017.1339759.

European Monitoring Centre for Drugs and Drug Addiction (EMCDDA) (2018): Drug consumption rooms: an overview of provision and evidence. www.emcdda.europa.eu/topics/pods/drug-consumption-rooms_en, 15.01.2024.

Haasen, Christian/Verthein, Uwe/Degkwitz, Peter/Berger, Juergen/Krausz, Michael/Naber, Dieter (2007): Heroin-assisted treatment for opioid dependence: Randomised controlled trial. In: British Journal of Psychiatry 191, No. 1, pp. 55–62. DOI: 10.1192/bjp.bp.106.026112.

Hampton, Gary/Buggy, Michael/Graves, Jenni/McCann, Lisa/Irwin, Jude (2017): Grappling with Realities: Policy and Practice in HIV Social Work. In: Australian Social Work 70, No. 1, pp. 92–103. DOI: 10.1080/0312407X.2016.1146313.

an der Heiden, Matthias/Marcus, Ulrich/Kollan, Christian/Schmidt, Daniel/Koppe, Uwe/Gunsenheimer-Bartmeyer, Barbara/Bremer, Viviane (2022): Schätzung der Anzahl von HIV-Neuinfektionen im Jahr 2021 und der Gesamtzahl von Menschen, die Ende 2021 mit HIV in Deutschland leben. In: Epidemiologisches Bulletin 47, pp. 3–18. DOI: 10.25646/10814.

Henrickson, Mark/Chipanta, David/Lynch, Vincent J./Muñoz Sanchez, Hernando/Nadkarni, Vimla V./Semigina, Tetyana/Sewpaul, Vishanthie (eds.) (2017): HIV and AIDS in the English-speaking Caribbean: social work responses. Auckland: Massey University Press.

Hossain, Ismail/Ahmad, Iftakhar/Mehedi, Nafiul/Akter, Rumina/Chipawe Cane, Tam Pheona (2022): Social stigma and vulnerabilities of HIV/AIDS-positive people: Reconsidering social work education and NGOs' role in Bangladesh. In: Journal of HIV/AIDS & Social Services 21, No. 3–4, pp. 167–193. DOI: 10.1080/15381501.2022.2060399.

International Federation of Social Workers (IFSW) (ed.) (2014): Global Definition of Social Work. www.ifsw.org/what-is-social-work/global-definition-of-social-work/, 22.02.2024.

Joint United Nations Programme on HIV/AIDS (UNAIDS) (2023): The path that ends AIDS. 2023 UNAIDS global AIDS update. www.unaids.org/en/resources/documents/2023/global-aids-update-2023, 22.02.2024.

Kaplan, Lauren M./Stöver, Heino/Leicht, Astrid/Schäffer, Dirk (2014): Integrated low-threshold services: Automated machines as an initiative for HIV and hepatitis prevention in Germany for people who use drugs: Den Weg zu Ende gehen! Deutscher STI-Kongress, Berlin, Germany, 19–21 June 2014.

Labra, Oscar/Ependa, Augustin/Chamblas, Isis/Gingras-Lacroix, Gabriel/Antoniadis, André/Biston, Cristine/Mukeshimana, Marthe/Giroux, Marie-Ève (2023): HIV/AIDS knowledge and attitudes among social work students: A comparative study. In: International Social Work 66, No. 4, pp. 1030–1044. DOI: 10.1177/00208728211004676.

Lazarus, Jeffrey V./Safreed-Harmon, Kelly/Hetherington, Kristina L./Bromberg, Daniel J./Ocampo, Denise/Graf, Niels/Dichtl, Anna et al. (2018): Health Outcomes for Clients of Needle and Syringe Programs in Prisons. In: Epidemiologic Reviews 40, No. 1, pp. 96–104. DOI: 10.1093/epirev/mxx019.

Lines, Rick/Jürgens, Ralf/Betteridge, Glenn/Stöver, Heino/Laticevschi, Dumitru/Nelles, Joachim (2006): Prison needle exchange: lessons from a comprehensive review of international evidence and experience. 2nd ed., Montréal: Canadian HIV/AIDS Legal Network.

Linsk, Nathan L. (2011): Thirty Years into the HIV Epidemic: Social Work Perspectives and Prospects. In: Journal of HIV/AIDS & Social Services 10, No. 3, pp. 218–229. DOI: 10.1080/15381501.2011.598714.

Mathers, Bradley M./Degenhardt, Louisa/Ali, Hammad/Wiessing, Lucas/Hickman, Matthew/Mattick, Richard P./Myers, Bronwyn et al. (2010): HIV prevention, treatment, and care services for people who inject drugs: a systematic review of global, regional, and national coverage. In: The Lancet 375, No. 9719, pp. 1014–1028. DOI: 10.1016/S0140-6736(10)60232-2.

Michels, Ingo Ilja/Stöver, Heino/Gerlach, Ralf (2007): Substitution treatment for opioid addicts in Germany. In: Harm Reduction Journal 4, No. 5. DOI: 10.1186/1477-7517-4-5.

Michels, Ingo Ilja/Stöver, Heino (2012): Harm Reduction – From a Conceptual Framework to Practical Experience: The Example of Germany. In: Substance Use & Misuse 47, No. 8–9, pp. 910–922. DOI: 10.3109/10826084.2012.663281.

Natale, Anthony P./Biswas, Bipasha/Urada, Lianne/Scheyett, Anna M. (2010): Global HIV and AIDS: Calling all Social Work Educators. In: Social Work Education 29, No. 1, pp. 27–47. DOI: 10.1080/02615470902810868.

Petersson, Frida J.M./Tikkanen, Ronny/Schmidt, Axel J. (2016): Party and Play in the Closet? Exploring Club Drug Use Among Swedish Men Who Have Sex With Men. In: Substance Use & Misuse 51, No. 9, pp. 1093–1103. DOI: 10.3109/10826084.2016.1160117.

Rosenbrock, Rolf (1987): AIDS kann schneller besiegt werden. Gesundheitspolitik am Beispiel einer Infektionskrankheit. Hamburg: VSA.

Schecke, Henrike/Lea, Toby/Bohn, Annette/Köhler, Thorsten/Sander, Dirk/Scherbaum, Norbert/Deimel, Daniel (2019): Crystal Methamphetamine Use in Sexual Settings Among German Men Who Have Sex With Men. In: Frontiers in Psychiatry 10, p. 886. DOI: 10.3389/fpsyt.2019.00886.

Schuller, Klaus/Stöver, Heino (1989): Die Zugänglichkeit zu sterilem Spritzenbesteck. Modelle der HIV-Prävention bei i.v. Drogengebrauch im internationalen Vergleich. Berlin: Deutsche AIDS-Hilfe e.V.

Sidibé, Michel (2017): Foreword. In: Henrickson, Mark/Chipanta, David/Lynch, Vincent/Muñoz Sanchez, Hernando/Nadkarni, Vimla/Semigina, Tetyana/Sewpaul, Vishanthie (eds.): Getting to zero: Global social work responds to HIV. Auckland: Massey University Press, pp. 5–6.

Stangl, Anne L./Lloyd, Jennifer K./Brady, Laura M./Holland, Claire E./Baral, Stefan (2013): A systematic review of interventions to reduce HIV-related stigma and discrimination from 2002 to 2013: how far have we come? In: Journal of the International AIDS Society 16, No. 2, p. 18734. DOI: 10.7448/IAS.16.3.18734.

Steinke, Ron (2005): „Ein Mann, der mit einem anderen Mann…“ Eine kurze Geschichte des § 175 in der BRD. In: Forum Recht 2, pp. 60–63.

Stöver, Heino (1991): Der tolerierte intravenöse Drogengebrauch in den Angeboten der Drogen- und AIDS-Hilfe. In: Deutsches Ärzteblatt 88, No. 27, p. A-2424–A-2425.

Stöver, Heino (2002): Consumption Rooms – A Middle Ground between Health and Public Order Concerns. In: Journal of Drug Issues 32, No. 2, pp. 597–606. DOI: 10.1177/002204260203200217.

Stöver, Heino (2012): Drogenabhängige in Haft – Epidemiologie, Prävention und Behandlung in Totalen Institutionen. In: Suchttherapie 13, No. 2, pp. 74–80. DOI: 10.1055/s-0032-1311600.

Stöver, Heino (2016): „Healthy prisons". Gesundheit und Gesundheitsversorgung Gefangener. In: Prävention und Gesundheitsförderung 11, pp. 251–258. DOI: 10.1007/s11553-016-0565-y.

Stöver, Heino (2018): Gesundheitliche und soziale Ungleichheiten in der Behandlung von Gefangenen. In: Bartsch, Tillmann/Görgen, Thomas/Hoffmann-Holland, Klaus/Kemme, Stefanie/Stock, Jürgen (eds.): Mittler zwischen Recht und Wirklichkeit: Festschrift für Arthur Kreuzer zum 80. Geburtstag. Frankfurt am Main: Verlag für Polizeiwissenschaft, pp. 429–472.

Stöver, Heino/Deimel, Daniel/Dichtl, Anna (2021): Der Prozess der Kriminalisierung und Inhaftierung drogenkonsumierender Menschen in Deutschland. Implikationen für eine gesundheitsbezogene Rehabilitation und Resozialisierung. In: Rechtspsychologie 7, No. 4, pp. 489–514. DOI: 10.5771/2365-1083-2021-4-489.

Stöver, Heino/Deimel, Daniel/Hößelbarth, Susann (2017): Social work and support of people who use drugs in Germany. In: Henrickson, Mark/Chipanta, David/Lynch, Vincent/Muñoz Sanchez, Hernando/Nadkarni, Vimla/Semigina, Tetyana/Sewpaul, Vishanthie (eds.): Getting to zero: Global social work responds to HIV. Auckland: Massey University Press, pp. 101–127.

Stöver, Heino/Knorr, Bärbel (2014): HIV und Hepatitis-Prävention in Haft – keine Angst vor Spritzen! Fachtagung 'HIV und Hepatitis-Prävention in Haft: Keine Angst vor Spritzen! Oldenburg: BIS-Verlag.

Stöver, Heino/Nelles, Joachim (2003): Ten years of experience with needle and syringe exchange programmes in European prisons. In: International Journal of Drug Policy 14, No. 5–6, pp. 437–444. DOI: 10.1016/j.drugpo.2003.08.001.

Stöver, Heino/Schäffer, Dirk (2014): SMOKE IT! Promoting a change of opiate consumption pattern - from injecting to inhaling. In: Harm Reduction Journal 11, No. 1, p. 18. DOI: 10.1186/1477-7517-11-18.

Stöver, Heino/Tarján, Anna/Horvath, Gergely/Montanari, Linda (2021): The State of Harm Reduction in Prisons in 30 European Countries with a Focus on People Who Inject Drugs and Infectious Diseases. In: Harm Reduction Journal 18, No. 67. DOI: 10.1186/s12954-021-00506-3.

Stroh, Kassian (2012): Maßnahmenkatalog gegen HIV: Als die CSU in den Krieg gegen Aids zog. www.sueddeutsche.de/bayern/massnahmenkatalog-gegen-hiv-als-die-csu-in-den-krieg-gegen-aids-zog-1.1292107, 22.02.2024.

Wicht, Holger (2012): Die Erfolgsgeschichte einer Katastrophe. Ein globaler Blick auf dreißig Jahre HIV und Aids. In: Dr. med. Mabuse 198, No. 4, pp. 24–26.

World Health Organization (WHO) (1986): Ottawa charter for health promotion. www.who.int/publications/i/item/WH-1987, 22.02.2024.

World Health Organization (WHO)/The Joint United Nations Programme on HIV/AIDS (UNAIDS)/United Nations Office on Drugs and Crime (UNODC) (2007): Interventions to address HIV in prisons: drug dependence treatments. www.iris.who.int/handle/10665/43759, 15.01.2024.

Zippel-Schultz, Bettina/Specka, Michael/Cimander, Konrad/Eschenhagen, Thomas/Gölz, Jörg/Maryschok, Markus/Nowak, Manfred et al. (2016): Outcomes of Patients in Long-Term Opioid Maintenance Treatment. In: Substance Use & Misuse 51, No. 11, pp. 1493–1503. DOI: 10.1080/10826084.2016.1188946.

Biographies

Zhyldyz Bakirova is deputy director of the Republican Center of Narcology in Bishkek, Kyrgyzstan and PhD student at Bishkek State University named after Karasayev. She is a psychiatrist by training and participated in a number of international research projects, including the CADAP annual report and the study "Needs and gaps in treatment and rehabilitation for people who use drugs in selected countries of EECA". Zhyldyz is an expert of the National Group of developers and pilots of the United Nations Office on Drugs and Crime (UNODC) quality assurance tools and has published articles on opioid overdose prevention and drug rehabilitation programmes in the Kyrgyz Republic. Her research interests include social work in the treatment continuum, drug treatment and psychoactive substances.

Alla Bessonova is the chairwoman of the Eurasian Women's AIDS Network and a Master student at the Faculty of Psychology at Bishkek State University named after Karasayev. She has participated in a number of gender research projects, including the women-led gender assessment "How countries address barriers to HIV services for women living with HIV, sex workers and women who use drugs". Alla is an expert in the regional drug policy group of the Eurasian Harm Reduction Association (EHRA). Her professional interests include advocating for the use and application of scientific approaches in drug treatment and working with people who use drugs.

Azizbek Boltaev, M.D., is a psychiatrist with 20 years of clinical and research experience in the field of addiction medicine, mental health and HIV. Azizbek Boltaev holds a position as director of the Human Research and Development Center in Bukhara, Uzbekistan. He participated in the development and management of programs aimed at treating people who use drugs in Central Asia and Eastern Europe. As an advisor to UKAID and PEPFAR-funded programs, he was actively engaged in the initiation and scaling-up of opioid substitution therapy in Kazakhstan, Kyrgyzstan, and Tajikistan. Dr. Boltaev served as technical expert for various international bodies including the UN Theme Group on injecting drug use (Austria), the Steering Committee of the Eurasian Harm Reduction Network (EHRA) (Lithuania), the Technical Review Panel of the Global Fund to fight AIDS,

Tuberculosis and Malaria (Switzerland). He regularly consults the World Health Organization (WHO), the United Nations on Drugs and Crime (UNODC), the United States Agency for International Development (USAID) and the Centers for Disease Control and Prevention (CDC). Azizbek Boltaev continues his daily clinical practice in Bukhara and sees patients with mental and substance use disorders.

Daniel Deimel is a social worker (Dipl.), addiction therapist (M.Sc.), health scientist (PhD), supervisor at the Deutsche Gesellschaft für Supervision und Coaching e.V. (DGSv) and Research Professor of Health Promotion and Prevention at the Technische Hochschule Nuremberg, University of Applied Sciences, Faculty of Social Sciences. He is also a visiting researcher at the University of Duisburg-Essen, Medical Faculty and LVR-Hospital Essen, Department of Addictive Behavior and Addiction Medicine. His work focuses on HIV and addiction research in the social sciences, project development and evaluation expertise, particularly in health promotion for vulnerable and marginalized groups, drug and HIV/AIDS services and evidence-based social work. He is part of the ESCAPE drug analysis project of the European Monitoring Centre for Drugs and Drug Addiction (EMCDDA) and a member of the Correlation European Harm Reduction Network (C-EHRN).

Jiang Du is a psychiatrist and research professor at the Shanghai Mental Health Centre. She holds a PhD and serves as a supervisor for doctoral and master students. Jiang Du has been engaged in basic and clinical research related to addiction for over ten years. She has been working on the assessment and clinical intervention of high-risk behaviors related to drugs for a long time, as well as on the research regarding the biological mechanisms of brain cognitive function changes caused by synthetic drugs. She has accumulated rich experience in the field of addiction research and evaluation. From 2007 to 2008, and in 2013, she received funding from the National Institutes of Health to visit and study at the University of California, Los Angeles. She studied under the guidance of professor Hser Yih-ing and was engaged in a long-term follow-up research and related statistical analysis of substance addiction patients.

Tynchtyk Estebes Uulu is a PhD student at the Department of Sociology and Political and Legal Disciplines of the Faculty of Social Psychology at Bishkek State University. He received a master's degree from the OSCE Academy in Bishkek, majoring in "Politics and Security (Central Asia)". His current research focuses on social work, NGOs, the probation system, drug addiction, drug trafficking and sustainable development.

Meryem Grabski is a postdoctoral researcher at the Frankfurt University of Applied Sciences. She completed her PhD on the role of craving in tobacco addiction and potential treatments for it at the University of Bristol in 2018. Before joining the SOLID project, she worked as a research associate at University College London and the University of Exeter in the UK. Here, she worked on a survey-based study investigating the substance use of young Europeans in the nightlife scene as well as a clinical trial investigating the effectiveness of ketamine as a treatment for problematic alcohol use. Her research interests include drug use and addiction as well as the investigation of novel treatment methods. She has been using different research methods to this end such as eye-tracking, pharmacological manipulations, online surveys and data collection using mobile phones (ecological momentary assessments).

Sandugash Ismagulova is a social work specialist in Kyzylorda city polyclinic No. 6. She is also a branch manager at the National Alliance of Professional Social Workers of Kazakhstan, for the city of Kyzylorda and Kyzylorda region.

Medet Kudabekov is a PhD student at the Department of Sociology and Social Work of the Eurasian National University named after L.N. Gumilyov in Astana, Kazakhstan. His main research interests include the professionalization of social work in the framework of the modernization of the social service system.

Ingo Ilja Michels, PhD, is sociologist and advisor for treatment of drug dependence. Since 2010, he was Project Leader of the EU Central Asia Drug Action Programme (CADAP), since 2020 he is the International Scientific Coordinator of the SOLID project at the Frankfurt University of Applied Sciences. He worked in a psychiatric clinic with drug dependent heroin users, as Head of the Drugs and Prison projects department of the German AIDS-Hilfe in Berlin, as Drug Commissioner of the Federal State of Bremen in northern Germany, and as Head of the Office of the Federal Drug Commissioner within the Federal Ministry of Health in Berlin. He is freelance advisor for drug services in PR China in Beijing and Shanghai and Guest Professor at the Department of Sociology/Social Work of the East China University of Science and Technology (ECUST), Shanghai.

He is author of several articles on prevention and treatment of drug dependents and on drug policy in International Journals on Substance Use.

Dalida Mukasheva is PhD student at the Department of Sociology and Social work of the Eurasian National University, named after L. Gumilyov. Her main research topics include health and social welfare in prisons, the situation of women with HIV and the professional roles of social workers. Before joining the SOLID Project, Dalida worked for development agencies in Kazakhstan. She has experience in education, science and research, and is member of the National Alliance of Professional Social Workers of Kazakhstan.

Nurgul Musaeva, PhD, is Associate Professor of Psychology at the Bishkek State University named after Karasayev. She holds a PhD in Social Philosophy. She is member of the Association of Social Workers of the Kyrgyz Republic and one of the developers of the State Educational Standards in the direction of "Social Work" and "Psychology" at Master's and Bachelor's level. Since 2020, she is National Scientific Coordinator of the SOLID Exceed SOLID project Kyrgyzstan, which is funded by the German Academic Exchange Service (DAAD). She is the author of more than 30 scientific articles, three books devoted to the philosophy of social work, the development of psychological thoughts among the Kyrgyz people and social psychology. Currently, she is studying the issues of training specialists to work with vulnerable population groups such as people living with HIV, people in prison and people using drugs.

Sona Orbelyan is Programme Manager for HIV and TB Programme at UNDP Tajikistan. She has been working as public health practitioner in programs and projects in HIV and TB with different donors and development partners in EECA region for 20 years. Her education background includes a Master's Degree in Public Health from the State University of New York (USA) and a Medical Degree from Yerevan State Medical University named after Mkhitar Heratsi (Armenia) with a specialization in Preventive Medicine. Ms. Orbelyan's research interests include HIV epidemiology, harm reduction and operational research.

Ulla Pape, PhD, is professor pro tempore for Comparative Political Science at the University of Greifswald and postdoc in the SOLID Project at the Institute of Addiction Research of the University of Applied Sciences in Frankfurt am Main. She holds a PhD in International Relations and International Organization from the University of Groningen. Before joining the SOLID project in 2022, Ulla was research associate at Freie Universität Berlin, University of Bremen, Radboud University Nijmegen, and Higher School of Economics in Moscow. Her research interests include international health and social policy, welfare state development and civil society in Eastern Europe and Central Asia. Ulla has published a book The Politics of HIV/Aids in Russia (2014) and several articles in international journals such as Europe-Asia Studies, the Journal of Civil Society, the International Journal for Sociology and Social Policy, and Voluntas. In the SOLID project, Ulla is responsible for the research on social work in the prisons and social work and infectious diseases (HIV, HCV and tuberculosis). Furthermore, she focuses on the participation with civil society actors in developing social work in Central Asia. In addition, Ulla is member of the editorial board of Voluntas and associate lecturer at the Freie Universität Berlin.

Tatsiana Pikirenia has a background in international relations and non-governmental organisations (NGOs). She is a dedicated and results-driven professional with over a decade of experience in leading and managing comprehensive initiatives in the public health and human rights sectors. She has created and supervised several project teams that implemented HIV-focused initiatives, including advocacy campaigns, community support, and capacity development programmes. She is an expert in strategic planning, team coordination, and programme implementation and also skilled in financial management, fundraising, and building partnerships, with a strong commitment to non-profit values and empathy.

Uladzimir Pikirenia, PhD, is a psychiatrist and researcher, currently serving as a Postdoc fellow in the SOLID project at Frankfurt University of Applied Sciences. He is also the head of the department at the psychiatric clinic "Inson" in Uzbekistan. Dr. Pikirenia's journey in psychiatry began with his graduation from Belarusian State Medical University in 2010, where he later served as an assistant and then associate professor at the Psychiatry and Medical Psychology department. His career spans over a decade of dedicated service in various capacities, including working at the Minsk City Clinical Narcological Centre and as an expert in Opioid Agonist Treatment at the NGO "Positive Movement". Dr. Pikirenia's expertise extends to international collaborations, having worked with UNAIDS, WHO, UNDP, UNODC, Doctors Without Borders and other notable organizations. He has contributed significantly to the field through scientific articles in peer-reviewed journals. His work focuses on social work with people living with HIV, substance use disorders, and harm reduction programs. He is deeply committed to improving mental health care and advocating for equitable access to healthcare. For correspondence: pikireniauladzimir@gmail.com

Mariya Prilutskaya, PhD, is a postdoc at the SOLID Project (Kazakhstan) and a research assistant at Semey Medical University (Pavlodar, Kazakhstan). She graduated from Astana Medical University in 2008 and has worked as a psychiatrist for ten years. The sphere of her professional interests is drug addiction. In the last seven years, she has focused on the problems of novel psychoactive substances in clinical practice of Kazakhstani doctors. Mariya Prilutskaya studies the epidemiological and clinical aspects of drug addictions caused by synthetic cannabinoids and cathinones in Kazakhstan. She is a member of International Society for the Study of Emergent Drugs and International Society of Substance Use Professionals. She participated in development of national clinical standards for management of addictions caused by novel psychoactive substances. Her research activities have been supported by CADAP and UNODC.

Safarkhon Sattorov is the Director of the Republican AIDS Center (Tajikistan) and has more than 15 years of experience on different positions at the Ministry of Health and the Republican AIDS Center. He received his master's degree from the Infectious Disease Department of the Avicenna Tajik State Medical University in 2008. Mr. Sattorov's research interests include public health, HIV, and epidemiology.

Jarkyn Shadymanova, PhD, is an associate professor at Bishkek State University and American University of Central Asia. She holds a PhD degree in Sociology. Her research interests include qualitative and quantitative research methods, social work, sociology of deviation, sustainable consumption issues, and gender studies. She was a postdoctoral researcher at the Sociology Consumption and Household Group, Wageningen University and the Department of Anthropology at the University of Amsterdam. Jarkyn is an author and co-author of numerous articles in peer-reviewed journals and book chapters on social issues. Jarkyn received several fellowship grants such as The Global Dialogues and Women's Empowerment in Eurasian Contexts Feminist Mentoring (WEF) Fellowship, IGS, LMH, Oxford University, 2018. 'Gendering the Youth: Representations of Gender in Contemporary Kyrgyzstan Media' Junior Fellowship Central Asia Research and Training Initiative, OSI, 2006–2008. Her research interests focus on sociology, gender studies and the role of NGOs in drug treatment.

Alijon Soliev is a graduate of the Avicenna Tajik State Medical University andhas been working as Deputy Director of the Republican AIDS Center (Tajikistan) since 2019. His research interests include HIV, viral hepatitis and size estimations of the key populations. Mr. Soliev has more than 15 years of experience in the implementation of projects in the areas of HIV and TB.

Larissa Steimle is a social worker currently working as a research assistant at the Institute of Addiction Research at Frankfurt University of Applied Sciences. Furthermore, she is completing her doctorate on the topic of professional, supportive relationships in the context of crisis interventions. As a social worker, she worked with people with mental illnesses for five years. Her main areas of research include topics related to mental illnesses and addiction, professional social work and harm reduction.

Heino Stöver, PhD, is a social scientist and Professor of Social Scientific Addiction Research, Faculty of Health and Social Work at the University of Applied Sciences in Frankfurt, Germany. since 2020 he is the project director of the DAAD project "Social work and strengthening NGOs in development cooperation to treat drug addiction" (SOLID) at the Frankfurt University of Applied Sciences. Since 1987, he is director of the Archive and Documentation Centre for Drug Literature and Research at the Frankfurt University of Applied Sciences (www.archido.info/), and the "Institute of Addiction Research of the University of Applied Sciences in Frankfurt". The main fields of his research and project development expertise are health promotion for vulnerable groups, drug services, prisons, and related health issues (especially HIV/AIDS, Hepatitis C, and drug dependence). He has been a consultant for the European Commission, United Nations Office on Drugs and Crime (UNODC), WHO, European Monitoring Centre for Drugs and Drug Addiction (EMCDDA), International Committee of the Red Cross (ICRC), and Open Society Institute (OSI) in various contexts. He has published several articles in international journals and books on preventing and treating infectious diseases adequately (HIV/AIDS, hepatitis, STIs, and TB), opioid substitution programs, and drug treatment in general.

Hang Su, PhD, is a postdoc researcher at Shanghai Mental Health Center, majoring in psychiatry and mental health. Since 2011, he has been engaged in basic and clinical research of drug dependence and substance addiction, and obtained knowledge about addiction medicine, psychology, epidemiology and sociology. Most of the time, he communicates with substance users in drug rehabilitation institutions and rehabilitation communities to understand their physical, mental state and social needs. At present, he is doing research focusing on the treatment of amphetamine-type stimulants and opioids addiction from several aspects: behavior, electrophysiology, molecular biology, neuroimaging, etc.

Umed Talbov is the head of the Dispensary Department at the Republican AIDS Center (Tajikistan). He has been working on HIV and infectious diseases for about 20 years. He has a Medical Degree form Avicenna Tajik State Medical University. Mr. Talbov's research interests include HIV, HIV/TB and HIV/HBV/HCV coinfections, as well as psychological support to PLWH.

Asel Tentigenova is a senior lecturer at the Department of Social Work and Practical Psychology at Bishkek State University named after Karasaev. She holds degrees in social work and psychology. She is a PhD student in psychology, and is writing a dissertation on the professional burnout of social workers. Her scientific and professional interests are related to the psychology of social work and the psychological counseling for people in difficult life situations. Asel has published more than 10 scientific papers and teaching aids. She is also an expert and consultant in projects to strengthen the professional potential of social pedagogues, school psychologists, responsible for home visits and socio-psychological contacts with families and children.

Mykyta Trofymenko is HIV Project Coordinator at UNDP Tajikistan. He has a Master of Laws Degree from National Taras Shevchenko University of Kyiv and currently works on a master thesis in public health at the University of Belgrade. In 2017–2018 he was a scholar-in-residence at the American University Washington College of Law. Mr. Trofymenko has nine years of experience in implementation of the projects in the healthcare area in EECA region and his research interests are focused on access to medical treatment.

Yifan Xu holds a Bachelor degree from Colorado State University, and currently serves as a research assistant in the Addiction Medicine Research Group at Shanghai Mental Health Center. Proficient in assessments, cognitive evaluations, and utilizing EEG and near-infrared methods for data collection, she has played a pivotal role in shaping addiction outpatient MDT services. Beyond this, her involvement in designing training courses and tackling various research responsibilities not only emphasizes dedication but also signifies a proactive contribution to advancing the field of addiction medicine.

Dinara Yessimova, PhD, is lecturer at the Department of Sociology of the Eurasian National University and executive director of the National Alliance of Kazakhstan's Professional Social Workers. To train competitive specialists, Yessimova Dinara pays attention to replenishing educational and methodological materials. Dinara has played an important role in the development and promotion of social work in Kazakhstan. She advises UN agencies in Kazakhstan on projects related to maternal and infant mortality, children's rights, and the development of social work in the health and justice systems.

Guzalkhon Zakhidova is a Phd student at Bukhara State Medical Institute and a psychotherapist at the City Psychoneurological Dispensary in Tashkent, Uzbekistan. Guzalkhon Zakhidova is a graduate from the Andizhan State Medical Institute. She has a degree in neurology, psychiatry, narcology and psychotherapy. With the SOLID project's support, Dr. Zakhidova is working on a PhD project on psychosocial interventions for users of new psychoactive substances (NPS).

Glossary

ADR	Acquired Drug Resistance
AFEW	Aids Foundation East West
AIDS	Acquired Immunodeficiency Syndrome
ANC	Antenatal Care
ART	Antiretroviral Therapy
ARV	Antiretroviral
ASSOR	Association of Schools of Social Work
BBS	Bio-Behavioural Survey
BZgA	Federal Centre for Health Education
CACT	Clinical Trial Network
CADAP	Central Asia Drug Action Programme
CARHAP	Central Asian Regional HIV/AIDS Program
CASWE	China Association for Social Work Education
CBO	Community-Based Organisation
CCM	Country Coordinating Mechanism
CCP	Chinese Communist Party
CDC	Centers for Disease Control and Prevention
CEDAW	Committee on the Elimination of Discrimination against Women
CFDA	China Food and Drug Administration
CI	Confidence Interval
CIS	Commonwealth of Independent States
CKD	Chronic Kidney Disease
CSW	Commercial sex worker
CUHK	Center for Liver Health of The Chinese University of Hong Kong
DAA	Direct-Acting Antiviral
DALY	Disability-Adjusted Life Years
DCR	Drug Consumption Rooms
e.g.	exempli gratia ("for example")
EACB	Eurasian Harm Reduction Association

ECDC	European Centre for Disease Prevention and Control
EECA	Eastern Europe and Central Asia
EHRA	Eurasian Harm Reduction Association
ELISA Test	Enzyme-Linked Immunosorbent Assay Test
EMTCT	Elimination of Mother-To-Child Transmission of HIV
ERST	Electronic Registry of Substitution Maintenance Therapy
FMC	Family Medicine Center
FPD	Former Plasma Donor
FSW	Female Sex Worker
GFATM	Global Fund to Fight AIDS, Tuberculosis, and Malaria
GIZ	German Technical Cooperation
GONGO	Government-Organised NGO
HAART	High Active Antiretroviral Therapy
HBV	Hepatitis B Virus
HCV	Hepatitis C Virus
HIV	Human Immunodeficiency Virus
i.e.	id est ("that is")
IASSW	International Association of Schools of Social work
IBBS	Integrated Bio-Behavioural Survey
ibid	ibīdem ("in the same place")
ICD-10	International Statistical Classification of Diseases and Related Health Problems, 10th Revision
IDU	Injection Drug Users
IEC	Information, Education, and Communication
IFSW	International Federation of Social Workers
INGO	International Non-Governmental Organisation
IOM	International Organization for Migration
iPMTCT	integrated Prevention of Mother-To-Child Transmission of HIV, Syphilis, and Hepatitis B programme
IQR	Interquartile Range
IUD	Intrauterine Device
IVDU	Intravenous Drug User
KP	Key Population

LM	Labour Migrant
M&E	Monitoring and Evaluation
MCH	Maternal and Child Health
MDT	Multidisciplinary Team
MMT	Methadone Maintenance Therapy
MOCA	Ministry Of Civil Affairs
MoH	Ministry of Health
MOIC	Ministry Of Industry and Commerce
MSM	Men who have Sex with Men
MSW	Men who have Sex with Women
MTCT	Mother-To-Child Transmission
MTOA	Maintenance Therapy with Opioid Agonist
n.d.	no date
NAPSW	National Alliance of Professional Social Workers
NCAIDS	National Center for AIDS/STD Control and Prevention
NEP	Needle Exchange Points
NFATP	National Free Antiretroviral Treatment Program
NGO	Non-Governmental Organisation
NIDA	National Institute on Drug Abuse
NPO	Non-Profit Organisations
NSP	Needle and Syringe exchange Program
OAMT	Opioid Agonist Maintenance Treatment
OHCHR	Office of the High Commissioner for Human Rights
OST	Opioid Substitution Therapy
PCR	Polymerase Chain Reaction
PEP	Post-Exposure Prophylaxis
PHC	Primary Health Care
PHIV	People with HIV
PLHIV/PLHA	People Living with HIV
PMTCT	Prevention of Mother-To-Child Transmission
PNSP	Prison-based Needle and Syringe Program
PrEP	Pre-Exposure Prophylaxis
PREP	Pre-contact Prevention of HIV Infection

PWID	People Who Inject Drugs
RAC	Republican AIDS Center (Kazakhstan)
RCPN	Republican Center of Psychiatry and Narcology
SDG	UN Sustainable Development Goal
SEP	Syringe/needle Exchange Point
SPA	Specially Affected Population
SPS	State Penitentiary Service
SSP	Syringe Service Program
STD	Sexually Transmitted Disease
STI	Sexually Transmitted Infection
SUD	Substance Use Disorder
SW	Sex Worker
TB	Tuberculosis
TDR	Transmitted Drug Resistance
TwHF	Tripterygium wilfordii Hook F
UN	United Nations
UNAIDS	The Joint United Nations Programme on HIV/AIDS
UNDP	United Nations Development Program
UNESCO	United Nations Educational, Scientific and Cultural Organization
UNFPA	United Nations Population Fund
UNICEF	United Nations Children's Fund
UNODC	United Nations Office on Drugs and Crime
USAID	United States Agency for International Development
USD	US-Dollar
USSR	Soviet Union
VCT	Voluntary Counseling and Testing
vs.	versus
WHO	World Health Organization